THE FALL AND RISE OF
ASPIRIN

THE FALL AND RISE OF ASPIRIN
THE WONDER DRUG

PETER SHELDON MD FRCP

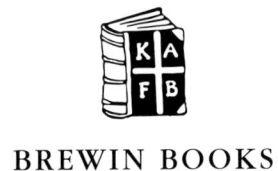

BREWIN BOOKS

First published by
Brewin Books Ltd, 56 Alcester Road,
Studley, Warwickshire B80 7LG in 2007
www.brewinbooks.com

© Peter Sheldon 2007

All rights reserved.

ISBN 13: 978 1 85858 403 4 (Paperback)
ISBN 13: 978 1 85858 281 8 (Hardback)

The moral right of the author has been asserted.

A Cataloguing in Publication Record
for this title is available from the British Library.

Typeset in Bembo
Printed in Great Britain by
Alden Press.

Contents

Preface		vi
Acknowledgements		vii
Foreword		viii
Introduction		x
List of Figures and Tables		xii
Chapter 1	Papyrus	1
Chapter 2	The Fevers	9
Chapter 3	The Herbals	66
Chapter 4	The Barks	89
Chapter 5	The Laboratory Chemists and Aspirin Manufacture	131
Chapter 6	The Fall of Aspirin	157
Chapter 7	Inflammation	173
Chapter 8	Aspirin Derivatives	202
Chapter 9	The Enlightenment	215
Chapter 10	The Rise of Aspirin	226
Chapter 11	The Future	243
Bibliography and References		262
Index		277

Foreword

Since the 1940s there has been an explosion of new drug development within the pharmaceutical industry. This has fuelled both the expectations of patients and clinicians alike in the hope that there will be a drug for every ailment and a cure for every disease. Modern drug development has several phases. Firstly the initial identification of a new chemical entity may require painstaking screening of hundreds of different compounds but happens often as much by luck as good judgment. There then follows a phase of careful scientific investigation with assessment of the efficacy and toxicity of the new entity prior to first use in man. This leads to the phase of clinical trials in patients and frequently at this stage the new drug is heralded as a major breakthrough or a 'wonder drug'. With more experience of its use and the likely emergence of unsuspected adverse effects the new drug then undergoes a phase of sceptical concern and reduced enthusiasm from the medical profession and patients alike. The final phase is one of consolidation and the emergence of a more focused use of the new agent usually associated with a fuller appreciation of its mechanism of action and the balance between benefits and harms.

The aspirin story mirrors closely these phases of modern drug development. The account of the fall and rise of aspirin is a combination of detective story and romance that has been astutely captured by Peter Sheldon. His book is at one extreme a fascinating chronicle of historical events and at the other provides the reader with insight into the scientific development and understanding of drug mechanisms and disease therapy. The numerous clinical vignettes of the use of 'herbals' and 'barks' by 18th and 19th century physicians are a window on the past which identifies both the careful observation of the human condition and the attention to detail of these clinicians as well as their serendipity.

A good example of the serendipitous approach is illustrated by the description of the observations of the Reverend Edward Stone with the 'lucky' discovery of the contaminating willow bark amongst the cinchona derived from the less available and more costly Peruvian bark. This may have been the first example of the use of a generic remedy of equivalent efficacy but at much less cost than the original product. The application of careful clinical observation is seen amongst others in the work of Dr. Thomas Maclagan who recognised the importance of the 'Doctrine of signatures' where remedies are often found in the locality of the greatest incidence of the 'malady' as for example the dock leaf and the stinging nettle. On this basis he evaluated the action of salicin derived from willow bark for the treatment of acute rheumatic fever and publication of his findings in the Lancet led to an upsurge of interest in the use of the agent.

There is an important synergism between the evaluation of the mechanisms of drug actions and the wider understanding of the physiology and biochemistry of the organs, tissues and cells which are the drug targets. This synergism frequently leads to a better understanding of disease and to the further development of novel therapies. So it is with the aspirin story. Thus the crucial elucidation by Sir John Vane and colleagues in the 1960s of the mechanism of the anti-inflammatory action of aspirin via inhibition of prostaglandin synthesis, some 200 years or so after the Reverend Stone's first serendipitous use of willow bark, has lead to outcomes as diverse as the improved understanding of the pathophysiology of inflammation and of gastro-protective mechanisms to most significantly the role of anti-platelet agents in the treatment of cardiovascular disease.

Salicin has been used to control fever, combat tuberculosis, treat inflammatory arthritis, help prevent and treat cardiovascular disease and possibly has a role in the management of colorectal cancer and even dementia. Where will it all end? The insight into this fascinating journey of discovery as provided by Peter Sheldon suggests that we may not be at the end of the story at all but still at the beginning.

Professor David Barnett MD FRCP
Professor of Clinical Pharmacology, University of Leicester Medical School, and Chair of the Appraisals Committee of the National Institute for Health and Clinical Excellence (NICE)

Introduction

Aspirin as we know it, was first used, albeit in a different form, as long ago as c.500 BC. Its use is documented in the Ebers papyrus, discovered at Thebes in the late 19th century, and contained in the writings of Hippocrates, Celsus, Pliny, and others. Subsequently it is mentioned in Dioscorides' *de Materia Medica*. Then, after more than a millennium, its use in treating a series of cases of patients suffering from 'agues' (fevers), was documented by the Reverend Edward Stone of Chipping Norton, in his letter to the Royal Society in 1773. It was prompted by the need for an anti-fever drug on account of a shortage of Peruvian bark, which, as its name implies, came from a species of tree called the Cinchona, and which was prevalent in Peru. Its use was for treating malaria, which was apparently common in Britain at the time. The doctrine of signatures implied that clues to the remedy for a disease were to be found in the vicinity of the agent that brought about the disease. The thinking at the time was that agues were due to the proximity of damp places. Reverend Stone perceived that willow trees were abundant in such areas. He tasted the bark, and thought it shared, to a degree, the bitterness of the Cinchona bark (which we now know is due to the quinine content of the latter). He proceeded to treat about fifty patients and claimed success in all but a few (who probably had real malaria, against which aspirin is ineffective). The next major step was the publication, in 1876, in the Lancet, of a paper by Thomas Maclagan, a physician in Dundee. He included the temperature charts of patients with acute rheumatism (rheumatic fever) successfully treated by aspirin.

Late in the 19th century, several chemists isolated the active ingredient – salicin – from three different sources – the willow bark, the meadowsweet flower, then called *Spiraea ulmaria*, and the wintergreen plant, *Gaultheria procumbens*. The German industrial giant Bayer, first in Elberfeld, and then Leverkusen, went into production with the acetylated form, called aspirin, from 'a' (acetylation), 'spir' from Spiraea, and 'in' which was the common suffix for many new drugs, e.g. heroin, insulin. Huge patent wars emerged after the first world war, as a consequence of which the Americans took over Bayer's plant in Rensselaer and sold it to Stirling products. In Australia, the firm of Nicholas was able to produce aspirin in a more soluble form – 'Aspro' – and in England, Reckitt in Hull introduced their product, again with the emphasis on solubility. Theirs was called 'Disprin'. But despite these 'improvements' side effects remained a major problem, mainly indigestion and bleeding from the gut. The interior of the stomach was viewable as early as 1938, using a rigid endoscope, and this revealed the obvious irritant effect of an aspirin tablet on the stomach lining.

Its popularity began waning with the introduction of paracetamol (acetaminophen in the USA), which appeared equally effective, and without the side-effects mentioned.

Surprisingly its mode of action remained a mystery until John Vane and Priscilla Piper published their findings in 1969, showing that it inhibited prostaglandin synthesis. This eventually spawned the cyclo-oxygenase story, and the rolling out by the pharmaceutical industry of the new 'safer' selective Cox-2 inhibitors, remarkably free from the irritant effects on the gut. The world was taken by storm, the National Institute for Clinical Excellence (NICE) was impressed, and advocated their use in patients over the age of 60 in whom the risk of stomach bleeding is known to be greater. Unfortunately, what the industry had kept quiet about was the disturbing effect on the cardiovascular system, in particular heart attacks. This led to the withdrawal of Vioxx by the manufacturer, Merck.

The rise of aspirin can be charted to the early 1950s, when Laurence Craven of Glendale, California, published his observations in the Mississippi Valley Medical Journal. He had noticed that post-tonsillectomy patients given chewing gum containing aspirin, 'Aspergum', had a greater tendency to bleed from the operation site. He thought aspirin was prolonging the prothrombin time (a measure of the rapidity of clotting of blood), and like other anti-coagulants of the time e.g. phenindione (Dindevan), might be of use in preventing heart attacks. He was wrong about the mode of action, but ahead of his time, because subsequent clinical trials carried out both in Britain and the USA, including meta-analyses of several trials, showed convincingly that aspirin in low dosage, prevented second heart attacks. Subsequently, great efforts have been made to see if it prevents first heart attacks, but the evidence is much harder to come by. It also reduces the risk of strokes when caused by clots in the brain.

More recently, evidence has been forthcoming of its possible benefit in reducing the risk of polyp formation in the colon, possibly of preventing cancer there, and also in slowing down the rate of progression in Alzheimer's disease.

It is a drug with a fascinating history, the full truth of which has not yet been unravelled.

List of Figures and Tables

Chapter 1 – Papyrus

1.1.	*Cyperus papyrus.*	1
1.2.	*Entrance to the valley of the kings.*	3
1.3.	*Portrait of George Ebers.*	3
1.4.	*Detail from the Ebers Papyrus.*	4
1.5.	*Days of the Ebers Papyrus.*	7
1.6.	*Egyptian postage stamp depicting the Ebers Papyrus.*	8

Chapter 2 – The Fevers

2.1.	*Remittent fever (hectic). Case of pulmonary tuberculosis.*	9
2.2.	*Intermittent fevers.*	10
2.3.	*Crisis. Case of lobar pneumonia.*	11
2.4.	*Lysis. Case of broncho-pneumonia.*	11
2.5.	*Portrait of Galen.*	12
2.6.	*The entire works of Dr. Thomas Sydenham.*	14
2.7.	*John Huxham MD (1692–1768).*	17
2.8.	*Huxham's essay on fevers.*	18
2.9.	*Portrait of William Heberden (1710–1801).*	26
2.10.	*Lettsom's reflections on fevers.*	36
2.11.	*Aitken's thermometer.*	50
2.12.	*Allbutt's thermometer.*	51
2.13.	*Glandular fever cell extracted from patient's blood, incubated with sheep red cells at 4^0C, then spun against a glass slide.*	60

Tables

2.1.	*Indexed mentions of fevers, amongst febrile diseases.*	55

Chapter 3 – The Herbals

3.1.	*Pedanius Dioscorides.*	66
3.2.	*Dioscorides, a scientist looks at drugs. Painted by Robert Thom (1915–1979).*	67
3.3.	*Illustration from the Wiener Dioskurides.*	68
3.4.	*Dioscorides' Materia Medica Book. Title page and description of the willow (Salix).*	69

3.5.	*Rubus fruticosus from the Apulonius Platonicus herbal.*	71
3.6.	*The herbal of John Gerard (1534–1612).*	75
3.7.	*Brunfel's Herbal (1530).*	76
3.8.	*Portrait of Leonhart Fuchsius (1501–1556).*	77
3.9.	*Colchicum autumnale, (1543), from "New Kreuterbuch," by Leonhart Fuchsius (1501–1566).*	77
3.10.	*The gout, as depicted by James Gillray (1756–1816).*	77
3.11.	*First page of the Ryff herbal, 1562.*	78
3.12.	*The Ryff Herbal, 1573.*	79
3.13.	*Wintergreen described in the Ryff herbal.*	80
3.14.	*Nicholas Culpeper (1616–1654). A Physicall Directory. Engraving by Cross.*	83
3.15.	*Portrait of Giambattista Della Porta.*	86
3.16.	*The herbs for the treatment of scorpion bite, note the articulated seed vessels.*	87

Chapter 4 – The Barks

4.1.	*Lacey Green – "a few miles south-east of the town" (Princes Risborough) in a "hollow of the hills" (Ralph Mann).*	92
4.2.	*Grounds of Horsenden Manor.*	92
4.3.	*Parish church of St. Michael in Horsenden, Stone's first Rectorship from c.1737.*	92
4.4.	*Church of St. Mary and St. Nicholas, at Saunderton, Stone's first Curateship, from March 1728.*	92
4.5.	*Church of St. Mary, Charlton-on-Otmoor, Stone's second Curateship, c.June 1728.*	93
4.6.	*Church of St. Peter, at Drayton, near Banbury, Stone's additional Rectorship from 1741, (together with Horsenden).*	93
4.7.	*Willow tree, in typically damp surroundings. Regent's Park, London.*	94
4.8.	*Sample of willow bark.*	95
4.9.	*Edward Stone's letter to the Royal Society.*	96
4.10.	*James' book on willow bark 1792.*	100
4.11.	*Title of White's book 1798.*	103
4.12.	*The common willow, Salix alba, from W. White's book.*	104
4.13.	*Goat broad-leaved willow, Salix caprea latifolia, from White's book.*	104
4.14.	*Wilkinson's book on willow bark, 1803.*	109
4.15.	*Goat broad leafed willow Salix latifolia (Wilkinson).*	109
4.16.	*Thomas Maclagan (1838–1903).*	116
4.17.	*Maclagan's paper on treatment of acute rheumatism.*	117
4.18.	*7 cases of acute rheumatism treated with salicin by Maclagan.*	118
4.19.	*Title page of Maclagan's book on Rheumatism, 1881.*	119
4.20.	*Fatal case of acute rheumatism – temperature chart.*	124

4.21.	Range of temperature in a case of acute rheumatism affecting many joints simultaneously.	124
4.22.	Chemical formula of quinine.	125
4.23.	Chemical formulae of aspirin and its sodium salt.	125
4.24.	Sebastiano Bado's 1663 opus on the fever bark (Cinchona).	127
4.25.	Cinchona officinale in the tropical hothouse at the Chelsea Physic Garden.	128

Chapter 5 – The Laboratory Chemists

5.1.	Simplified formula of acetylsalicylic acid (aspirin).	131
5.2.	Meadowsweet. (Filendipula ulmaria, previously Spiraea ulmaria).	132
5.3.	Wintergreen. (Gaultheria procumbens).	132
5.4.	Historical overview of production of aspirin from natural sources.	133
5.5.	The founder, Friedrich Bayer (1825–1880).	135
5.6.	Premises of Friedrich Bayer & Company in Heckinghauser Strasse, in the Rittershausen section of Barmen.	136
5.7.	Felix Hoffmann (1868–1946).	136
5.8.	Hoffmann's description of the preparation of acetylsalicylic acid, 1897.	137
5.9.	Heinrich Dreser, Head of the Experimental Pharmacology Department.	138
5.10.	Arthur Eichengrun, colleague of Hoffmann.	138
5.11.	First page of company circular 23rd January 1899. The baptism of aspirin.	139
5.12.	Second page of company circular, Elberfeld, 23rd January 1899.	140
5.13.	Hoffmann's patent announcement from the patent office of the USA.	141
5.14.	Official description of aspirin issued from the Bayer Company.	142
5.15.	The Bayer factory at Rensselaer in the USA before World War I.	143
5.16.	Bayer Document, trade mark renewal application, 18th June 1909.	144
5.17.	Where it all happened, Bayer's aspirin research laboratory, c.1900.	145
5.18.	Early example of Bayer aspirin in powder form.	146
5.19.	500 grams, presumably powder, Bayer Leverkusen. Note new Bayer logo.	147
5.20.	25 grams Aspirin powder for the French market.	147
5.21.	Early aspirin tablets in tubed glass container, from Bayer Leverkusen.	148
5.22.	Tin of Aspirin tablets from Bayer Leverkusen.	148
5.23.	Some other Bayer products of the time.	149
5.24.	Bayer advertising.	149
5.25.	Like the greatest works of art, so is Aspirin for headaches, colds and rheumatism. (Presumably Tutanchamon found them useful too!)	150
5.26.	The Bayer cross, 1933, Leverkusen headquarters.	150
5.27.	Hot air balloon hovering over the Leverkusen factory.	151
5.28.	Locomotive advertising aspirin plus vitamin C.	151
5.29.	ASPRO advertisement, The Times, Saturday March 11th, 1939.	152

5.30.	Genasprin advertisement, from Genatosan of Loughborough From The Times, Tuesday, November 13th, 1923.	152
5.31.	Disprin from Reckitt of Hull.	153
5.32.	Disprin for headache, from The Times, Friday November 25th, 1955.	154
5.33.	From The Times, Friday September 10th, 1954.	154
5.34.	From The Times, Friday October 21st, 1949.	155
5.35.	Chemical reaction for producing acetylsalicylic acid.	156

Chapter 6 – The Fall Of Aspirin

6.1.	View through rigid endoscope (a) adherent barium, (b) Hyperaemia around aspirin tablets, (c) Gastric tube and pool of mucus, (d) Hyperaemia due to mustard.	158
6.2.	Gastric ulcer (depicted by arrow) in a barium meal examination, with clear dramatic evidence of healing.	159
6.3.	Duodenal ulcer, showing the typical trefoil or shamrock deformity.	160
6.4.	A gastric ulcer viewed through a modern endoscope, equipped with a TV camera.	164
6.5.	Reye's original paper, from the Lancet, 12th October 1963.	166
6.6.	Pre-hospitalisation salicylate consumption by children with Reye's syndrome, related to stage of Reye's syndrome at most severe point. Increasing dose of salicylate and severity of Reye's syndrome are directly related.	167
6.7.	Cases of Reye's syndrome reported 1977–1985.	168
6.8.	Rates of mention of aspirin or acetaminophen (paracetamol) by age groups by year.	168
6.9.	Rates of physician mentions of aspirin and acetominophen (paracetamol) for flu and chickenpox, by age group by year.	169
6.10.	Purchases of adult aspirin and acetominophen (paracetamol) by drugstores.	169
6.11.	Purchases of children's aspirin and acetominophen (paracetamol) by drugstores.	171

Tables

6.1.	NSAIDs most unlikely to be followed by any adverse event.	162
6.2.	Unlikelihood for gastro-intestinal adverse events due to NSAIDs.	162
6.3.	Major NSAIDs prior to designer Cox-2 selective inhibitors.	165

Chapter 7 Inflammation

7.1.	Celsus (25BC–50AD).	173
7.2.	Hippocrates of Cos, (470BC–410BC).	174
7.3.	Acute gout involving mainly the big toe. Also termed 'podagra'.	180

7.4.	This slide shows the muscle coats and peritoneum of a normal appendix. The peritoneal surface runs diagonally across the upper right hand corner. It is covered by a layer of mesothelial cells (not apparent in this picture) underlying which is a layer of pale staining fibrous tissue in which are a few small blood vessels. The outer longitudinal and inner circular muscle coats consist of smooth muscle with a few small blood vessels.	182
7.5.	This slide shows the same area in an acutely inflamed appendix. The changes are striking. The peritoneum is widened by an increase in tissue fluid (oedema) and by many inflammatory cells. In addition, the blood vessels are dilated. The muscle coat also shows oedema which has caused separation of the muscle fibres. There are numerous inflammatory cells between the muscle fibres.	182
7.6.	This slide shows a higher magnification view of the muscle coats of the normal appendix.	182
7.7.	This slide shows a high magnification view of the same area in an acutely inflamed appendix. The muscle fibres have been separated by oedema and numerous inflammatory cells. At this magnification it can be seen that most of the inflammatory cells are neutrophil polymorphs having the characteristic lobed nucleus.	182
7.8.	Fibrinous inflammation.	186
7.9.	Haemorrhagic inflammation.	186
7.10.	Suppurative inflammation.	187
7.11.	Necrotising (gangrenous) inflammation.	188
7.12.	This slide shows the peritoneal surface of an acutely inflamed appendix. The pink layer on the peritoneal surface consists of fibrin in which cells are enmeshed.	193
7.13.	This slide shows pink staining threads of fibrin with leucocytes in alveoli of the lung, in a case of pneumonia (pneumonitis in current terminology).	193
7.14.	High-magnification of pus in the lumen (inner cavity) of the appendix. Pus consists of living and degenerate neutrophil polymorphs together with liquefied debris.	194
7.15.	A capillary surrounded by polymorphonuclear leucocytes in an area of inflammation in the lung. Leucocytes are adherent to the vascular endothelium (margination), from here they will migrate into the surrounding tissue.	195
7.16.	Pavementing of neutrophilis.	196
7.17.	Neutrophil emigration.	196
	Chapter 8 – Aspirin Derivatives	
8.1.	Cavitating tuberculosis of the lung.	204
8.2.	Jurgen Lehmann, (1898–1989).	205
8.3.	4-aminosalicylic acid (para-amino salicylic acid syn. 'PAS').	206

8.4.	Temperature chart in case 1, showing the effect of the third course of para-aminosalicylic acid.	207
8.5.	5-aminosalicylic acid linked to a sulphonamide gave salazopyrin (sulphasalazine).	212

Chapter 9 – The Enlightenment

9.1.	Erythema marginatum.	215
9.2.	Early rheumatoid arthritis.	216
9.3.	Advanced rheumatoid arthritis showing deviation of the fingers, and dislocation of the knuckle joints after several years.	217
9.4.	Inflamed rat paw in experimental arthritis.	219
9.5.	Effect of aspirin treatment in experimental arthritis.	219
9.6.	Portrait of the late Sir John Vane. (1927–2004).	221
9.7.	Prostaglandin inhibition by aspirin. Contraction of male rabbit thoracic aorta.	223

Tables

9.1.	Piper and Vane's experiment. Simplified scheme detecting histamine.	220
9.2.	Piper and Vane's experiment. Simplified scheme detecting prostaglandin.	220
9.3.	Relative Cox-2 selectivity.	224

Chapter 10 – The Rise Of Aspirin

10.1.	Platelets form a plug to stop bleeding.	228
10.2.	Craven's paper which won third prize in the 1952 Mississippi Valley Medical Society's essay contest.	231

Tables

10.1.	Usage of aspirin among patients admitted for heart attacks ('acute infarction'), or for other reasons.	234
10.2.	The Physicians' Health Study. 325 milligrams aspirin on alternate days, versus placebo.	236
10.3.	Aspirin in the prevention of a first heart attack – an overview of several clinical trials.	241

Chapter 11 – The Future

11.1.	A large polyp, in the lower left portion, as seen through a colonoscope.	244
11.2.	Alois Alzheimer (1864–1915).	257
11.3.	Histology of Alzheimer's disease.	257
11.4.	Nurse Sykes' powders advertisements c.1960.	261
11.5.	Fennings Junior Aspirin.	261

11.6.	Proprietary brand of willow bark extract.	261
11.7.	Willow bark extract, 2006.	261

Tables

11.1.	Effect of prior aspirin, vitamin A and Vitamin C on cancer (unclassified) showing significant differences between cases and controls (P<0.001 for females, and males plus females combined. For males, P=0.02) (388 male cases, 398 controls; 713 female cases, 727 controls).	246
11.2.	Effect of exposure to aspirin and non-aspirin NSAIDs during the study period on the appearance of colorectal cancer.	247
11.3.	Results showing number of polyps during the period of observation in the patients previously diagnosed with colorectal cancer and receiving either aspirin or placebo.	252
11.4.	Aspirin at 2 doses v. placebo. Incidence of adenomas and advanced tumours appearing in patients previously diagnosed with colorectal adenoma.	252
11.5.	Estimates of numbers needed to treat (NNT) for some benefits and harms from aspirin.	253
11.6.	Risk reduction for development of colorectal adenoma, looking at duration and number of aspirin tablets taken weekly.	254
11.7.	Showing reduction in risk of colorectal cancer with years of consuming aspirin.	255

Chapter One

PAPYRUS

"Those about to study Medicine, and the younger physicians, should light their torches at the fires of the Ancients".

Rokitansky

In tracing the history of the ubiquitous, and possibly most widely consumed drug ever, namely aspirin, our story begins in the mists of antiquity. Wisdom and knowledge in ancient times was passed from generation to generation by word of mouth, by song, by painting and other works of art, and by writing. We now of course take writing on paper for granted, but before paper was invented, other methods were in use. And of course, leaping ahead in time, as we all know, in the future we may do without hard copy, and use electronic means to record writing. Ancient writing material included wood, ostraka (see explanation below), wax tablets, papyrus, and later, parchment and then paper. Also used were pottery and animal hides. As mentioned **wood** was one of the first. It was cheap, and could easily be written upon using ink. Additionally, much

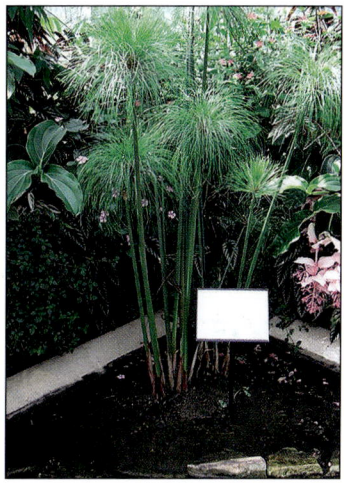

Figure 1.1. Cyperus papyrus.

as we use large key-holders for some hotel rooms, so wooden tags, appropriately inscribed, were used as mummy tags. Wooden tablets were often used in education, and were re-usable because the water-based ink could be washed off. They also had a military use, as exemplified by the writing tablets of a Roman settlement called **Vindolanda**, found near Hadrian's Wall. They were written by soldiers, merchants, women and slaves. **Wax tablets** could also be erased. They were made by depositing a thin layer of wax onto wood, and were used both in education and for official documents such as birth certificates. Another medium used was the broken fragment of pottery, known as a **pot-sherd**, or **ostrakon**. These were written upon in ink, or else scratched. One common use of pot-sherds was as tax receipts. The word ostrakon has given rise to the term 'ostracism', which derived from the practice of exiling one person from a city each year. The person to be exiled was determined by voters naming their choice on an ostrakon. **Papyrus** was made from the pith of the papyrus plant, *Cyperus papyrus,* see figure 1.1.

This is a wetland sedge growing to 15 ft and used to be plentiful in the Nile Delta of Egypt. The word is derived from the Greek *papuros,* and was also used when papyrus was used as a foodstuff. An alternative word was *bublos*, when the plant was used for making cord, basketry or as a writing surface. From this origin, have arisen the words *bibliography*, and *bible*. Vellum was preferred to papyrus in northern regions, whose climate was unsuitable for the preservation of the latter. Parchment was generally favoured over papyrus from 300 AD. Additionally, it could be produced anywhere with access to animals, whereas papyrus depended on the papyrus reeds found growing in Egypt. Papyrus was (and still in some places is) made from the plant stem, using the pith after stripping off the outer rind. Strips of pith were laid side by side on a hard surface, edges slightly overlapping, after which a second layer was applied at right angles. Subsequent hammering resulted in the two layers being mashed into one. A period of drying followed, after which the papyrus was polished using a rounded object, possibly a stone. Text was applied by the ancient Greeks on the main surface such that the lines followed the horizontal fibres which ran parallel to the long strip of united sheets, constituting a scroll.

In the world of the ancients, writing on tablets of stone became replaced by writing on papyrus. The word "papyrus" means, "that which belongs to the house" (in this case the ancient Egyptian bureaucracy). Papyri are triangular reeds found at that time growing along the banks of the Nile. The word "paper" derives from papyrus. Interestingly, the ancient Egyptians used papyrus as recycling bins in their offices, often after having written on them. The papyri themselves were also recycled and used to wrap mummies. The corpses were first covered using linen cloth. Next they received layers of papyrus (cartonnage), which was coated with plaster, and painted in bright colours. Few papyri outside Egypt have survived. This is probably due to the climate within ancient towns and their cemeteries. Papyri were written in many languages, depending on the time. They include Hieratic, Demotic and Coptic Egyptian; Latin, and Arabic.

One might imagine that all papyri contained writing of great literary merit. This was not the case. They included tax receipts, letters, administrative documents, religious or magic texts, stories, or medical recipes. In the first century AD, papyri were put into leaves, constituting codices, where previously they were put into rolls (up to thirty five feet long). Because papyrus was expensive, it was recycled and re-used. It could be inscribed on both sides. It was usually manufactured and sold in rolls, 20–40 cm high, and up to 30 metres in length. For major works, the rolls would be left intact, but for lesser more mundane uses, such as for letters, could be cut into sheets. The text was written horizontally along the roll, and divided into columns.

The **Papyrus Ebers** is the longest and most famous document relating to medical practice as far back as 3000 BC and was written by scribes about 1500 BC. It consists of snippets of folk-lore, and has presented enormous problems in comprehension and

Chapter One – Papyrus

translation. The most significant translation is that by Dr. H. Joachim. From this, Dr. Cyril Brian has translated to English, whilst not slavishly following the German version.

The Ebers papyrus was found in a tomb at Thebes (nowadays Luxor, in the Valley of the Kings – see figure 1.2), together with another text, the Edwin Smith Papyrus, about 1862. The writings include descriptions from as far back as the first dynasty (c.3400 BC). They are magical and mystical. It was most likely written about 1500 BC but was probably copied from much older works. It states that one passage dates from the First Dynasty (c.3400 BC) and another is associated with a queen of the 6th Dynasty. It is not a book but a miscellaneous collection of extracts and jottings collected from at least 40 sources. In 1862, the Ebers papyrus (though not yet thus named), was purchased by Edwin Smith, an American living in Cairo. It was said to have been found between the legs of a mummy in the Assassif district of the Thebes necropolis. The papyrus was sold by Smith to **George Ebers**, a German explorer – see figure 1.3, in 1872. It consisted of a single solidly-rolled sheet of yellow brown papyrus of finest quality, 0.3 metres wide, and 20.23 metres long. There are a multitude of

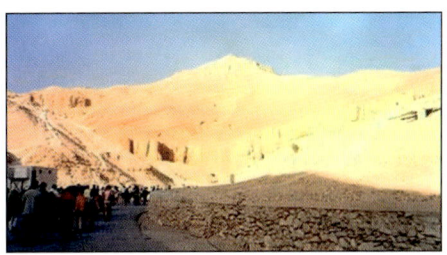

Figure 1.2. Entrance to the valley of the kings.

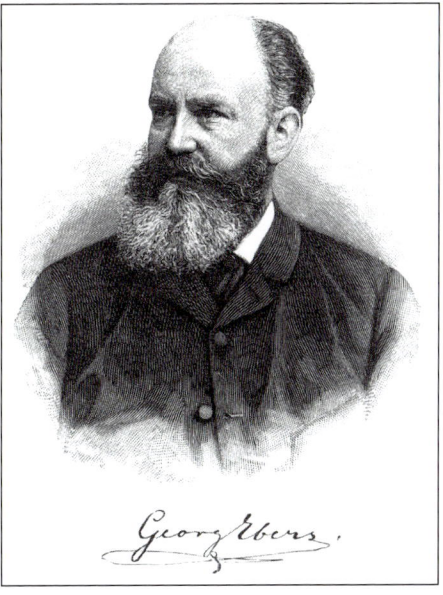

Figure 1.3. Portrait of George Ebers.

prescriptions for named ailments, together with the names of the drugs, the quantities required and the method of administration. There are 110 large columns (each of 22 lines) in the original roll. For purposes of preservation and exhibition it has been cut into several lengths. It is written partly in black, and partly in red ink, the latter at heads of sections and in the expression of weights and measures. The characters are known as Hieratic, being a cursive form of the Hieroglyphic. Hieratic is a simplification, a combination of picture writing and phonetics. Hieroglyphic in ancient Egypt was the written language, and was confined to the sacerdotal caste, see figure 1.4.

The Fall and Rise of Aspirin

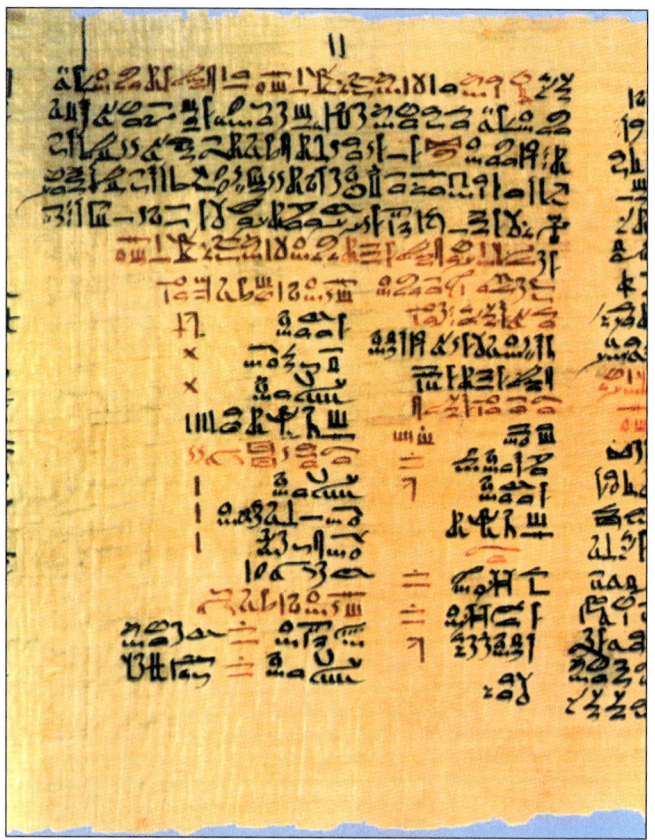

Figure 1.4. Detail from the Ebers Papyrus.

Ebers, from a consideration of palaeographic investigation of the form of the written characters, the occurrence of the names of Kings, and examination of a calendar in the bark of the first page, assigned the writing to 1552 BC. It is one of the ancient Hermetic (i.e. ascribed to the god Hermes/Thuti) writings. A quote "from the late Librarian of the Astor", is as follows:

"It is hardly possible to exaggerate the literary, scientific and historical importance of this remarkable document. It is the largest, best preserved, and most legible text in the language of the hieroglyphics, and does not speak vaguely of incomprehensible and fantastic ideas, but furnishes indubitable insight into different phases of the life of the ancient Egyptians".

Within 3 years, a facsimile in two volumes appeared, plus a German and a Hieroglypho-Latin glossary. 50 years later, this English translation appeared. George Ebers acquired the papyrus at great cost in the winter of 1872. The huge roll was in an incredible state of preservation. In Joachim's opinion, the papyrus "– surpasses in importance all other medical papyri in the richness of its contents and its completeness and perfection. It is the largest, the most beautifully written, and the best preserved of all the medical papyri".

It deals with the following complaints:

Headache, migraine, giddiness, constipation, diarrhoea, indigestion, colic, dysentery, melaena, piles, inflammations of the anus, tumours and inflammations of the abdomen, tapeworms, roundworms, guinea-worm, hookworm, polyuria, frequency of micturition, accumulation and obstruction of urine, cystitis, enlarged prostate, stricture, stone, cardiac pain and weakness, palpitation, disorderly action of the heart, atheroma, debility, diseases of the liver, glandular swellings, tumours innocent and malignant, fat tumours, skin tumours, tumours of nerves and vessels, baldness, alopecia, scurf, eczema, impetigo, scabies, stings of wasps and tarantulae, bite of a crocodile, burns of the first, second, third, fourth and fifth day, wounds, abscesses, gangrene, pustules and suppurations, menstrual irregularities, amenorrhoea, leuocorrhoea, aids to delivery, abortion and lactation, diseases of the breasts, falling of the womb, ulcers and diseases of the female genitalia, teeth irregularities, gumboils and abscesses, coryza, catarrh, diseases of the tongue, deafness, discharges from, and ulcerations of, the ear, and eye diseases, of which Ebers has described blindness, blepharitis, cancer, chemosis, chalazion, cataract, ectropion, entropion, granulations, haemorrhage, hydrophthalmos, inflammations, iritis, leucoma, ophthalmoplegia, pinguecula, pterygium, staphyloma, trichiasis.

811 prescriptions appear. Some treatments have not changed wildly in the course of a few thousand years. For instance, raw meat is recommended to be applied to a black eye, and:

'Remedy to clear out the body and to get rid of the excrement in the body of a person. Berries of the castor oil tree. Chew and swallow down with beer in order to clear out all that is in the body'.

The willow tree is mentioned, as is berry of the willow tree and splinters of the willow tree. However, recommendations for the use of the willow are rather disappointing. Splinters of the willow tree, are recommended for making the met supple. Unfortunately, it is not entirely clear what is meant by 'met'. It may apply to nerves, or to blood vessels. Also, willow is only one of 35 other ingredients needed to make a poultice for making the met supple.

The willow or parts of the willow are mentioned as follows:

In section 293, willow is mentioned as a remedy to allow the heart to accept nutrition. In section 582, berries or possibly catkins are for treating swelling (which as will be described in chapter 7, is one of the cardinal features of inflammation). In Section 663, splinters for softening blood vessels. In section 766, fruits of the willow, catkins, are for treating the ears.

The age of the papyrus was, Bolton (1884) states, determined by a consideration of three points:

1. Palaeographic investigation of the form of the written characters.
2. Occurrence of names of kings.
3. Examination of a calendar which occurs on the back of the first page.

Taking the above into account, the date of the papyrus Ebers was determined to be 1552 BC, which was prior to the exodus of the Israelites, and when Moses was aged 21 years. The authorship of the papyrus is not revealed, but it is believed to be one of the six Hermetic Books on Medicine named by Clement of Alexandria (200 AD).

The receipts and prescriptions are evidently collected from various sources, some from even more ancient writings. Ebers believed the compilation was made by the College of Priests at Thebes. Among its contents are the following:

Page 1.	The preparation of medicines.
Page 25.	Salve for removing the uhav (? meaning of this).
Page 47.	Catalogue of the various uses of the Tequem tree.
Page 48.	Medicines for curing the accumulation of urine and diseases of the abdomen.
Page 65.	Medicaments for preventing the hair turning grey, and for the treatment of the hair.
Page 66.	Medicines for forcing the growth of the hair.
Page 79.	Salves for strengthening the nerves, and medicines for healing the nerves.
Page 85.	Medicines for curing diseases of the tongue.
Page 89.	Medicines for the removal of lice and fleas.
Page 91.	Medicines for ears hard of hearing.
Page 99.	The Secret Book of the Physician. The science of the beating of the heart, and the science of the heart as taught by the priestly physician, Nebsecht.

Translation, by Ebers (1875) of the first four lines of Plate 1:

"The book begins with the preparation of the medicines for all parts of the body of a patient. I came from Heliopolis with the Great Ones from Het aat, the Lords of Protection, the Masters of Eternity and Salvation. I came from Sais with the mother goddesses who extended to me protection. The Lord of the Universe told me how to free the gods from all murderous diseases".

As an example of a prescription:

Chapter One – Papyrus

"Beginning of the Book of Medicines. To remove illness from the stomach. Rub up the seed of the Thehui; plant with vinegar, and give the patient to drink.

The same for sick bowels.		Boil, stir, and eat The same:	
Caraway seed	1/64 dram	Pomegranate seed	1/8 dram
Goose fat	1/8 dram	Sycamore fruit	1/8 dram
Milk	1 tenat (0.6 litres)	Beer	1 tenat
		Treat as above".	

The Ebers papyrus contains a particularly apposite description of both the inflammatory condition and the efficacy of willow extracts:

'When you examine a man with an irregular wound – and that wound is inflamed – (there is) a concentration of heat; the lips of that wound are reddened and that man is hot in consequence – then you must make cooling substances for him to draw the heat out – the leaves of the willow'.

The pharmaceutical preparation of remedies has been beautifully illustrated by **Robert Thom** (1915–1979), as shown in the accompanying figure 1.5, "Days of the Papyrus Ebers."

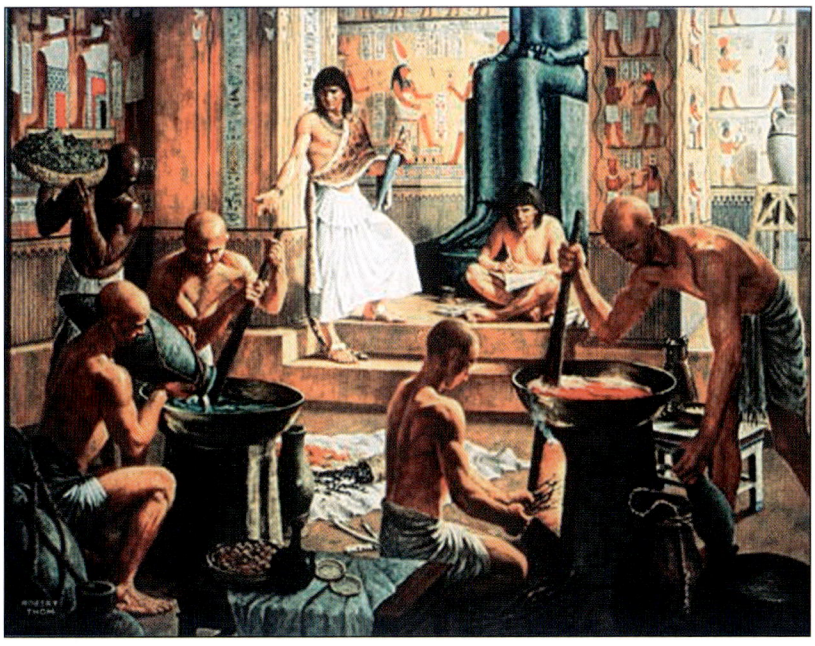

Figure 1.5. Days of the Ebers Papyrus.
(Reproduced with permission of the Pfizer Corporation).

Pharmacy at the time in ancient Egypt involved the gatherers and preparers of the drugs, and the chiefs of fabrication, or head pharmacists, who would dictate to the preparers the quantities of the various constituents required, and who would supervise the actual procedure.

(As an aside, Thom was born in Grand Rapids Michigan and at one time worked with the Art and Chart department of Chevrolet. In World War II, he supervised the illustrations for the service manuals of Pratt and Whitney engines. Subsequently he set up the Robert Thom studio, one of the largest commercial facilities in Detroit. In 1949, he was approached by the Parke Davis pharmaceutical company to illustrate a series of 40 paintings depicting the history of pharmacy. Examples of his work may be viewed in the Birmingham (Michigan) Historical Museum).

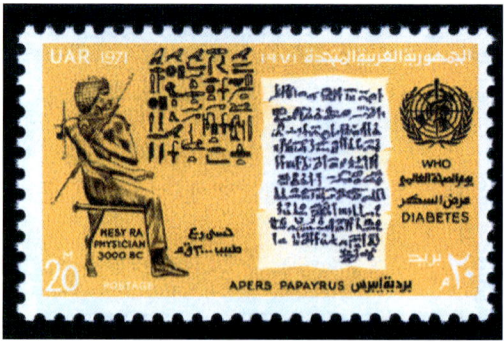

Figure 1.6. Egyptian postage stamp depicting the Ebers Papyrus.

Hippocrates, over 2400 years ago is reputed to have prescribed willow tree leaves for eye disease and childbirth. Dioscorides (40–80 AD) – see chapter 3, advised:

"The leaves (of the willow) being beaten small and dranck with a little pepper and wine doe help such as are troubled with the Iliaca Passio (colic)… The decoction of ye leaves and barck is an excellent fomentation for ye Gout…"

In 23–79 AD, Caius Plinius Secundus listed many uses for salix (i.e. willow) species, including use for removal of corns and callosities, having produced a paste from the ash of willow bark, an infusion of poplar bark for sciatica and willow tree juice as a diuretic. Remedies based on willow have also been recorded in China, Burma, South Africa and in North America.

Parchment is a specially treated form of leather, and when of particularly high quality, is known as **vellum**. It was in vogue during the Ptolemaic period, (Ptolemy, the Greek astronomer and geographer lived from c.85–165 AD). Papyrus was stable in the dry conditions of Egypt, but under more humid damp conditions, was prone to attack by moulds, which is the reason so few remain. By 800 AD it had largely been replaced by parchment and vellum. Initially papyrus was produced in rolls, but later was produced in pages, as was parchment. These were bound together, each being known as a **codex**. They were introduced in Rome in the first century AD, and were widely prevalent by the fifth century.

In 1971, a postage stamp commemorating the Ebers papyrus was produced, and is seen in the figure 1.6.

Chapter Two

THE FEVERS

As everyone knows, fever is a sign of illness. These days, having access to all sorts of sophisticated tests, the diagnosis of the cause is made easier. In most cases, fever is due to a viral infection, and disappears within the course of a week to ten days, causing no great concern, although we feel pretty ropey at the time. However, in past times, much was made of the fever, its magnitude, and its frequency. By discerning different patterns, clues emerged as to the diagnosis. Below are shown several types of fever. These are taken from the author's medical bible of 1960, Hutchinson's Clinical Methods, 13th Edition Cassell, London 1959. Broadly speaking, there are three types of fever, see figures 2.1.–2.4. below. (Please note, all attempts to trace the copyright holders of these charts have been unsuccessful). Following this are the enumerated writings of historical authorities on the subject.

1. Continuous
In which the body's temperature varies by no more than 1.5 degrees Fahrenheit, or 1 degree centigrade, and is above the upper limit of "normal", i.e. 99 degrees Fahrenheit, or 37.2 degrees centigrade.

2. Remittent

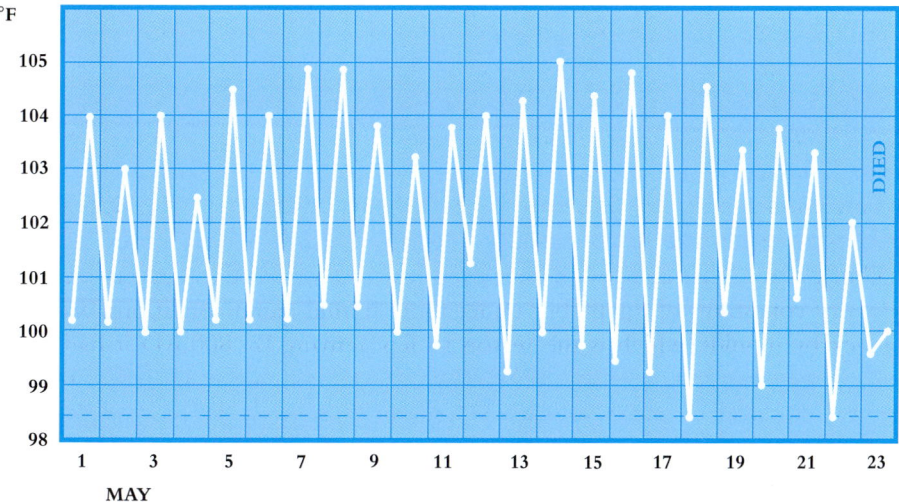

Figure 2.1. Remittent fever (hectic). Case of pulmonary tuberculosis.

As can be seen, a remittent fever is elevated above normal rising each day several degrees and falling, but never to normal, until the illness passes.

3. Intermittent

By contrast, an intermittent fever, as illustrated below, rises and falls several degrees, and when falling, comes down to normal. Sub-types of intermittent fever are shown, and include quotidian (up and down each day), tertian (up every other day), and quartan (up every alternate day plus one). Another way to describe it is to say that in a tertian fever, there are two spikes every third day, and in a quartan, two spikes every four days. Tertian and quartan fevers we now know are typical of malaria, a disease caused by parasites spread by the bite of the female anopheline mosquito.

Before the days of antibiotics, it was not uncommon for people with acute lobar pneumonia, (each lung is divided into lobes, and in this condition, only one lobe is involved) to run a high fever, and then, having for a while appeared to be at Death's door, suddenly experience a fall in temperature to normal, and with it would come a rapid recovery. This phenomenon was called recovery by *crisis*, see figure 2.3. In contrast, patients with broncho-pneumonia, (in which parts of several or all lobes are involved), would recover more gradually, as shown in figure 2.4, this pattern being termed resolution by *lysis*. In acute fevers there is a disturbance in heat regulation, with a re-setting of the body's thermostat. This is situated in an area of the brain known as the hypothalamus. In order to achieve a higher core body temperature, it is necessary

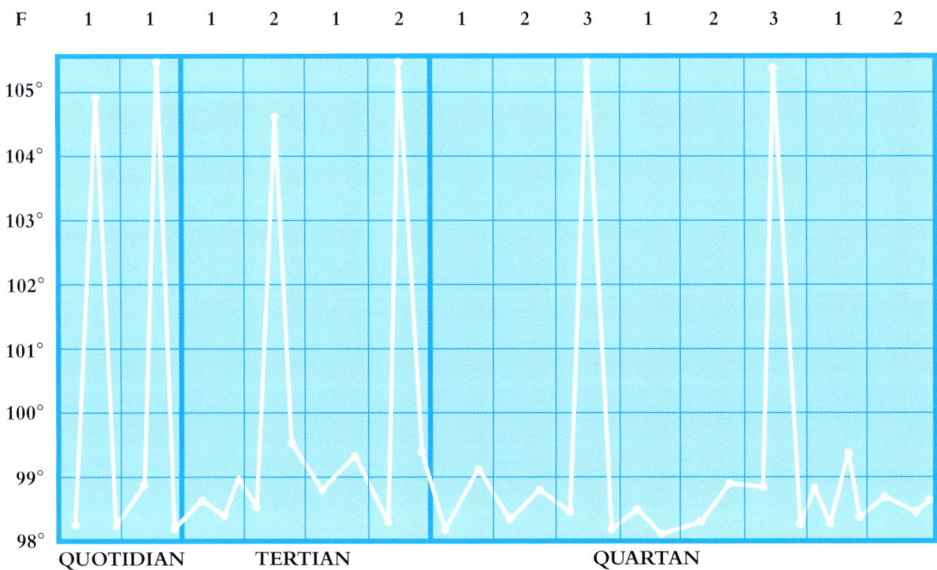

Figure 2.2. Intermittent fevers.

Chapter Two – The Fevers

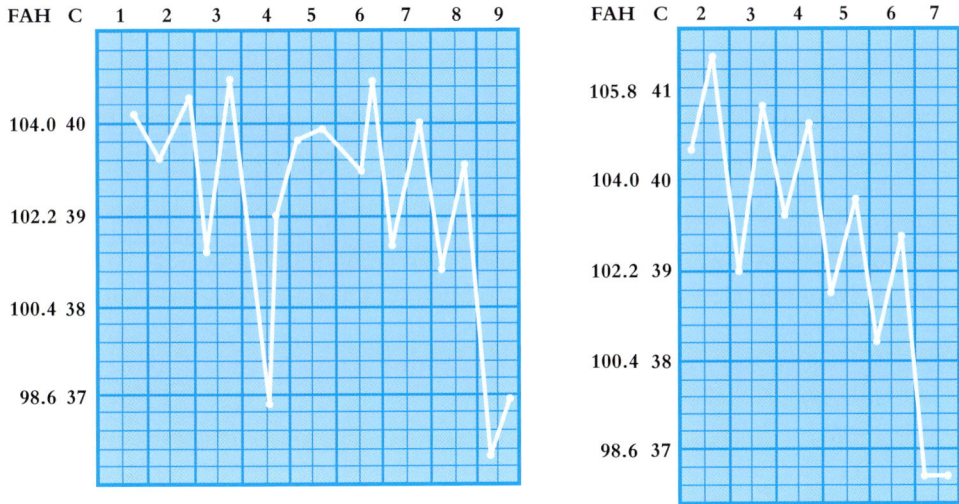

Left: Figure 2.3. Crisis. Case of lobar pneumonia.
Right: Figure 2.4. Lysis. Case of broncho–pneumonia. (Figures 2.1. to 2.4. inclusive are taken from Hutchinson's Clinical Methods, Publisher Cassell PLC, a division of the Orion Publishing Group (London). All attempts at tracing the copyright holder of the temperature charts aforementioned have proved unsuccessful).

during the build up phase to conserve heat in the periphery, and this is why we feel cold initially. This may set off reflex shivering, which is designed to generate more heat. Shivering is also called "ague", a term frequently met in older literature.

4. Galen (131–201 AD)

Early writers went to considerable length in describing fevers, and then prescribing. Early writings include those of Galen, see figure 2.5, full name **Claudius Galenus of Pergamum** (131–201 AD), a city famous for its statue of Asclepius. Pergamum is now called Bergama, in Turkey. Galen studied medicine for 12 years. Upon his return to Pergamum in 157 AD, he worked as a physician in a gladiator school for about 3 years. Naturally, he witnessed an enormous amount of gruesome conditions, which he later described as "windows into the body." From his vivisection experiments on animals, he discovered some of the workings of the kidneys and spinal cord. Galen was a firm exponent of Hippocratic medicine, whose influence held sway until the Renaissance. He generally ignored the writings of Celsus. His own writings included a seventeen volume opus titled "On the Usefulness of the Parts of the Human Body." Like Plato, he believed in a purposeful creation, a view acceptable both to Christian and Muslim. The fundamental principle of life was *pneuma* (air, or breath). Also there was *pneuma physicon* (animal spirit), in the brain, which accounted for movement, perception, and senses. *Pneuma zoticon* (vital spirit) in the heart controlled blood and body temperature. "Natural spirit" in the liver affected nutrition and metabolism. Essentially, he was right – no-one would argue that breath was essential to animal life, that the brain was involved in motor and sensory functions, together with cognition (learning), that the heart exerted control over the blood circulation (though this was not adequately described until William Harvey's epic work, "De motu cordis" in 1628), and that the liver was important in nutrition and metabolism (the nutrients absorbed from the intestinal tract, are absorbed and pass via the mesenteric veins to the liver via the portal vein (which also receives input from the spleen and pancreas). He also was of the opinion that the mind resided in the brain, not the heart, in which respect his view differed from that of Aristotle. Most of his views of anatomy were based on dissection of pigs, apes and dogs.

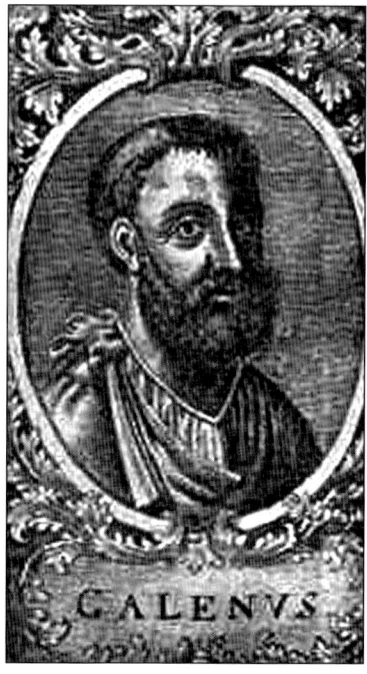

Figure 2.5. Portrait of Galen.

(Dissection of humans was not permitted). As a consequence, those areas in which there were differences, were not recognised as such until dissections carried out centuries later. And because Galenic medicine was held in such high regard, medical knowledge remained flawed until the 16th century and the Renaissance. In his third book, he wrote about fevers:

"These then are the things to be done by those, who, being in health, have cause merely to be apprehensive. Now there follows the treatment of fevers, a class of disease which both affects the body as a whole, and is exceedingly common. Of fevers, one is quotidian, another tertian, a third quartan. At times certain fevers recur in even longer cycles, but that is seldom. In the former varieties both the diseases and their medicines are of various kinds.

Now quartan fevers have the simpler characteristics. Nearly always they begin with shivering, then heat breaks out, and the fever having ended, there are two days free; this on the fourth day it recurs.

But of tertian fevers there are two classes. The one, beginning and desisting in the same way as a quartan, has merely this distinction, that it affords one day free, and recurs on the third day. The other is far more pernicious; and it does indeed recur on the third day, yet out of forty-eight hours, about thirty six, sometimes less, sometimes more, are in fact occupied by the paroxysm, nor does the fever entirely cease in the remission, but it only becomes less violent. This class most practitioners term *hemitritaion*.

Quotidian fevers, however, vary and have many forms. For some begin straightaway with a feeling of heat, others of chill, others with shivering. I call it a chill when the extremities become cold, shivering when the whole body shakes. Again, some desist so that complete freedom follows, others so that there is some diminution of the fever, yet none the less some remnants persist until the onset of the next paroxysm; and others often run together so that there is little or no remission, but the attacks are continuous. Again, some have a vehement hot stage, others a bearable one; some are every day equal, others unequal, and the paroxysm in turn slighter one day, more severe another: some recur at the same time the day following, some either earlier or later; some take up a day and a night with the paroxysm and the remission, some less, others more; some set up sweating as they remit, others do not; and in some, freedom is arrived at through sweating, in others the body is only made the weaker. But the paroxysms also occur sometimes once on any one day, sometimes twice or more often. Hence it often comes about that daily there are several paroxysms and remissions, yet so that each corresponds to one which has preceded it. But at times the paroxysms also become so confused together, that neither their durations nor intermissions can be observed. It is not true, as some say, that no fever is irregular unless as the outcome either of an abscess or of inflammation or of ulceration; for if this were true, the treatment always would be the easier, but what evident causes bring about, hidden ones can bring about also. And men are not arguing about facts but about words if, when during the same illness fevers come on in different ways, they say that these are not irregular returns of the same fever but other different ones in succession; even though it were true, it would have nothing to do with the mode of treatment. The duration of remissions also is at times considerable, at other times scarcely of any length.

Such for the most part is the account of fevers; but there are different sorts of treatment in accordance with what is held by the several authorities. Asclepiades said that it is the office of the practitioner to treat safely, speedily, and pleasantly. That is our aspiration, but there is generally danger both in too much haste and too much pleasure. But what moderation must be shown, in order that as afar as possible all those blessings may be attained, the patient's safety being always kept first, will be considered among the actual details of the treatment."

There then follows a lengthy discourse on how to care for the patient.

"The ancients tried to ensure assimilation by administering certain medicaments, because they dreaded indigestion most of all; next by the repetition of clysters" (enemas) —"they extracted the matter which appeared to be doing harm. Asclepiades did away with medicaments; he did not clyster the bowel with such frequency but still he generally did this in every disease; but the actual fever, he professed to use as

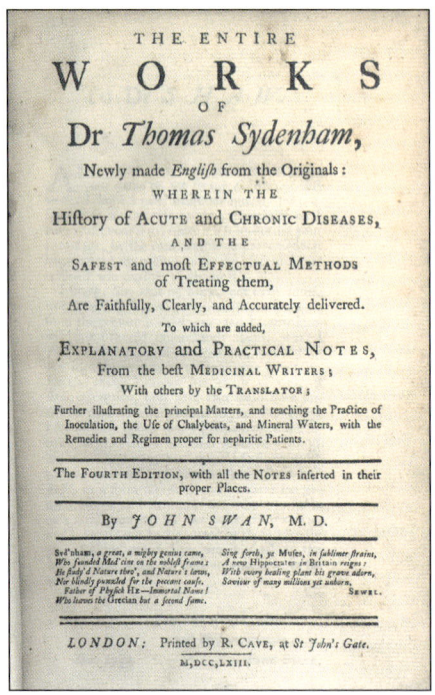

Figure 2.6. The entire works of Dr. Thomas Sydenham.

a remedy against itself: for he deemed that the patient's forces ought to be reduced by daylight, by keeping awake, by extreme thirst, so that during the first days he would not allow even the mouth to be swilled out. Therefore those are quite wrong who believe that his regimen was a pleasant one in all respects; for in the later days he allowed even luxuries to his patient, but in the first days of the fever he played the part of the torturer." (It would appear that Asclepiades was adopting a strict 'nil by mouth' regimen, as would be the case today in a patient suspected of intestinal obstruction, or perforation of the bowel, or when awaiting a general anaesthetic). An alternative view might be that he was demonstrating control, and rewarding the patient for surviving several days!

After this there is a prolonged discussion about when to administer food, with a perceived mysticism over the actual day numbers after onset of illness when food should be allowed.

Next the pulse is considered, and Galen makes a very pertinent observation:

"On the contrary, the bath and exercise and fear and anger and any other feeling of the mind is often apt to excite the pulse; so that when the practitioner makes his first visit, the solicitude of the patient who is in doubt as to what the practitioner may think of his state, may disturb the pulse. On this account a practitioner of experience does not seize the patient's forearm with his hand, as soon as he comes, but first sits down and with a cheerful countenance asks how the patient finds himself; and if the patient has any fear, he calms him with entertaining talk, and only after that moves his hand to touch the patient".

To this day, medical students are taught how important it is to put the patient at ease before commencing history taking.

5. Sydenham (1634–1689)

Fast-forwarding about 1,500 years, another eminent physician was **Thomas Sydenham** who was born in 1634 at Windford Eagle, in Dorset. His father, William, we gather was a wealthy man, but there is little information on Sydenham's education. In 1642, he went to Oxford university, to Magdalen Hall, as a commoner, but it appears his education there was interrupted by the English Civil War (1642–1649). It is hinted that he had a commission in the King's army. However, and by whatever means, by 1648 he obtained the degree of Bachelor of Physic. He subsequently travelled to other seats of learning, including Montpellier. Eventually he became a resident in Westminster, attaining the degree of Doctor of Physic from Cambridge, and receiving a licence from the College of Physicians. Sadly, at age 52 years, he developed frequent attacks of gout, and a kidney stone. He died at his house in Pall Mall on 29th December 1689, and was buried in the church of St. James, in Westminster. He was highly regarded by all, including Boerhaave (see below). His collected works were translated from their originals into English, the frontispiece of the fourth edition, in 1763, being shown, see figure 2.6.

This work, extending to nearly 700 pages, includes a description of fevers under the following headings:

Fever continued	Fever, a winter one
Fever depuratory	Fever hectic
Fever erysipelatous	Fevers
Fever malignant	Fevers epidemic
Fever morbillous	Fevers intercurrent
Fevers pestilential	Fevers intermittent
Fever pleuritic	Fevers quartan
Fever putrid	Fevers quotidian
Fever scarlet	Fevers tertian
Fever stationary	

His main methods of treatment included bleeding and purgation. Sydenham cites the following fevers:

Scarlet; stationary; a winter one; hectic; epidemic; intercurrent; intermittent; quartan,; quotidian; tertian. From the number of pages devoted to each of these fevers, it will be seen that by far and away the types of fevers receiving the most attention were intermittents.

With regard to a stationary fever, Sydenham states:

"The matter seems to stand thus: there are various general constitutions of years, that owe their origin neither to heat, cold, dryness, nor moisture; but rather depend upon a certain secret and inexplicable alteration in the bowels of the earth, whence the air becomes impregnated with such kinds of effluvia, as subject the human body to particular distempers, so long as that kind of constitution prevails, which, after a certain course of years, declines, and gives way to another. Each of these general constitutions is attended with its own proper and peculiar kind of fever, which never appears in any other; and therefore I call this kind of fever stationary".

He goes on:

"There are also certain particular constitutions of the same year, in which, tho' such kind of fevers as follow the general constitution of the year, with regard to the manifest qualities of the atmosphere, may prove more or less epidemic, and rise either earlier or later; yet the fevers that appear in all years (which we therefore call intercurrents) do proceed from some one or other manifest quality of the air; for instance, pleurisies, quinsies, and the like, which generally happen when an intense and long continued cold is immediately followed by a sudden heat. It may therefore be, that the sensible qualities of the air have some share in producing those intercurrent fevers, –"

Much to Sydenham's credit, when managing a case of fever:

"– we may by degrees find out a way to secure the patient provided we do not hurry on too fast, which indeed I esteem to be most particularly pernicious, and to have destroyed more persons in fevers, than any other thing whatsoever. Nor do I think it below me to acknowledge, with respect to the cure of fevers, that when no manifest indication pointed out to me what was to be done, I have consulted the safety of my patient, and my own reputation, most effectually, by doing nothing at all – ***But it is much to be lamented that abundance of sick persons are so ignorant, as not to know that it is sometimes as much the part of a skilful physician to do nothing at all, as, at others, to exhibit the most effectual remedies –***" (italics and bold type by this author, who feels strongly as did Sydenham).

Unfortunately, when discussing the "Winter fever" Sydenham spoils it all.

"I have found a certain fever prevail from the beginning of winter to the beginning of spring, which, both in the symptoms and method of cure, manifestly differs from the then reigning *stationary*, or *epidemic* fever of the general constitution, and is therefore to be reckoned amongst those fevers I call *intercurrents* – To cure this fever, I endeavour to make a revulsion of the copious serum collected by the

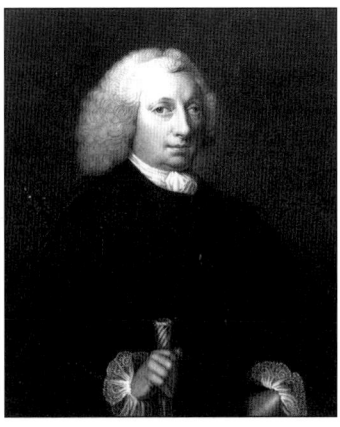

*Figure 2.7. John Huxham MD (1692–1768).
(Reproduced with permission of the National Portrait Gallery).*

diminution of insensible perspiration in the winter, by bleeding, and to carry it off by repeated purgation. With this view, as soon as I am called, I order nine or ten ounces of blood to be taken away from the arm; and the next day I exhibit my common purging potion. – I repeat this potion twice more, interposing a day between each purge, providing all the symptoms do not go off before –"

In fact, and upon reflection, when investigating patients today, (and particularly where a patient presents with a protracted fever whose cause is unknown), it would be by no means unusual to extract 40 millilitres, or say two ounces, of blood for investigatory purposes. Not infrequently further tests are requested depending on the patient's progress, and the degree of enlightenment (or otherwise) of the attending doctors, such that it would not be unusual for the process of drawing blood to be repeated several times, and the total amount removed might easily equal, or even exceed the amount removed by Sydenham.

Though Sydenham describes hectic fevers in children, and his treatment method, he does not define what he means by a hectic fever.

6. Huxham (1692–1768)

Another physician of the time was **John Huxham**, see figure 2.7. He was a student of the renowned Dutch physician **Herman Boerhaave**, a great medical teacher at the University of Leiden. Huxham practised in Plymouth. He had to cope with a great restraint on his medical practise (and income) because, as a religious dissenter, he was only permitted to treat non-conformists. He found this too hard to bear, and converted. Rapidly his practise improved, and he was admitted to the Royal Society. He is well known for his description of the "Devonshire colic" (lead poisoning), his

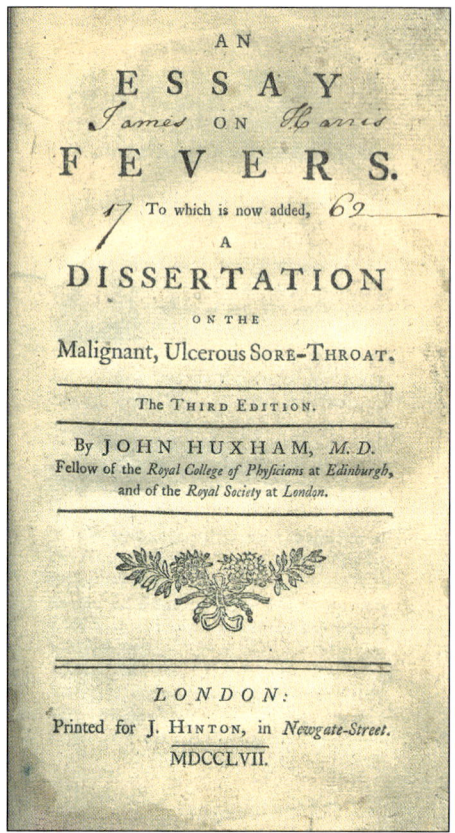

Figure 2.8. Huxham's essay on fevers.

preparation of cinchona bark ('Huxham's tincture'), and his advocacy for the use of citrus fruits to prevent scurvy. His best known work was his **'Essay on fevers'** first published in 1739. In great detail he described the appearance of the throat in diphtheria. The title page is shown in the figure 2.8, and it will be seen that a previous owner has written in ink, 'James Harris 1762'. This might possibly have been James Harris the first Earl of Malmesbury (1746–1820). He was educated at Winchester. Quite what he would have thought of Huxham's book is difficult to decide, as he later went into politics. Perhaps at the age of 16 or thereabouts he had an interest in medicine?

In the preface to his book, Huxham says:

'Though I have all along strictly kept close to Facts and repeated Experience, (and where I have reasoned from these, I have aimed at the justest Analogy); yet I have supported my Doctrine and Practice very frequently by the Authority of the Ancients,

Chapter Two – The Fevers

particularly *Hippocrates*. – And this I have the rather done, as well knowing of what great Use they were to me in the Course of my Studies and Practice; and also with a View of recommending their frequent Perusal to young Physicians. – But although my Advice perhaps, in this Matter, may have no great Weight; yet I hope, the concurrent Judgment of the greatest Masters in our Profession will be duly regarded. I will not take upon me to say, a Person cannot be a good Physician, without consulting that great Oracle of Physic, and reading the Ancients; but this let me say, He will make a much better Physician for so doing: And I believe, few, if any, ever made any considerable Figure in their Profession, who had not studied them.– Indeed *Hippocrates* hath been accounted the very Father of Physic, and the Plan, which he laid down, as the *Basis* of all true and solid Medicine – The Reason of which is evidently this, that he studied Nature with the greatest Care and Assiduity –'

It is interesting that in Huxham's book, devoted to fever, there is no definition of it, or any reference to any means of measuring it. He describes three causes of fever:

The consequence of violent exercise such as running. This he stated would increase the velocity, heat and friction of the blood.

Exposure to cold, moist air, which would suppress perspiration.

Drinking too largely of Wine, or other spirituous liquors.

In fact, none of these would, by current understanding cause fever. It is more likely the consequent red appearance due to any of the aforementioned activities was mistaken for fever. The treatment, based on their misguided concepts, would appear obvious, namely bleeding. In addition to bleeding, he recommended cooling, emollients and laxatives. Purgation was thought to be of great value.

He then went on to describe intermittent fevers ('intermittents'). These he believed were due to a moist foggy *Atmosphere* exhaling from a 'swampy morass soil, or a Continuance of cold, rainy thick Weather; hence in low fenny Countries Agues are *endemic*, and in such seasons *epidemic* –' The fever is thus believed to be affected by the ambient conditions acting on 'the Fibres' which are thought to be 'too much relaxed, and regular Perspiration obstructed, which soon generate a *Lentor* –?, of the Blood, and that Obstructions and some Degree of Stagnation in the ultimate branches of the sanguineous Arteries; as is manifest from the Coldness, Paleness, and Lividity of the Fingers, Nails, Lips, &c. which immediately precede and begin the *Rigor* of *an aguish Paroxysm*. – The blood hence recoils upon the Heart, and all the Powers of Nature rouse up to remove the Obstructions; which are soon carried off by the hot Fit, in Sweats, turbid urine, &c. – We see a Kind of aguish paroxysm brought on by Bathing in very cold Water; Paleness, Coldness, Shivering, a Stoppage of the Blood in the cutaneous Arteries, and Repulsion towards the Heart; you are no sooner out of the Bath than the Heart, Arteries &c. overcome the Resistance from the precedent Constriction, and bring on an universal *Glow* of Heat. But if the Person bathed be weak, the Water very cold, and the Continuance in it long; he may die in the cold Bath, as a weakly Patient may in the cold Fit, (which commonly happens, when the Disease proves mortal) the Heart not being able to overcome the Resistance.' Huxham goes on to state that cures follow if the 'fibres' are strong, but if not, there is a risk of these fevers turning into continued forms, which may be turned into quotidians or tertians by wrong treatment leading to pneumonia. He recalls the *'catarrhal Fever'* of 1743 which spread through Europe and which was known by the name *Influenza*. He goes on to say;

'The invigorating Power of the advancing Spring, and the encreasing genial Warmth and Dryness of the Air, by rarefying and attenuating the heavy fizy Humors, and opening the Pores, are the Reasons why vernal Agues go so easily off at the Approach of Summer. And probably the enlivening, attenuating Influences of the growing Spring, actuating the Powers of Nature to throw off the heavy, ropy *Colluvies*, that in some may be considerably amassed during a cold moist Winter, may be one Reason, at least, of the Frequency of Agues in the Spring Season.– It is certain, all Nature at that Time of the Year undergoes a Kind of *Orgasm*; even the torpid Vegetables regain fresh Life, and their concreted Juices resume new Motion'.

One can immediately sense how subjective by today's standards these statements are, in fact verging on the poetic. Huxham then mentions that too hasty use of the bark (by which he means the Peruvian bark, the source of quinine) may change a tertian to a quotidian or a remittent fever. One wonders whether such cases were not in fact true cases of malaria, and were instead due to some other cause which we now know would not have responded to quinine anyway.

He proceeds on the conviction of a profound division of fevers into two fundamentally different types, the **'slow nervous fever'** and the **'malignant putrid fever'**. Slow nervous fever has its origin in disease of the 'lymphatic and nervous juices', whereas putrid malignant fever affects primarily the blood. The former type of fever tends to be more chronic (i.e. longer lasting), and the latter associated with signs of sepsis. He also stated that these fevers could be artificially induced by diet or 'regimen'. Hot, acidic, salty, spicy food or hot air, amongst other things, could produce a putrid malignant fever. By contrast, cold watery slimy things like cucumber, melon, 'crude trashy fruit', damp cold air etc could bring on the other sort of fever. His imagination is ever to the fore when he likens the slow nervous fever to the effect of a virus transmitted from a mad dog which has a very slow onset of effect, and which affects the lymph and the nervous juices, with no sign of sepsis or putrefaction until very late. The latter he likens to the effect of a poison from a viper "which immediately affects and destroys the blood globules". In the analogy quoted for the slow nervous type of fever, he exhibits astonishing perspicacity. Viruses were not visible, bacteria only just, using the microscope of Leuvanhoek. And the mad dog bite we now know to be the mode of transmission to humans of rabies virus, which ascends to the brain via nerve sheaths. The word slow is apposite, as the incubation period can be many months. He then proceeds to a description of the slow nervous fever over the ensuing 18 pages. This, as its name implies, is of gradual onset:

"The Patient at first grows somewhat listless, and feels slight Chills and Shudders, with uncertain sudden flushes of Heat, and a kind of weariness all over, like what is felt after great Fatigue: This is always attended with a Sort of Heaviness and Dejection of Spirit, and more or less of a Load, Pain, or Giddiness of the Head; a *Nausea* and Disrelish of every Thing, soon follows, without any considerable Thirst, but frequently with urging to Vomit, tho' little but insipid Phlegm is brought up.

– In this Condition the Patient often continues for five or six Days, with a heavy pale sunk Countenance, seeming not very sick, and yet far from being well – The Pulse, during all this Time, is quick, weak and unequal, sometimes fluttering, and sometimes for a few Minutes slow, nay intermitting; – About the seventh or eighth Day the Giddiness, Pain, or Heaviness of the Head, become much greater, with a constant Noise in it, or *Tinnitus Aurium*, which is very disturbing to the Sick, and frequently brings on a Delirium. – Frequently profuse Sweats pour forth all at once about the ninth, tenth, or twelfth Day, commonly coldish and clammy on the Extremities: – Now Nature sinks apace, the Extremities grow cold, the Nails pale or livid, the Pulse may be said to tremble and flutter rather than to beat, the Vibrations being so exceeding weak and quick, that they can scarce be distinguished – The Delirium now ends in a profound *Coma*, and that soon in eternal Sleep. All Persons grow deaf and stupid towards the End of the Disease – This is a Description, (tedious indeed, but pretty exact) of the slow nervous Fever in its most aggravated Circumstances – It most commonly attacks Persons of weak Nerves, a lax Habit of Body, and a poor thin Blood – and also those, who have used much crude unwholesome Food, vapid impure Drinks, or who have been confined long in damp, foul Air; that have broken the Vigor of their Constitutions by Salivations, too frequent Purging, immoderate Venery, &c. – Whence I think it is evident, this Disease, arises from a too relaxed State of the Solids, a poor weak blood, and a *Lentor and Vapidity of the lymphatic and nervous Juices*: The very Method of Cure shews this, which consists in mild stimulating, attenuating and proper Cordial, Strengthening Diet and Medicines. *Hippocrates* somewhere notes, that the successful Method of Cure shews the Nature of the Disease".

Huxham then discusses treatment of the slow nervous fever, including use of rhubarb, milk, sugar salt, mild diaphoretics (substances that induce perspiration), Wine-whey, Gruel, thin chicken broth, "Juice of Sevile Orange, or Lemon, – Towards the Decline of the Fever, where the Sweats are abundant and weakening, I moreover give small Doses of the Tincture of the Bark with Saffron and Snake Root – which makes the Remissions, or intermissions, – more distinct and manifest, and gives a fairer Opportunity for Preparations of the *Bark*. – I have more than once known Patients sink under this Fever, after having been kept in a sweating Method for five or six Weeks together, and after having gone thro three or four successive Crops of miliary Eruptions (as they were called) they all the while melting away, and weltering in their own Sweat, and the Bed rotting under them –"

Next Huxham turns his attention to a description of the putrid, malignant, petechial fever.

"Let us next take a View of the putrid, malignant, or pestilential, petechial Fevers, and then proceed to offer some few Directions as to the Method of Cure.

The highly putrid, malignant, and even petechial Fevers many Times arise from mere antecedent Acrimony of the Blood, agitated by the supervening Fever, yet generally the pestilential and petechial have their Origin from Contagion; and may therefore affect Persons of all constitutions –

In general however these Fevers attack with much more Violence than the slow nervous, the *Rigors*, if any, are greater – The Head-ach, Giddiness, *Nausea* and Vomiting are much more considerable – Commonly the temporal Arteries throb much".

(The author would here interpose the observation that nowadays we recognise a condition called "Temporal Arteritis", or "Giant cell Arteritis". It chiefly affects patients over the age of 60 years and is characterised by severe pain and tenderness in the region of the temporal arteries. If a 2 centimetre strip ("biopsy") of the temporal artery is removed under anaesthesia and examined under the microscope after appropriate staining, it will reveal a characteristic pattern of inflammation with the presence of giant cells, which give rise to the name of the disease. Many patients have a fever during active phases of this disease, which requires steroid treatment to prevent its most dreaded complication, – blindness. Originally described in 'modern' textbooks in the early 1960s, it is possible Huxham had seen cases in the 18th century).

The account continues with reference to the prostration of spirits, weakness and faintness, lumbago, limb pain changes in the colour of the tongue from white to exceedingly black, thirst commonly very great, urine pale at onset growing ever darker even black.

"The Stools, especially near the State, or in the Decline of the Fever, are for the most Part intolerably stinking, green, livid or black, frequently with severe Gripes and Blood –

Sometimes about the eleventh or fourteenth Day, on the coming on of profuse Sweats, the Petechiae disappear, and vast Quantities of small *white, miliary Pustules,* break out – Vibices, or large black and bluish Marks resembling Bruises, are frequently seen towards the Close of the Fever; and, when attended with Lividity and Coldness of the Extremities, are certain Tokens of approaching death –" (This might perhaps be a situation nowadays described as 'Defibrination syndrome', in which overwhelming septic infection results in the body's immune defences going berserk, and invoking mass coagulation – a desperate primitive response to staunch bleeding. In the course of bleeding and coagulation, or clotting, fibrin is produced. However, when the process is prolonged and generalised, all the fibrin gets used up. Then the patient starts bleeding everywhere, from all the body orifices, and under the skin, resulting in the bruises mentioned).

"– I am very sensible, the Word malignant, as applied to Fevers, hath of late Years fallen into very great Disrepute, and probably it hath been often made Use of to cover Ignorance, or magnify a Cure. – But there is really a Foundation in Nature for such an Appelation, at least for some Word, that may distinguish such a Disease, as I have been describing, from a common inflammatory Fever; indeed the very Term inflammatory Fever supposes there are other Kinds of Fevers. – It is perhaps indifferent whether you call them putrid, malignant or pestilential; – when *Petechiae* appear, every one calls them spotted or petechial, – and, if from Contagion, contagious".

He goes on to prepare the reader for his difference of opinion to that of Sydenham, as follows:

" – I will contend with nobody about Words, but it is necessary we should have some to communicate our Ideas, and, where they are well defined, no one hath great Reason to quarrel with them.

I have the utmost Honour for the Memory of the great Sydenham; and yet, I must say, had he not treated all Fevers as merely inflammatory, even the Plague itself, his Practice had been more universally just and imitable, as being extreamly well adapted to those, that depend on an inflammatory Lentor. – But surely it is not always to be followed, even in the Small-pox, which in general he hath admirably well described and most judiciously treated. – Without all Doubt, there are Fevers, that require something more than the Lancet, small Beer and a Purge. – But Honour to whom Honour is due: He justly opposed and exploded the hot, sweating, fiery Regimen, which was then commonly used in all Kinds of Fevers – But Opposition is commonly carried too far, and a favourite Notion may sometimes lead one to *extinguish almost the vital Flame*, and *another* to fire the Fabric, lest the *deleterious Miasmata* should make a lodgement in it.

If a Fever be an Effort of Nature to throw off some offending, or morbid Matter, as most certainly it is, surely it will not always be proper to check it. –"

Here Huxham is displaying a commendable approach of attributing the fever to part of the body's means of combating its cause. We now know that fever is beneficial in speeding the blood flow, which brings antibodies and immune cells quickly to sites of infection, and also permits body cooling by radiating away the heat through the skin. Anti-pyretics by lowering the body temperature will make a patient feel better but not necessarily alter the natural course of the disease, except where the fever is so high that permanent damage could occur. This is seen occasionally in heat stroke, where sweating has failed, and also in cases of cystic fibrosis, where there is defective sweat.

" – In Truth Bleeding in a contagious Disease, as arising merely from Contagion, seems not indicated; because the contagion is intimately mixed with the Humors, and, by drawing off a small Part of the Blood, you very little lessen the whole Contagion, which will have its Effect, more or less, whether you bleed, or bleed not".

One should point out at this stage, that sterility could never be guaranteed, its whole concept was woolly, and therefore the risks of bleeding by their very nature, i.e. by risking the introduction of infection by dirty equipment, were very poorly understood.

"And we find, by the Experiment of Inoculation, that the least Quantity of the variolous Matter, introduced into the Blood, will produce the Small-pox – When you have intimately mixed any Ferment with a Liquor to be fermented, you cannot destroy the Fermentation by drawing off Part of the Liquor; for every Part of the Liquor, when in Fermentation, is a Ferment; so Contagion received into the Blood operates on and in every Part of it. – By cooling indeed, adding Acids, &c. you may moderate the Fermentation; and when it is too violent, you may prevent the Splitting of the Vessel (if too full and close shut) by giving proper Vent; So in contagious Fevers, by drawing off Blood you may lessen its Quantity, and prevent it from over-distending, inflaming and rending the Vessels, and lessen the Heat – But if, to carry on the *Simile*, you cool the fermenting Liquor too much, and prematurely suppress the Fermentation, you render the whole vapid and ropy, and it never purifies itself by a proper *Despumation* – Thus when Contagion is received, if you weaken the Powers of Nature too much by Bleeding &c. and hinder her Operations in *despumating* (as *Sydenham* calls it) the morbid Humors; you concentrate the Disease –

But let us finish this Chapter with a few Words on the curative Intentions, proper in the Fevers, which it particularly treats of – yet Bleeding to some Degree is most commonly requisite, (nay necessary in the strong and Plethoric) not only to lessen the *Moles movenda*, and give a freer Play to the oscillating Vessels –.

Tho' Hippocrates advises in general against purging off the crude Humors, in the Beginning of Diseases, before they are concocted; yet he allows we may purge in the Beginning –"

Most of what Huxham says on the subject of bleeding and purging is nowadays untenable, though it doubtless permitted doctors the luxury of being seen to take some sort of action, and to pontificate over the different (as they saw it) types of fever, and action of the vessels. To the author's knowledge there is only one situation in which bleeding is beneficial in a direct sense i.e. other than to provide a sample for laboratory analysis, and that is in the disease haemochromatosis, where weekly bleedings of up to a pint may be required for prolonged periods to leech out excess iron that has accumulated in the body owing to a genetic failure to control its absorption from the intestine.

Several pages later, we at last perceive something of credible interest:

"Here I beg Leave to insert the following Preparation of the Bark, which I have used for many Years with Success, not only in intermittent and slow nervous Fevers, but also in the putrid, pestilential, and petechial, especially in the Decline; and that too many Times though the Remissions have been very obscure, and yet with a very good Effect –" The bark he is referring to is of course the Peruvian Cinchona, as he does not appear aware of the earlier writings of Rev. Edward Stone (see chapter 4).

The use of Peruvian bark in the treatment of Gangrenous angina (syn. Malignant ulcerous sore throat, Pestilential and child strangling abscess disease of the throat, et al) is described in the MD thesis of William Withering (1641–1799). He states;

"– But as soon as the macules appear, Peruvian bark must be called into assistance. Of the various preparations of it none is more suitable for the sufferers, or more efficacious for health, than the decoction –"

It is of interest that Peruvian bark, quinine, was often being used, and with some success, in the treatment of diseases that in no way resembled malaria. No current medical practitioner would consider administering quinine for a high fever, (non-malarial), paracetamol being the drug of choice nowadays.

7. Heberden (1710–1801)

Another authority early in the 19th century was **William Heberden**, who was born in Southwark on 13th August 1710, the fourth of six children, see figure 2.9. His father was an innkeeper in the parish of St. Saviours. Together with three brothers, William attended the Free Grammar School, which stood in the precincts of St. Saviours church, now Southwark Cathedral. At this time, life for most was harsh and brutal, **only 25% of children attaining their fifth birthday**. Life in the city meant being subjected to smoke from countless fires, people living in extremely cramped surroundings, and with the added hazard of almost complete lack of sanitation. The contrast in early education and environment enjoyed by **William Withering** (1741–1799), the son of a well-to-do apothecary in rural Wellington, a town situated at the foot of the Wrekin in Shropshire, and that of Heberden is extreme. Withering enjoyed the personal tuition of a local curate, and went on to describe the use of foxglove leaf in the treatment of the dropsy. Like Withering, we unfortunately have no record of Heberden's early life. His educational prospects would have been unremarkable had he not shown himself to be an extremely able pupil whose headmaster at Southwark, William Symes, wanted him to continue his education at university. This would have presented no problem had not Heberden's father died intestate, and with financial affairs that remained unsettled for four more years. This delay meant that William Heberden had insufficient funds to proceed to university. However, his school awarded him an exhibition, value £7 per annum, which he was to receive for seven years, and with this assistance he was able to matriculate at Cambridge. He attended St. John's College from December 1724, aged

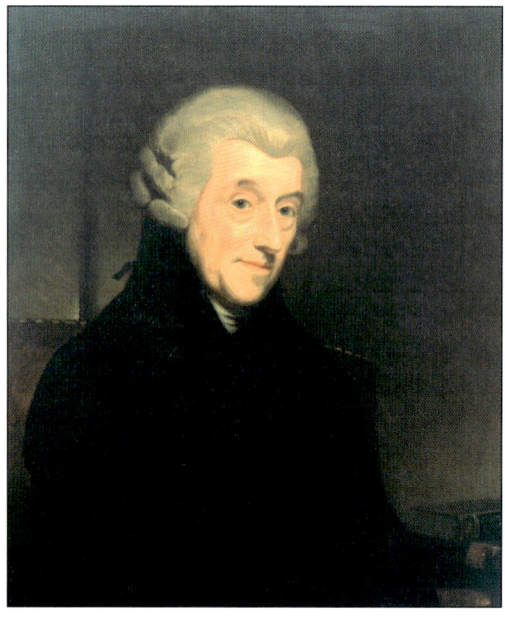

*Figure 2.9. Portrait of William Heberden (1710–1801).
(Copyright, The Royal College of Physicians of London. Reproduced with permission).*

a mere 14 years. At this time, subsequent to the accession of William and Mary, all Fellows of the college were expected to swear allegiance to the House of Orange.

Many who refused were ejected. Students were categorised as either:

- **'Sizars'** (too poor to pay normal fees), therefore were in receipt of free accommodation, free or cut price tuition, a small allowance for food, but were required to perform certain duties such as waiting in hall.
- **'Pensioners'** (the majority), who enjoyed no special privileges, but were required to pay modest fees for board, lodging and tuition.
- **'Fellow-commoners'**, (sons of the wealthy and of the aristocracy), enabling them to take their meals at the Fellows' table in hall.

Unlike Withering who went up to Edinburgh to read Medicine from the start, Heberden studied for a Bachelor of Arts degree, comprising mainly classics, divinity and philosophy. He obtained his degree in 1728. In 1731, he was elected to a Fellowship at St. John's which required him to take Holy Orders. In 1732 he obtained his MA, and in 1734, obtained a medical Fellowship, which meant he was no longer required to take Holy Orders. In the same year, he was made Linacre Lecturer in

Physic, though apparently there were no specified duties. The medical faculty at this time was small, and commanded little respect, being stuck with pre-enlightenment doctrine. He obtained his MD in 1738, having at some stage also trained in a London hospital, probably St. Thomas's. He prepared a course consisting of no fewer than twenty six lectures on **Materia Medica**, the first lecture being delivered on 9th April, 1740. This series of lectures he gave annually until 1748. Included in his course was a description of Peruvian Bark, obtained from the South American cinchona tree, and which we know to be the source of quinine, which at the time was used extensively in the control of fevers. Included also was Heberden's view on how to ascertain whether or not a drug was of use:

"....the first of these is Experience, with which Mankind, as we have seen, set out, but soon grew weary of this tedious but safest method of finding the true effect of medicines. Tho' this may justly be called the most unerring guide, yet even this may prove an useless or dangerous one unless followed with caution. Experience is either that of our own, or what we receive from the testimony of others. In original experience many have been misled by coming to a conclusion before they had a sufficient number of tryals to ground it upon. Almost everyone thinks himself able to pronounce what was the cause of a disease, & to what the recovery was owing. But those who are aware of the difficulties of coming at truth in this matter will agree that it may be very false reasoning to conclude that such a medicine cured a man because he took it and recovered. It is not therefore a single fact, but facts repeated in a variety of circumstances that can establish the just reputation of a remedy..." This clearly shows that Heberden was aware how misleading anecdotal experience can be, and how much more likely the truth will be revealed by proper clinical trial.

We are told Heberden never ventured overseas, but no reason is given. Given his poor origins this is understandable, but later in his career, it might have been extremely interesting to have done the 'Grand Tour'. Nevertheless, he did travel in England, collecting specimens of possible medical interest. During vacations, he was fond of visiting spas, particularly Scarborough, where he met many well-to-do patients, which contributed to his financial success.

Heberden was involved in the publication by the Royal College of Physicians of London, of the **London Pharmacopoiea**. Most of the remedies included were useless, many were dangerous, and nearly all consisted of mixtures of many things e.g. Theriaca Andromachi (Venice Treacle) comprised 65 ingredients including dried vipers, and Mithridatium had 50 components. In 1746 appeared the new edition of the **Pharmacopoiea**, in the introduction of which, appeared Heberden's writings taken from his Materia Medica lectures. His influence was quite clear.

"It would be a disgrace and a merited reproach to us if our Pharmacopoiea abounded any longer in discordant and random mixtures introduced by primitive ignorance or thrust into it by fear of poison and perpetual suspicion...."

In 1746, having satisfied the censors the previous year, Heberden was elected to Fellowship of the Royal College of Physicians, (FRCP).

He was very interested in the medicinal properties of vegetables, and attempted to establish a garden at Cambridge for the culture of plants of medicinal value, which would lend themselves to research. It took 15 years however before this was achieved.

What did Heberden have to say on the subject of fevers?

"A FEVER, or general languidness with a quick pulse, is sometimes an attendant upon other disorders, and will retreat in proportion as they are mitigated by their proper remedies. When it is itself the only distemper, it is still so various in its nature, that very different methods of cure must be employed for different fevers; and some part of the treatment must be learned from knowing the patient's age, and constitution, and manner of living, as well as from a due attention to the season of the year and the peculiar nature of the reigning disease.

Where the fever is evidently inflammatory, as in the inflamed sore throat, peripneumonies, pleurisies, and inflammations of the bowels, there can be no doubt of the necessity of bleeding; and repeated bleedings are often required. The jail-fever," (typhus) – "and others which resemble it, seldom appear to stand in need of bleeding; but it is often of great importance in the beginning of these fevers to clear the stomach and bowels, which is pointed out by the sickness which at that time teases the patient. This may very properly be done by one scruple of ipecacuanha, joined with one grain of emetic tartar, which, beside vomiting, will generally occasion a few stools. The sickness is usually so perfectly removed by one dose of this medicine, that a second is very rarely wanted. A head-ach is a very distressing symptom in the beginning of fevers, for which a blister between the shoulders is an almost certain remedy. In the inflamed sore throat, pleurisies and peripneumonies, blisters are likewise of great use in abating (perhaps by diverting) the inflammation, and in all stages of low fevers, where they act as cordials, and stimulate the power of life to exert themselves, and to shake off the languor with which they are oppressed. The strangury which they are apt to occasion is certainly cured by a clyster made of water and oil, each two ounces, and fifteen drops or more of tincture opii. In the progress of the illness, if a purging should come on, the helps mentioned under the article of diarrhoea, must be employed to check it. The contrary state of too great costiveness will be best removed by a clyster of half an ounce of salt, and twelve ounces of water, with two ounces of oil. Restlessness, and want of sleep, will often yield to fomenting the head and feet frequently with flannels wrung out of hot water; and two or three drops of tincture Thebaica may be given every six hours. Heat, and thirst, may be allayed with lemonade, or toast and water. Languor, and excessive lowness, may safely be teated with wine or cider mixed with water, or a spoonful of the camphor julep. Hiccups, and convulsive twitchings, and agitations, have appeared to be relieved by frequently taking a spoonful of the musk julep; but though musk may have some virtue in quieting spasms, and camphor has in some cases procured sleep, yet their effects are neither great nor constant. I have seen one scruple of camphor given every six hours, and, together with this, one scruple of musk as often as in the intermediate hours; they were both of them borne well by the stomach, but had no perceivable effect in abating the convulsive catchings, or composing the patient to rest. While the sick person in his senses, his own inclination, and strength, will best determine whether he should sit up, or keep his bed, even in the eruptive fevers, as well as in all others.

A specific in continual fevers is, I fear, still one of the desiderata in physic, though it have been much sought after, particularly among the preparations of antimony. In the beginning of fevers, the safe antimonial emetics and cathartics are unquestionably useful; but I have never yet been able to satisfy myself that they do more good, than would be done by any other equally strong purges and vomits. Many judicious physicians are persuaded that, in the succeeding stages of a fever, antimonial medicines, given in such a dose as just not to vomit or purge, are efficacious in abating the fever, either by bringing on a sweat, or by some specific power. In deference to their judgement, have directed four grains of emetic tartar to be dissolved in four ounces of some simple distilled water, of which solution I have given two drams, which contain a quarter of a grain, mixed with three spoonfuls of water, every six hours. This quantity is as much as an adult can usually bear without being sick; and where it is more than the stomach can be easy with, the draught may be divided into two parts, to be taken at the distance of half an hour from one another, instead of the whole being taken at once. Of this medicine I have had considerable experience; but not enough to convince me that antimony possesses any specific virtue of curing continual fevers.

The Peruvian bark has been much dreaded, except in a clear and perfect intermission; but the free use which has been made of it, notwithstanding the height of the fever, in mortifications, and in other cases, where a good suppuration was wanted, has taught us, that this dread is groundless as the many other fears which people have had of this valuable simple; of which the more we know, the less danger we find of its doing any harm, and the more powers of it doing good. Accordingly it has been tried in high continula fevers, in which I am not so sure of its being useful, as I am of its being innocent, not only when two ounces of the decoction have been given every four hours, but when two scruples or a dram of the powdered bark have been directed to be taken as often.

In every fever, it is of the utmost consequence to keep the air of the patient's chamber as pure as possible. No cordial is so reviving as fresh air; and many persons have been stifled in their own putrid atmosphere by the injudicious, though well meaned, care of their attendants. The English seem to have a very extraordinary dread of a person's catching cold in fevers, and almost all other illnesses; the reason of which I could never rightly comprehend. The sick do not appear to me to be particularly liable to catching cold; nor do I know that a cold would be so detrimental, as not to make it worth while to run the risk of it for the sake of enjoying fresh air. I remember one, who, being delirious at the eruption of the small-pox, was so unmanageable, that by frequently throwing the clothes off, and being frequently naked, he catched a great cold, as appeared by all the common signs of one; yet I could not observe that it had any effect in retarding the maturation, or heightening the fever, or preventing his recovery.

It is often useful not only to keep the room well ventilated, but likewise to correct the bad air, by pouring vinegar on a red-hot shovel, and making the room full of the acid vapour which arises from it. Very pale urine, unless the patient have drunk a great quantity of small liquors, is a bad sign in fevers, and it is very desirable to see it become thick, and deposit a sediment; but I know of no other use of it, than the giving us hope that the distemper is beginning to abate: nor am I aware that any important purpose can be answered by examining the faeces; for I know of no state of them which would direct us to employ, or to forbear, any particular method of cure.

For the use of observing the pulse in fevers, see the Medical Transactions, vol.ii, art. 2.

In the long and dangerous fevers of children, it is very common for them to lose all powers of speaking for many days; this is no bad sign, and as the fever abates, the voice always returns.

Adults, as well as children, are sometimes rendered deaf for a time, without any bad consequence.

Concerning the wry neck of children, see chap. 91, *on spasms*.

Chapter 38. *Febris Intermittens*

THE fit of an intermittent fever seldom lasts above twenty four hours, and often not so long. The shivering, and sense of coldness, with which it begins, will continue from half an hour to two hours; then succeed the heat, and restlessness; and these yield to a sweat, the degrees of which, are very various, according as they are more or less promoted by lying in bed and drinking warm liquors. The fit will be a quotidian, returning every day; or a tertian, and return every other day; and if there be the interval of two days between the fits, it is called a quartan. Much longer intervals have been known; but these happen so seldom, that they have been distinguished by no name, and are not of any importance to deserve our notice.

Besides the common appearances of fever, every fit has been sometimes accompanied with other complaints; in some with rheumatic pains; in several with a light delirium; in others with an eruption of the skin, or colic, or faintings, with a pain and swelling of the testicles, a languidness, and almost paralytic weakness of the limbs. These have regularly come and gone with the fever, and with the cure of that have finally disappeared.

Chapter Two – The Fevers

It is a question, or rather perhaps it was a question before men knew well how to cure an intermittent, whether they might safely attempt to cure it. For it was supposed to be an effort of the body to relieve itself from some latent seeds of mischief, which would shew themselves if the intermittent were cured. Some respectable names in physic have patronised this opinion, and I began to practise with a persuasion of its truth: but every year's experience weakened my belief of this doctrine, and I have long since, by numberless proofs, been convinced of the safety of stopping this fever as soon as possible: nor can I doubt of having observed ill consequences where the fever has been suffered to remain, by delaying to use the effectual means of preventing its returns. The Peruvian bark is the well-known specific, with which Providence has blessed us for the cure of this disorder; and if the first fit have been marked so clearly, as to leave no doubt of its being a genuine intermittent, this remedy should be immediately given in such a manner, as to prevent, if possible, a second. If six drams of powdered bark can be got down, by taking a dram at a time, before the hour of its return, the patient will find the fever at least much weakened, if not entirely removed; and the same quantity taken four times a day for six days will usually free the patient from all danger of relapse. But if this medicine be not uncommonly disgustful, there may be good arise, but there can be no harm, from his taking it twice a day for ten days longer. This way of using the bark I think is the most to be depended upon; but where the bark in substance cannot be taken, or borne, there two ounces of a strong decoction used as often will generally be successful. The success would be made less uncertain, if there were no objection from the patient's palate, or stomach, to the dissolving in each dose one scruple, or half a dram of the extract. Bark is a difficult medicine to be got down children's throats, especially in such quantities as would cure their agues. One scruple of the extract, and as much sugar, first mixed with half a spoonful and a half of milk, is a form which will disguise its nauseousness sufficiently for many children to take it without any unwillingness. But wherever either in them, or in adults, it cannot be taken or borne in any form upon the stomach, they may still have the benefit of it by having three or four ounces of the decoction with one or two drams of the powder injected at least twice a day as a clyster; and if this should not be readily retained, ten drops of tincture of opium may be added. It has been proposed to cure an intermittent by keeping the feet immersed in a strong decoction of bark: this I have known tried without success. Cases sometimes occur in which the bark, though properly taken, will not hinder the returns of the fever: this is suspected to be owing to a foulness of the stomach, which hinders the bark from making a due impression upon it; and therefore an emetic is given, and afterwards the bark is repeated as at first. If it still fail, a scruple of chamomile flowers powdered may be given in the same manner as the bark, and I have known this method more than once succeed: I have also given in some extraordinary cases two scruples of calamus aromaticus, and have found it more efficacious than a variety of other means which had been previously directed.

Sometimes it has been of use to take twenty drops of tincture of opium when the fit is coming on.

A quartan ague is far more obstinate than a quotidian, or tertian, and will for a long time elude the power of the bark given in the usual manner, and with all other remedies. I have found several of the inveterate quartans yield to a quarter of an ounce of the bark taken just before the coming on of the fit. From a persuasion that the bark is dangerous, if taken before the fever has perfectly subsided, many begin to take it with very uneasy apprehensions, and sometimes will too long delay taking it, to their great detriment. Now the only harm which I believe would follow from taking the bark even in the middle of the fit, is, that it might occasion a sickness, and might harass the patient by being vomited up, and might set him against it; but in my judgement it can never be taken too soon after the fever begins to decline, provided the stomach will bear it.

Chapter 39. *Febris Hectica*

A HECTIC fever is frequently mentioned in the writings of physicians, and likewise in common conversation; but the precise meaning of the term hectic has not been well settled, and generally acknowledged; so that probably, by different authors, it is not always used to express the same illness. I understand by it that fever which passes under the name of the irregular intermittent, or symptomatic, and what usually attends great suppurations; of which it may not be useless to give a short description, with some mention of the causes by which it is brought on.

This fever very much resembles the true intermittent, from which it must be carefully distinguished; for their nature is totally different, requiring a very different treatment, and the two distempers are extremely unlike in the degree of danger with which they are attended.

In the intermittent the fits are longer, and the three stages of cold, and heat, and perspiration, are more exactly defined, and in all the fits continue nearly the same length of time, after which there is a perfect cessation of the fever. But in the clearest remissions of the hectic there is still some quickness of the pulse, so as to beat at least ten strokes more in a minute than it should in a healthy state. The fits also of the hectic vary from one another, seldom continuing to return in the same manner for more than three times together. Shivering is sometimes succeeded immediately by perspiration, without any intervening heat, without any preceding cold; and the patients sometimes experience the usual chilliness without any following heat or sweat. The fit therefore of the hectic is usually shorter, not only because the whole three stages are shorter, but because one of them is often wanted, and sometimes even two.

The hectic patient is very little, or not at all relieved by the breaking out of the sweat; but is often as restless and uneasy after he begins to perspire, as he was while he shivered, or burned. All the signs of fever are sometimes found the same after the perspiration is over; and during their height the chilliness will in some patients return, which is an infallible character of this disorder. Almost all other fevers begin with a sense of cold; but in them it is never known to return and to last twenty minutes, or half an hour, while the fever seems at its height; which in the hectic will sometimes happen.

However, it is not very unusual for the hectic to have two fits, and even three, as exactly resembling one another, as those of a genuine intermittent; but afterwards they never fail to become totally irregular; so that I hardly remember an instance in which the returns continued regular for four consecutive fits.

The hectic in some cases comes on so seldom, and is so slight, as scarcely to be perceivable for ten or twelve days; but in other instances, where the primary disorder is very great, the fever will be strongly marked, and will attack the patient several times on the same day, so that chilliness of a new fit will begin as soon as perspiration of the former is ended. Several little threatenings of a cold fit have been known to return within a few hours.

In a regular intermittent, the urine during the fever is pale, and thick in the intervals; but its appearance in the hectic is governed by no rules; so that it will be either clear, or loaded, equally during the fits and in the intervals; or even muddy in the fever, and clear in its absence; and will now and then, as in common fevers, be pale during the attack, and muddy afterwards.

Beside the usual distress of a fever, the hectic patient is often harassed with pains like those of the rheumatism, which either wander through the whole body, or remain constant and fixed in one part; and, what is rather strange, often at a great distance from the primary malady, and in appear unconnected with it. These pains have been so great, as to make no small part of the patient's sufferings, and to be not tolerable without the assistance of opium. They are chiefly observable, as far as I can judge, in those whose hectic has been occasioned by ulcers in the external parts, as in cancers of the face and breast, and in other places open to the outward air. In some few hectic cases it is remarkable that considerable tumours will instantly arise upon the limbs, or body, lasting only for a few hours, without pain, or hardness, or discolouring of the skin.

There have been those who when they thought themselves tolerably well have suddenly and vehemently been sized with a fever, not unlike an inflammatory one; and, like that, seeming very soon to bring the life into danger. However, after a few days, the distemper has abated, and the patients have had hopes of a speedy recovery: but these hopes have not improved upon them; for though the first commotions have subsided, and but little fever remain, yet this little, being kept up by some deep and dangerous cause, resists all remedies, and gradually undermining the health, ends only in death. But this is one of the rarer forms of this malady; for in the beginning it most usually dissembles its strength, making its approaches so slowly, that the sufferers feel themselves indeed not quite well, but yet for some months hardly think themselves in earnest ill; for they complain only of a slight lassitude, and that their strength and appetite are a little impaired. This state of their health may be judged not very alarming; but yet if at the same time the pulse be found half as quick again as it should be, there will be a great reason for solicitude about the event. There are not many diseases in which an attention to the pulse affords more instruction than it does in this; yet even here, whoever relies too confidently upon the state of the pulse, will in some cases find himself misled: for it happens, as well as I can guess, to one among twenty hectic patients, that while all the powers of life are daily declining, with every sign of an incurable mischief, the artery will to the last minute continue to beat as quietly, and as regularly, as it ought to do in perfect health.

Great suppurations in any part of the body will bring on this fever; and it will particularly attend a scirrhous gland, while it is yet very little inflamed, and in the very beginning of the inflammation. It increases in proportion as the gland becomes more inflamed, or ulcerous, or more disposed to a gangrene. Glandular diseases are of such a nature, that some patients will linger in them, not only for many months, but even for a few years.

When a scirrhous inflammation is in any external part, and obvious to the sight, or touch, or when its seat is in the lungs, or in any of the viscera, whose functions are well known and cannot be disordered without shewing manifest signs of the disease, in all such cases we can be at no loss about the cause of the fever. But if an internal part, the uses of which are not clearly known, happen, by being diseased, to bring on hectic symptoms, there the fever, which is only symptomatic, may be mistaken for the original and only distemper.

Lying-in women, on account of the mischief arising from difficult births, are liable to this fever, and it often proves fatal. The female sex in general, after they have arrived at their fiftieth year, are in some danger of falling into this irregular intermittent: for in that change which their constitution experiences about this time, the glands of the womb, or ovaries, or of the breasts, are apt to become scirrhous, and as soon as they begin to inflame, the hectic comes on; and not only these, but all the glandular parts of the abdomen, seem at this time particularly liable to be diseased, and to bring on this, of which we are speaking, as well as all other signs of a ruined constitution. The same evils are the portion of hard drinkers, arising from the scirrhous state of the liver in particular, and often of the stomach, and other viscera, which are the well-known effects of an intemperate use of wine and spirituous liquors.

The slightest wound from a sharp instrument has been the cause of many distressful symptoms, and such as have even proved fatal. For after such an accident, not only the wounded part has been in pain and has swelled, but other parts of the body, and those at a great distance from the wound, have been affected with pain and swelling, and have shown some tendency to suppuration. These symptoms never fail to be joined by the irregularly intermittent fever, which continues as long as any of them remain. The time of their continuance is uncertain: some have been harassed with them for two or three weeks; and others for as many months; and, in a few, they have ended only in death.

The hectic fever is never less formidable, than when it is occasioned by a well-conditioned suppuration, in which all the injured parts are resolved into matter so circumscribed as to be readily discharged from the body.

Inflammations of scirrhous glands in the breasts, or in the interior parts, sometimes yield to remedies, or to nature, and together with their cure, the fever, which depended upon them, ceases. But these diseased glands much oftener end in cancers and gangrenes; and the fever continues as long as any life remains.

It cannot be supposed, that a fever arising from so many different causes, and attended with a great variety of symptoms, should always require, or bear to be treated in the same manner.

As the hectic is always occasioned by some other disease, whatever most effectually relieves the primary malady must be the best means of relieving all its natural attendants. When the fever has been the consequence of some small wound, a mixture of opium and asafoetida will prove a useful remedy. In almost all other cases, the attention of the physician must be chiefly, if not wholly employed, in removing the urgent symptoms. A cooling regimen will temper the heat, when it is excessive; the bowels must be kept nearer to a lax than a costive state; sleep, if wanted, must be procured by opium; profuse sweats may be moderated by a decoction of bark and elixir of vitriol; beside which, the greatest care must be taken that the air, and food, and exercise, may be all such, as will be most conducive to putting the body into the best general health. After doing this, the whole hope must be placed in that power, with which all animals are endowed, not only of preserving themselves in health, but likewise of correcting many deviations from their natural state. And in some happy constitutions this power has been known to exert itself successfully, in cases that have appeared all but desperate. For some patients have recovered from this fever, after there had appeared very great signs of its arising from some viscus incurably diseased, where every assistance from medicine had been tried in vain, and where the strength and flesh were so exhausted, as to leave no hopes of any help from nature. In this deplorable state, a swelling has been known to arise, which, though not far from the seat of the primary disorder, yet could not be found to have any immediate communication with it. This tumour has at length suppurated, in consequence of which the pulse has grown calmer, some degree of appetite has returned, and all appearances of distemper have gradually lessened, till the strength and health were perfectly restored. What in some very few instances I had observed nature thus to effect, I have endeavoured to imitate, by applying a blister, or by opening an issue, or seton, near the apparent seat of the internal mischief; but the success has not answered my expectations.

Not many years ago, in some fortunate recoveries from mortifications, the Peruvian bark had been prescribed, and had the credit of the cure; since which time it has been very generally used by practitioners in all tendencies to gangrenes, and where suppurations had not proceeded in a kindly manner. There is every reason to believe, that it may safely be employed in such cases; and no other remedy is known, which has any pretence to rival it for these purposes. Besides, as the hectic fever is so very like an intermittent, even where there was no suspicion of any gangrene or ulcer, the desires of the sick, or of their friends, for trying the bark, have been too importunate to be controlled; and physicians have sometimes prescribed it from their own judgement. But it has greatly disappointed all expectations of benefit to hectic patients; for it seems to have no efficacy, where there is no ulcer; and indeed it has often been useless in mortifications, that there may be some doubt, whether in the prosperous cases the cure were not owing to other causes.

But though I dare not be confident that the Peruvian bark has any extraordinary virtues in stopping the progress of mortifications; yet I can have no doubt that it may safely be used; for neither in these cases, nor in any other, have I ever had reason to suspect its doing harm, unless it can be said to do so when it occasions a sickness or

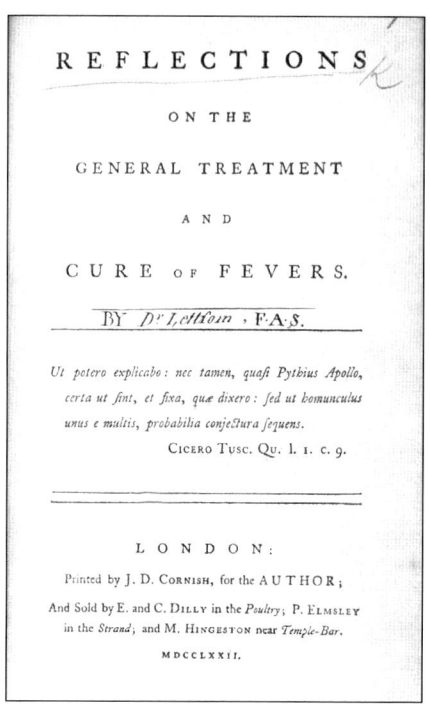

Figure 2.10. Lettsom's reflections on fevers. (Reproduced with permission of the British Library).

diarrhoea, where the stomach happens to be weak, or the dose has been too great, or where it has been taken in hard boluses, which were not readily dissolved in the stomach: and I remember to have heard Sir Edward Hulse say the same, who had for above forty years been giving as much of it as any physician in England, and probably much more than any one had given in all the countries of Europe. Experience every day more and more confirms this testimony in favour of the bark: and hence it must have happened, that the quantity of it used in England for the last ten years, is ten times greater than it was in the same length of time in the beginning of the eighteenth century. It is evident therefore that the more we know of this noble simple, the less reason we find for those suspicions with which it was at first calumniated; so that it affords some exception to the general rule, *ubi virtus, ibi virus*. Yet we are told, that many physicians are still afraid of ever giving it in the beginning of an intermittent; and some are afraid of ever curing it at all with this remedy. They may perhaps adhere to the doctrine (which I believe is founded in error), that an intermittent is an effort of nature, by which the constitution frees itself from many hurtful humours, and from the rudiments of many impending disease; and consequently where these friendly exertions are checked, those dangerous maladies will fall upon the internal parts, terminating in fatal dropsies. I suspect these groundless fears have had their origin from those fevers, which were falsely judged to be intermittent, when in reality they were hectic; and that the obstructions in the abdominal viscera were not owing to the bark, but were the original cause of the illness.

In all chronical disorders which yield to no other remedies, it is usual for the sick to be urged by their own hopes, and by the advice of their friends, to make trial of the Bath waters. Now the inconveniences of travelling, and of missing the comforts of their own houses, must occasion some additional sufferings to the sick; and for these the hectic patients can have no just hopes of having any amends made them by going to Bath: on the contrary, those waters would not fail, by heightening the fever, to aggravate all their complaints, and to hasten their death."

8. Lettsom (1744–1815)

Another authoritative writer on fevers was **John Coakley Lettsom**. He was born 22nd November 1744 in Little Jost Van Dykes, near the main island of Tortola, West Indies, and died 1st November 1815, in Sambrook Court, London.

He was an English Quaker on his father's side, his mother was Irish. There was a high mortality rate among the Tortola population, possibly due to its inclement weather and fevers. In 1772, he wrote three books. They were:

(a) Reflections on the General Treatment and Cure of Fevers, see figure 2.11.
(b) The Natural History of the Tea Tree.
(c) The Naturalist's and Traveller's Companion.

In the Preface he wrote:

"The subject of the following essay is of the greatest moment in medicine; a method of curing FEVERS at their commencement, is what the author has attempted to lay before the public, in as concise a manner as possible, to render it intelligible. The great fatality annually arising from fevers, and the simplicity of the cure proposed, may probably induce some to neglect the treatment recommended; but there are doubtless others, who may reason more liberally, and be induced at least to suspend an unfavourable opinion, till experience may enable them to decide.

Judicio perpende, et si tibi vera videtur, Dede manus; aut si salsa est, accingere contra. LUCRET. Lib. II

In this country, the apothecaries are usually first employed to visit the sick; and the trust thus reposed in them should be considered as sacred; in which not an individual solely, but families likewise are immediately concerned. I mean not to convey the most distant reflection against the part of the faculty; I know too many gentlemen of Character in the profession, to suppose that inclination or interest could induce them to protract a disease, tho' insinuations to their prejudice, in this respect, have often been suggested against them.

I am, however, persuaded, that no man engaged in the divine art of healing, can acquire the cool deliberate baseness of prolonging the miseries of a fellow-creature, who places him in the light of a guardian angel, and with confidence, relinquishes every thing that respects health and life to his disposal; under these circumstances no being, less unfeeling than a demon, could be capable of acting such a tragedy.

However, it is a general and just remark, that all degrees of the faculty, as soon as they attain much employment in their professions, are too apt to fall into a certain routine of form of practice, which afterwards prevents the necessary exertion of the mind, to discover more powerful remedies, or a better method of applying them in the cure of diseases. If physicians acquire habits of this tendency, it is not to be expected that much deviation will be made by other practitioners, who are liable to follow received opinions, and established forms of prescribing; but as physicians are consulted principally in the later periods of a disease, what might be proper then, may not be so at commencement; and therefore it particularly behoves those, who are first employed by the sick, to be anxiously concerned to administer the most suitable remedies as early as possible; by attention to which, many a painful hour in a sick chamber, would be shortened or alleviated; and many agreeable sensations would animate the breast of a man, thus laudably engaged, while every care would be amply compensated by the gratitude of a family thus relieved from distress and painful suspence.

It might have been expected, that the hospitals established in this city, would have contributed more generally to extend the knowledge of medicine; but the public have been mistaken: and the cause will evidently appear, from a candid review of their oeconomy and management. Many of the hospitals in *London* contain four hundred patients; half of which number are usually divided amongst three physicians, who visit them thrice a week, each time requiring about two hours attendance: hence it appears, that one patient with another, two minutes at the most are allotted to each, in order for the physician to hear their complaints, to understand their different symptoms, and to prescribe proper remedies. Does any physician think, that two hours are sufficient to allow him to visit upwards of sixty patients conscientiously? Does any man of reflection expect, that the medical art will improve by the practice in hospitals? Or is the great end of humanity answered in such receptacles of distress? But the faculty are not blameable, while the general oeconomy of hospitals is so deficient. The situation of the practitioners in the *West Indies* affords them frequent opportunities of seeing the sick, and prescribing remedies, at the first attack of the disease. I had there many occasions of observing the success of the practice recommended in the succeeding sheets, when applied in the beginning of fevers, particularly of such as often prove fatal within the *Tropics*, and in warm climates and seasons in general, if not cured in their earlier stages; to stop the progress of these fevers is more necessary, because the longer they continue, the more difficult of cure; and the same remedies which prove efficacious in their commencement, are often unavailable in their advanced periods, as I have experienced with concern. A few days lost are too frequently irremediable; in spite of every endeavour, the fatal preludes of dissolution succeed. My view, therefore, has been the most effectual in curing fevers at their commencement. If it should not always be attended with success, and it undoubtedly will not universally, I presume it never will injure any patient in the fevers I have described, nor prolong the disease where it may not cure. If I have any apology to make respecting this publication, it is for its brevity; but this I hope to remedy at a future period, and to compensate for the present deficiency, I have been induced to make several referrals to writers, and quotations from such of them as have treated most judiciously as the particular subjects I have considered, that the reader might consult further authorities with greater facility".

In section IV of the text that follows, he goes on to say;

"Of the actual sources of FEVERS.

All the varieties of intermittent, and those called continued fevers, probably derive their origin from *marsh miasmata*, and common contagion, differently modified and combined, or acting with various degrees of violence, upon different constitutions; but these causes will be considered more particularly in their subsequent sections...........

Section XI. Of the GENERAL REMEDIES in the CURE OF FEVERS. Emetics............"

He also used powdered bark (Peruvian, not willow, of which he had apparently not heard, though Stone's letter to the Royal society (see chapter 4), had been published nine years earlier).

Peruvian Barks
"It has already been copiously discussed and is a subject at present under the investigation of a physician of eminence and ability in his profession." He was referring to Sydenham. In respect of general remedies, such as saffron, valerian, contrayerva, castor, and neutralised vegetable acids, these he rejected as ineffective.

Bleeding
Lettsom states that here the purpose is:

1. To take off the fever by removing the spasm.
2. To strengthen the system against the recurrence of fever.
   " – it is therefore necessary to procure a general relaxation of the capillaries or extreme vessels, and thereby an universal perspiration.
   The most relaxing topical application – is – warm water, followed by early emetics (tartar), –"

So here we have it, the grand finale of his remedy for the treatment of a fever was – warm water! Of course we all know that tepid sponging of a febrile child will help lower its temperature, but to see the need to write a book on the subject in 1772, suitably dressed up with the experiences of others, whilst omitting the only worthwhile paper (read on behalf of Edward Stone to the Royal Society, in 1763), was little short of ridiculous.

His book on fevers was dedicated to the Earl of Dartmouth, Colonial secretary and connected with the Aldersgate Dispensary, of which Lettsom was President. The book was concerned with the treatment of malaria and yellow fever. They were believed to arise from "miasmas." To quote;

"From this source chiefly, if not solely, all kinds of intermittent fevers at last are produced. These miasmata arise from marshy ground, lakes and woods, when acted upon by certain degrees of heat, particularly in warm climates, and in warm seasons, where the ground is liable to inundations, and is therefore left in a moistened state." Mosquitoes, in the 18th century, were not suspected of causing disease. Lettsom felt that both heat and moisture were needed together to cause fevers, since he observed that in hot dry weather, fevers were less likely than when hot weather was accompanied by dampness. Insofar as treatment of fevers was concerned, he did not subscribe to the prevailing custom of bleeding (a method which, together with purgation, was the mainstay of treatment of yellow fever), as espoused by Benjamin Rush, in his classic account of the 1793 yellow fever outbreak in Philadelphia (see below).

He felt that heat and moisture were essential, as intermittent fevers hardly ever occurred in cold weather.

9. Rush (1745–1813)

An epic struggle against fever (in this case **yellow fever**), was waged by **Benjamin Rush** who was born near Philadelphia, and received his education at the College of New Jersey, later to be known as Princeton University. After this he was apprenticed to Dr. John Redman, the leading medical practitioner in the city. This was followed by a period of study at Edinburgh, where he received his MD in 1768. Next, he stayed in London, receiving further training from William Hunter, then on to Paris, where he visited the Hôtel de la Charité and the Hôtel Dieu. He returned to Philadelphia in 1769, establishing his own medical practice, and was made professor of chemistry at the University of Pennsylvania Medical College. In 1789 he was awarded professorship in the practice of medicine, and in 1791, in physiology. About Rush it has been said:

"Rush's theory of illness appears idiosyncratic and antiquated to modern readers. Devoutly religious, he saw God's unifying hand in everything earthly and consequently viewed all disease as having a unitary character. In the human body, he made this a question of excitability, stimulus, and the production of excitement. In his thinking, he followed Albrecht von Haller's proposals for the basic responsive capacities of the body (irritability and sensibility) and William Cullen's and John Grown's development of a simplified medical theory of energetic response. Rush differed from Cullen, who had made the nervous system central to his responsive theory, by going back to the circulatory system. This arose from and simultaneously justified his great belief in the efficacy of bleeding in the treatment of a wide variety of illnesses".

He is best known for his book 'An account of the bilious remitting yellow fever, as it appeared in the city of Philadelphia, in the year 1793'. It was printed by Thomas Dobson, at the Stone-House, No. 41 South Second Street, Philadelphia, in 1794.

The book starts with an account of the diseases which preceded the yellow fever. There follows a blow by blow account, detailing the cases as they arose, the ambient weather conditions, and the results of Rush's administrations – chiefly bleeding and purging.

"........The weather was uniformly warm in July. The scarlatina continued during the beginning of this month, with symptoms of great violence. A son of James Sharswood, aged seven years, had with the common symptoms of this disorder, great pains and swellings in his limbs, accompanied with a tense pulse. I attempted in vain to relieve him with vomits and purges..........The next day he was nearly well."

Rush builds up the tension as he chronicles the appearance of the epidemic.

"There was something in the heat and drought of the summer months, which was uncommon, in their influence upon the human body. Labourers everywhere gave out (to use the country phrase) in harvest, and frequently too when the mercury in Fahrenheit's thermometer was under 84°. It was ascribed by the country people to the calmness of the weather, which left the sweat produced by heat and labour, to dry slowly upon the body.

The crops of grain and grass were impaired by the drought. The summer fruits were as plentiful as usual, particularly the melons, which were of an excellent quality....

I now enter upon a detail of some solitary cases of the epidemic, which soon afterwards spread distress through our city, and terror throughout the United States.

On the 5th of August, I was requested by Dr. Hodge to visit his child. I found it ill with a fever of the bilious kind, which terminated (with a yellow skin) in death on the 7th of the same month."

Rush went on to describe more cases.

A colleague, Dr. Hodge, told Rush that a malignant fever had carried off four or five people within sight of Le Maigre's house. From these facts, Rush was able to list several of the index cases and come to the conclusion that they had been in the vicinity of some putrid coffee in a dockside area, and that this was the likely source of the outbreak which he named the 'bilious remitting yellow fever.' He had previously witnessed an epidemic in Philadelphia in 1762, and had taken notes at the time:

"In the year 1762, in the months of August, September, October, November and December, the bilious yellow fever prevailed in Philadelphia, after a very hot summer, and spread like a plague, carrying off daily for some time, upwards of twenty persons."

Rush let it be known that in his opinion, the city was in the grip of a 'malignant and contagious fever.' But there were many who expressed doubt, feeling that this was just the usual annual fever, albeit with a higher than expected mortality, and sought to discredit him. Nevertheless, the governor of the state directed Dr. Hutchinson, the inspector of sickly vessels, to inquire into events. He wrote to Rush:

"Dear Sir,

A considerable alarm has taken place, in consequence of the appearance of an infectious disorder in this city; from which the governor has been induced to direct me to make enquiries relative to the existence and nature of such disorder. In executing this duty, I must rely on the assistance of such of my medical brethren as may have been called to attend any of the persons supposed to have been infected: as I understand you have had several of them under your care, I would be much obliged to you to communicate to me (as speedily as can be done with convenience to yourself) such facts as you have been able to ascertain relative to the existence of such disorder; in what part of the city it prevails; when it was introduced; and what was the probable cause of it.

Chapter Two – The Fevers

I am, Sir,
With the greatest respect,
Your obedient servant,
AUGUST 24th, 1793
J. HUTCHINSON"

Rush replied,

"Dear Sir,
A MALIGNANT fever has lately appeared in our city, originating I believe from some damaged coffee, which putrified on a wharf near Arch-street. This fever was confined for a while to Water-street, between Race and Arch-streets; but I have lately met with it in Second-street, and in Kensington; but whether propagated by contagion, or by the original exhalation, I cannot tell. The disease puts on all the intermediate forms of a mild remittent, and a typhus gravior. I have not seen a fever of so much malignity, so general, since the year 1762.

From, dear sir,
Yours sincerely,
August 24th,
1793
BENJ. RUSH"

J. Hutchinson, the physician of the port, replied with his information, to Nathaniel Falconer, the health-officer of the port, to the effect that the current death toll was about 40, and that the disease originated from some damaged coffee, or other putrified vegetable and animal matter. It was felt not to be an imported disease, as no foreigners or sailors had been affected. Clinically, it exhibited great variation, from mild remittent fever to the worst type of typhus.

On 25th of August, the local college of physicians met in order to plan their strategy for coping with this disease. Their recommendations based on fragmentary data, pre-conception of ideas, and a well motivated intention to avoid panic were as follows:

1st   People should avoid mixing with those affected.
2nd   Houses containing sufferers should be marked.
3rd   Infected persons should be placed in the centre of large and airy rooms, abed, without curtains, with strict regard to hygiene etc.
4th   That a large and airy hospital be provided in the neighbourhood of the city. (One wonders if some people saw the disease as a heaven sent opportunity to acquire a hospital!)
5th   Stop tolling the bells. (Bad for morale!)

6th   Burial to be kept as quiet and private as possible.
7th   Keep the streets and wharves clean.
8th   Avoid all fatigue of body and mind. (One wonders how this was to be achieved given the circumstances).
9th   Avoid standing or sitting in the sun; also to have moving air, especially the evening air.
10th   Dress appropriately, and keep warm.
11th   Avoid inebriation, but to take wine, beer and cider in moderation.

"The college conceives **fires** to be very ineffectual, if not dangerous means of checking the progress of this fever. They have reason to place more dependence upon the burning of **gun-powder**. The benefits of **vinegar and camphor**, are confined chiefly to infected rooms, and they cannot be used too frequently upon handkerchiefs, or in smelling bottles, by persons whose duty calls them to visit or attend the sick.

Signed by order of the college,

WILLIAM SHIPPEN, JUN.
Vice President
SAMUEL P. GRIFFITHS
Secretary"

However doubt was expressed in various quarters both in regard to the actual existence of an epidemic outwith the usual seasonal crop of fevers, and whether the present one which Rush was treating so enthusiastically by bleeding and purging had in fact originated from the putrefying coffee.

He made the interesting observation, revealing an understanding of human psychology in regard to the denial of the possibility of serious disease.

"The answers to the first question upon visiting a patient, were calculated to produce a belief in the mind of the physician, that the disease under which the patient laboured, was not the prevailing malignant epidemic – I was particularly struck with this self deception in many persons, who had nursed relations that had died with the yellow fever, or who had been exposed to its contagion in families –"

He noted the tendency to haemorrhage, but went on to remark how few signs there were of damage to the liver. He also stated that he wished to record that the yellow fever "like all other diseases" is influenced by climate and season. He believed the vomiting and constipation to be due to the morbid state of the brain in the first stage of the fever, but on day 4 or 5 he believed it to be the effect of inflammation. Under the heading "Secretions and excretions" he mentioned that on the 4th and 5th days there was "a discharge of matter from the stomach, resembling coffee impregnated with its grounds". He attributed this to "a modification of vitiated bile, but I was led afterwards by its resemblance to the urine – to suspect that it was produced by a morbid secretion in the liver, and effused from it into the stomach. Many recovered who discharged this coffee-coloured matter". (This as any medical student would know, was in fact the presence of blood that had been acted upon by acid in the stomach – commonly described as "coffee ground vomit").

"A total deficiency of the urine took place in many people for a day or two, without pain. – It generally accompanied or portended great danger. I suspected that it was connected in this disease, as in the hydrocephalus internus, with a morbid state of the brain".

Rush described many other symptoms of doubtful specificity including lymphadenopathy (swollen lymph glands). He went on to discuss the skin colouring – "The yellow colour from which the fever has derived its name, was not universal. It seldom appeared where purges had been given in sufficient doses. The yellowness rarely appeared before the third, and generally about the fifth or seventh day of the fever – The eyes seldom escaped a yellow tinge; and yet I saw a number of cases in which the disease appeared with uncommon malignity and danger, without the presence of this symptom. Two very different causes have been supposed to produce this colour of the skin. By some it has been attributed to the dissolution of the blood; but I shall say hereafter, that the blood was seldom dissolved in this fever. The yellow colour, moreover, occurred in those cases where the blood exhibited an inflammatory crust, and it continued in many persons for five or six weeks after their recovery. From these facts it is evident, that the yellowness was in all cases the effect of an absorption and mixture of bile with the blood."

"Many persons had eruptions which resembled moschetto bites. They were red and circumscribed. They appeared chiefly on the arms, but they sometimes extended to the breast. Like the yellow colour of the skin, they appeared and disappeared two or three times in the course of the disorders."

"Petechiae were common in the latter stages and in most cases were the harbingers of death."

With use of Rush's remedy – purging and bleeding – "putrefaction did not take place sooner after death than is common in any other febrile disease, under equal circumstances of heat and air."

His inability to discern a clear pattern in the majority of cases was explained thus:

"It was my misfortune to be deprived by the great number of my patients, of that command of time which was necessary to watch the exacerbations of this fever under all their various changes, as to time, force, and duration. From all the observations that were suggested by visits, at hours that were seldom left to my choice, I was led to conclude, that the fever exhibited in different people all that variety of forms which has been described by Dr. Cleghorn in his account of the tertian fever of Minorca..... I think I observed the fever to terminate on the third day more frequently in August, and during the first ten days of September, than it did after the weather became cool..... The danger seemed to be in proportion to the tendency of the disease to a speedy crisis, hence more died in August in proportion to the number who were affected than in September, or October, when the disease was left to itself. But, however strange after this mark it may appear, the disease yielded to the remedies which finally subdued it, more speedily and certainly upon its first appearance in the city, than it did two or three weeks afterwards."

Rush went on to describe three classes of patients:

1. Those in whom the disease produced symptoms of indirect debility e.g. coma, languor, sighing, syncope and a weak or slow pulse.
2. Those in whom the disease, acting with less force, resulted in headache, and pain elsewhere (unspecified), delirium, vomiting, heat, thirst, and a quick, tense or full pulse, with remittent or intermittent fever.
3. Mild manifestations of disease, insufficient to confine the patient to bed, or to remain housebound. This third class was very numerous, and many recovered without medical aid. Many were (allegedly) saved by "moderate bleeding and purging", whilst some died (these were patients who ascribed their symptoms to a common cold, and neglected to take proper care (i.e. bleeding and purging). Rush went on to point out that this was an area of controversy, many authorities being of the opinion that the yellow fever was not the most likely cause of fevers at that time, whereas Rush was prepared to diagnose the condition in many more cases. He went on to state:

"I have before remarked, that the influenza, the scarlatina, and a mild bilious remittent, prevailed in the city, before the yellow fever made its appearance. In the course of a few weeks they all disappeared, or appeared with symptoms of the yellow fever; so that after the first week of September, it was the solitary epidemic of the city". Rush went on at length to cite others who had observed similar phenomena in other disorders: smallpox (Sydenham, and Huxham). He went on:

"I beg pardon for the length of this digression. I did not introduce it to expose the mistakes of those physicians who found as many diseases in our city, as the yellow fever had symptoms, but to vindicate myself from the charge of innovation, in having uniformly and unequivocally asserted, after the first week in September, that the yellow fever was the only febrile disease which prevailed in the city. I shall hereafter mention some facts upon the subject of the extent of the contagion, which will add such weight to the assertion, as to render the disbelief of it, as much a mark of a deficiency of reason, as it is of reading and observation.

Science has much to deplore from the multiplication of diseases. It is as repugnant to truth in medicine, as polytheism is to truth in religion. The physician who considers every different affection of the different systems in the body, or every affection of different parts of the same system, as distinct diseases, when they arise from one cause, resembles the Indian or African savage, who considers water, dew, ice, frost, and snow, as distinct essences: while the physician who considers the morbid affections of every part of the body, (however diversified as they may be in their form or degrees) as derived from one cause, resembles the philosopher, who considers dew, ice, frost, and snow, as different modifications of water, and as derived simply from the absence of heat....."

Rush here displayed a quaint naivety in attempting to make all-encompassing pigeon-hole diagnoses, whereas we now recognise multiple pathology as the norm, and the brilliant all-encompassing diagnosis as pretty unusual. Thus, a patient with diabetes, liver disease, and arthritis, is more likely to have diabetes (common), *plus* portal cirrhosis, (common), *plus* osteoarthritis (very common), i.e three diseases, than haemochromatosis, one disease which can cause all three clinical features, as a consequence of abnormal absorption of iron and its deposition in the pancreas, liver and joints. On the other hand, it could be argued that to treat peripheral vascular disease, retinopathy, and obesity as separate when all may be linked by diabetes, would be wrong. By optimising the treatment of diabetes, one would improve the prognosis of the other complications, but in actual practice, one would treat each complication as well as the underlying disease. So when Rush stated;

"The sword will probably be sheathed for ever, as an instrument of death, before physicians will cease to add to the mortality of mankind, by prescribing for the names of diseases," he was probably right insofar as the prescribing habits of the profession are concerned, though incorrect in assuming that thereby mortality would be increased. This is a reflection of Rush's reductionist theory, whereby his critical faculties were not to the fore when confronted with the outbreak of yellow fever, which he almost certainly over-diagnosed. As a consequence, he could claim remarkable success in cure rates, as a result of his bleeding and purging regimen.

Rush described many (to him) possibly relevant associations, or lack of associations of the disease. Included in the former were servant maids, families living in wooden houses, people who frequented narrow streets and alleys; whereas the latter included those living on board ships moored in the bay, people confined to the House of Employment, the hospital, the jail (ascribed to the airiness and remoteness of these places).

He continued;

"A meteor was seen at two o'clock in the morning on or about the twelve of September. It fell between Third-street and the Hospital, nearly in a line with Pine-street. Moschetoes (the usual attendants of a sickly autumn) were uncommonly numerous...."

How ironic that he did not at any time consider the mosquito as in any way relevant, yet all manner of other things attracted his attention — mainly things that were obvious to the special senses – if not to a scientific sixth sense. He described the post-mortem findings, again without anything conclusive emerging. However, his best achievement was in counting the numbers of deaths on each day from August 1st to November 9th. He compared this data with the register of the weather. In all, there were four thousand and forty four deaths in this time.

The effect of wet and (relatively) cold weather was not lost to Rush, but as to why this was the case was not obviously addressed. When deaths per week was plotted against mean daytime temperature during the months of August, September and October, it was apparent that the number of deaths increased with falling temperature.

The remainder of Rush's book is devoted to detailed descriptions of his experiences with bleeding and purging. The mosquito is not subsequently given mention though we now know that yellow fever is a viral infection spread by the bite of the mosquito. The elucidation of the cause of this disease was to take many years, notwithstanding a period of time during which it was confused with leptospirosis (a bacterial infection spread by sewer rats).

But how and when was the presence of a fever objectively detected and measured?

The earliest method of recording changes in body temperature was made by **Philo** of Byzantium, 200 BC. This was a thermoscope. **Sanctorius** introduced the thermoscope into medicine – recording the temperature of the hand, the breath, and the inside of the mouth. One needs to bear in mind that the measurement of fever was not routinely carried out before the 18th century, although the concept was apparent to **Galileo** in about 1603. **Benedetto Castelli** wrote in 1638:

'He took a small glass flask, about as large as a small hen's egg, with a neck about two spans long (perhaps 16 inches) and as fine as a wheat straw, and warmed the flask well in his hands, then turned its mouth upside down into a vessel placed underneath, in which there was a little water. When he took away the heat of his hands from the flask, the water at once began to rise in the neck, and mounted to more than a span above the level of the water in the vessel. – Galileo then made use of this effect in order to construct an instrument for examining the degrees of heat and cold.' The liquid in glass thermometer was developed in the 1630s but there was as yet no established standard scale of temperature. It was Fahrenheit, Celsius and de Reaumur who used a mixture of ice and brine, ice and water, the boiling point of water, and body temperature to develop a scale. These instruments were called thermoscopes.

Boerhaave (1668–1738), a famous physician in Leiden, exerted a tremendous influence on medical education, and as part of his research program, doctors from abroad used Fahrenheit thermometers to study patients under his care. Earlier, Boerhaave had suggested to Fahrenheit (1686–1736), originally from Danzig, that he make a mercury thermometer, taking the temperatures of ice and boiling water as fixed points. Within this scale, the temperature in the axilla (armpit) was 96°. Through strong academic connections between Leiden and Edinburgh, the mercury thermometer was introduced to Great Britain. Wilson produced thermometers in London. In 1797, **Dr. James Currie** of Liverpool (1756–1805), studied the effects of cold and warm water in fevers. He used a thermometer which was not self-registering i.e. it had to be read whilst it was still inserted under the tongue of the patient, whilst they were undergoing treatment for typhus or typhoid by dunking them in cold baths! The thermometer had a right angle bend, thus enabling it to be read whilst projecting from the mouth. **Carl Wunderlich** (1815–1877), professor of medicine at the university of Leipzig, assiduously kept human temperature records, and by 1868 had amassed data from 25,000 patients! He was able, consequently, to describe the temperature pattern of many fevers. It was said of him, that he found fever a disease, but left it a symptom.

In 1864, Professor **William Aitken** (1825–1892) of Netley hospital published his book on the Science and Practice of Medicine. In it, he gave a detailed discussion of the theory and practice of medical thermometry. He acknowledged the earlier work of Wunderlich, and had a thermometer made for his use in 1852. Subsequently, Aitken's thermometers went on sale in London, imported from Leipzig. There were two types, one a straight model 25.4cm long, and able to self-register the maximum temperature attained. The other had a curved end designed to fit the axilla, with a length of 30.5 cm and was not self-registering, so had to be read whilst in place, see figure 2.11.

These examples having been made by L. Casella of London, were in general use between 1867 and 1885. The time needed to reach maximum temperature was twenty to twenty five minutes! An interesting little anecdote alludes to a day, sometime in 1867 at St. Thomas's hospital in London. A nurse, Rebecca Strong, was asked by a surgeon to take a patient's temperature. The sister on the ward discovered what she was doing, and severely reprimanded her for doing what was perceived as the work of a medical student. Nevertheless, as we all know, this eventually fell within the remit of the duties of nurses.

Clearly, such a time consuming procedure limited its practicality in everyday use, and so it fell to **Thomas Clifford Allbutt** (1836–1925) to design a thermometer in 1866, which was small and which required only five minutes placement in the axilla (armpit) of the patient, see figure 2.12, this example having been made by Maw, Son & Thompson. He worked in the Leeds House of Recovery, (a fever hospital opened in 1802). Allbutt was elected a physician to the Leeds Infirmary. In 1867 he wrote:

"I wanted a thermometer which would live habitually in my pocket, and be as constantly with me, or more constantly, than a stethoscope. Such a one Messrs. Harvey and Reynolds, of 3, Briggate, Leeds, have had made for me. It is scarcely six inches in length, and being slipped into a strong case, not much thicker than a stout pencil, is carried in the pocket easily and safely. It is made as I proposed – namely, by slightly widening the thread above the bulb, so as to allow the mercury to expand for

20 degrees of heat without rising much in the thread. The graduation begins a little above this widened portion at 80°, and runs up to 115°." Apparently, he had initially requested Casella, an instrument maker from Hatton Garden in London, to make the thermometer, but no interest was shown. The first thermometers made by Harvey and Reynolds cost seven shillings and six pence, and came in a case. It was graduated in Fahrenheit. Allbutt preferred the centigrade scale, but when this was produced, sales plummeted.

He was also a distinguished medical historian. In his latter years he was Regius Professor of Physic at Cambridge.

Although the mercury thermometer had been invented in 1714 by **Daniel Fahrenheit** (1686–1736), a German physicist, it was not until Allbutt invented the pocket sized mercury thermometer in 1866 that it came into general medical use.

The thermometer was critically evaluated by **Thomas Maclagan** (1838–1903), in the Edinburgh Medical Journal of 1867. He wrote as follows:

"That the exact value of the thermometer as a guide to the diagnosis, prognosis, and treatment of disease is as yet undefined, is abundantly proved by the diversity of opinion regarding its utility which is found among medical men. By some it is lauded as an infallible guide to the attainment of a proper knowledge of many diseases; whilst others regard it as an unnecessary and fallacious attempt at refinement – 'a mere scientific toy.' Extreme views are apt to be erroneous, and probably are so in the present case. An instrument which has been found valuable in the hands of men noted for professional, and scientific attainment cannot be a mere toy: at the same

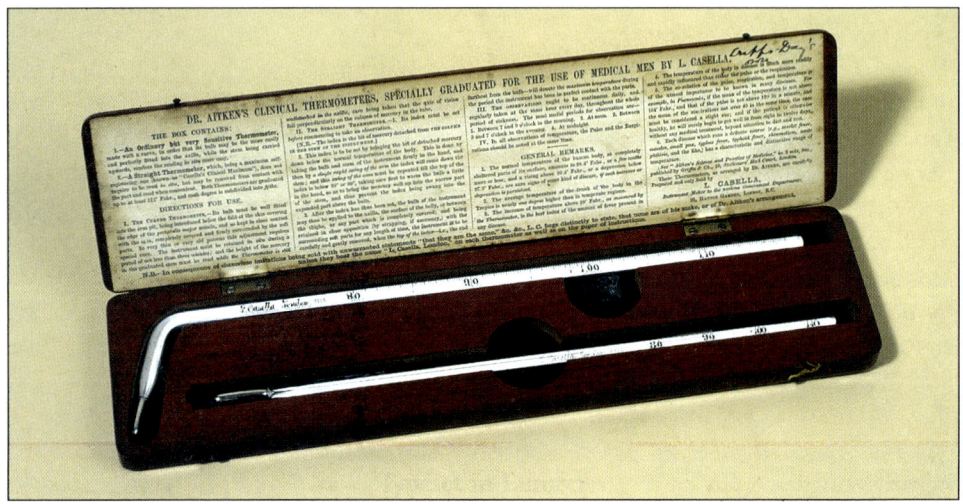

Figure 2.11. Aitken's thermometer.
(Reproduced with permission of the Science Museum, London).

Chapter Two – The Fevers

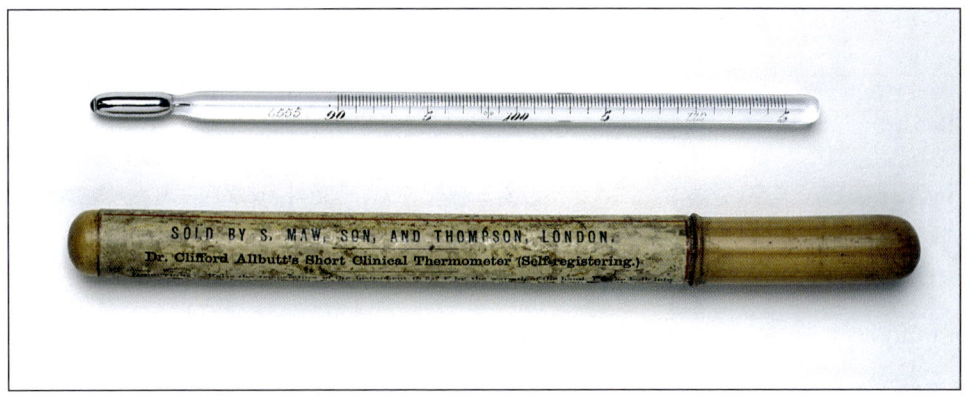

*Figure 2.12. Allbutt's thermometer.
(Reproduced with permission of the Science Museum, London).*

time, it does not become us, as honest searchers after truth, to accept the conclusions of even such men as Wunderlich, Ringer, Aitken, etc., without submitting them to the proof, and testing, by further observation, the value and accuracy of the conclusions at which they have arrived. Imbued with this impression, I began to observe for myself, and was, ere long, led to regard the thermometer as a very valuable aid in acquiring a knowledge of various diseases, but as not possessing those high virtues which some have ascribed to it."

He used the thermometer as designed by Casella – a straight self-registering type. He took his observations from the axilla, initially four times a day, namely at 10 am, 2 pm, 7 pm, and at midnight. Subsequently (and perhaps to make life a little less onerous), he confined his observations to morning and evening. At the same time he observed pulse rate and respiratory rate. He then gave an account of his observations in several cases of typhus, a disease caused by intra-cellular Gram negative bacteria, and spread to man by tick or mite bites. It is highly dangerous, as evidenced by the 'Black Assize' at the Old Bailey in 1750. Typhus was also called "Gaol fever" and at the assize in question, one prisoner's infection was transferred by body lice or fleas to the Lord Mayor, a justice of the Common Pleas, a Baron of the Exchequer, an alderman, a barrister, a number of attendants, several of the jury, and forty members of the public sitting in the court that day – which was the day they all incurred a fatal dose!

These were his findings in 58 cases which recovered, the days at which the fever began falling being recorded alongside the numbers of cases corresponding. After day 9, all cases had begun recovery, but in those cases where recovery, though commenced, nevertheless were still febrile, the morning and evening readings were still noted.

			Morning	*Evening*
In 1 case the temperature was on the	1st day			100.8
In 3 cases	"	2nd day	102.4	102.5
In 10 cases	"	3rd day	102.7	103.2
In 20 cases	"	4th day	103.1	103.5
In 30 cases	"	5th day	103.3	104.0
In 41 cases	"	6th day	103.1	103.3
In 47 cases	"	7th day	103.0	103.5
In 54 cases	"	8th day	102.8	103.4
In 58 cases	"	9th day	102.8	103.1
In 55 cases	"	10th day	102.8	103.1
In 37 cases	"	11th day	102.4	103.4
In 28 cases	"	12th day	102.6	103.1
In 17 cases	"	13th day	102.7	103.0
In 13 cases	"	14th day	102.5	102.9
In 7 cases	"	15th day	102.6	102.9

The findings are intriguing in their own right. Certainly the point is well made that taking the average of all the cases, the mean morning temperature was 102.77°, and the evening temperature excluding day 1, (for which there were no paired data), was 103.21°. He continued:

"It would seem that the temperature gradually and steadily rose, showing little or no tendency to a morning fall, till it reached its highest point on the 5th evening, that it then fell somewhat, and did not again reach the same height; and that on the 6th day commenced those morning falls which characterised the remaining course of the case, and which, though occasionally slight, were generally quite appreciable. The range above the average on the 6th, 7th, and 8th evenings I am inclined to attribute to the fact, which I have several times noted, that in those cases in which the appearance of the eruption is delayed for a day or two beyond the usual time, the temperature does not reach its maximum so early as in those in which it is out on the 5th day. It seems, in fact, that the febrile disturbance, as indicated by the temperature, reaches its height about the time at which the rash is fully developed."

Maclagan attempted to convey his impressions as to the utility of the thermometer in an established febrile illness:

"For the sake of illustrating what has already been said, and of conveying a better idea of the exact place and value of the thermometer, I shall give examples –" He went on to describe the clinical course of a man of 22 years, with a fever and rash. He charted the temperature, pulse and respirations up to the 16th day.

"What, then, was the use of the instrument in this case, which has been instanced as one tending to prove its utility? *It was the first thing which gave certainty to the unfavourable opinion which had been formed of the nature of the case.* The rise of the temperature at midnight of the 7th day, and the continued high range on the 8th, gave a stamp of precision and certainty to the prognosis which at that stage of the illness would otherwise have been wanting – On the 13th morning, the temperature fell from 103.6° at midnight of the 12th to 102.1°; in the evening it was 101.1°; and at midnight 100.5°; thus showing that defervescence had fairly set in; the pulse fell at the same time, and though the general aspect of the case was only slightly if at all improved, there was no hesitation in pronouncing the greatest danger to be past. From that time improvement was progressive. In this case the thermometer gave the first certain sign of impending danger, and likewise the first indication that the danger was past. –

The great use of the thermometer, so far as treatment is concerned, is to point out, during the first week, the cases in which the head-symptoms are likely to be a source of danger, and so enable us to adopt proper precautionary measures sooner than they would be indicated by the other symptoms. It is useful in treatment in the same cases in which it is useful in prognosis. Where death is threatened by asthenia or asphyxia, it is of little or no service; the general symptoms, and condition of the heart and lungs being in such cases the best guides to the proper line of treatment. –

The following statement shows that the thermometer is the best index of commencing defervescence:

In 81 cases, in which the fact was specially noted, the fall of the temperature *alone* gave the first indication of commencing improvement in 18; the temperature and pulse declined simultaneously in 82; improvement in the general aspect and symptoms occurred simultaneously with a fall of pulse and temperature in 27; improvement in the general symptoms and a fall of the temperature preceded a fall of the pulse in 4: thus a fall of the temperature was one of the earliest indications in 100 per cent of the cases; a fall of the pulse in 72.8; and improvement in the general symptoms in 38.2 per cent. –

I do not think that age has much influence in increasing the range of the temperature in typhus;

Neither does sex have any appreciable influence; –

I have never found the temperature of the ward have any effect on that of the body during the height of the fever.

My experience quite accords with that of other observers, when they say that the temperature invariably falls below the normal standard during convalescence, and remains so for some time. My own observations lead me to regard the generally adopted standard, 98.4°, as being, as nearly as possible, correct. –

In the formation of a diagnosis, the thermometer gives, at an early stage of the disease, no evidence sufficient to enable us to distinguish typhus from any other forms of continued fever. –

In conclusion, I would repeat, that the chief use of the thermometer in practice is to enable us, during the first week, to recognise and pick out with greater precision those cases in which the head-symptoms are likely to run high; later on in the case, when all the symptoms are fully developed, its chief use is to give an early indication of commencing defervescence –"

The practicality of thermometry at the time was still somewhat elusive, as a letter to the Editor of the Lancet, in 1916, vol. 1, page 317 showed.

"Sir,

In reference to the introduction of the thermometer into clinical practice in this country, my own recollections are definite. I held the appointment of house-physician in the clinical wards of the Royal Infirmary of Edinburgh, from October 1866, to the end of July, 1867. These wards were for the teaching of clinical medicine to University students. The professors of clinical medicine were Dr. (later Sir) Douglas Maclagan, Dr. Hugh Bennett, and Dr. Laycock; who each held office for three months. When I entered upon my duties as house-physician I found, amongst other apparatus for use in the ward, a case containing two clinical thermometers, one straight, and the other somewhat bent. Each was about ten inches or more in length and took about five minutes or more to reach the temperature of the body when it was placed in the axilla. This thermometer case I used to carry under my arm as one might carry a gun, and most of the thermometric readings I took myself, rarely entrusting the thermometer to the clinical clerks. The thermometers were known as Aitken's thermometers in the hospitals. The clumsy character of these thermometers and the long time they took to rise prevented them from coming into general use, and it was only after their reduction in size, at Sir Clifford Allbutt's suggestion, that their use became common.

I am, Sir,
Yours faithfully,
LAUDER BRUNTON
New Cavendish St, W.
January 31st 1916"

Maclagan's meticulous methodology does him great credit. Determination of the temperature, pulse and respiratory rate, together with testing the urine and measuring the blood pressure, remain the *sine quae non* of clinical assessment. Unfortunately, these are frequently not all carried out as a routine in the busy hospital out-patients.

It is not uncommon for patients to develop a fever for no apparent reason. By this is meant a fever which is not accompanied by the usual features e.g. sore throat,

Chapter Two – The Fevers

Author and date of publication	Sydenham 1763	Osler 1892	Cecil & Loeb 1958	Davidson 1978	Harrison 1983	Kumar & Clark 2002
Book length (pages)	666	1050	1660	938	2400	1320
Diseases listed with fever suffix	17	41	158	19	10	15
Pages on fever	152 (22.8%)	43 (4.1%)	167 (10%)	20 (2%)	13 (0.5%)	16 (1.2%)

Table 2.1 Indexed mentions of fevers, amongst febrile diseases.

cough, muscle pains etc. Instead, the fever continues possibly for weeks or months. When the cause is not obvious, it acquires the accolade **"fever of unknown origin"** commonly referred to as "FUO", or "PUO", (same thing except that the word pyrexia is substituted for fever). There are many possible causes, and it is a favourite examination topic for medical students and doctors in training to master. Amongst the many possible causes is infection of the heart valves ("endocarditis"), tuberculosis, malignancy, overactive thyroid, drug reaction, malignancy, and even, in the most puzzling cases, the patient warming up the thermometer by placing it in a mug of hot tea! The traditional mercury thermometer is now being replaced by a thermocouple placed in the mouth, which gives a more rapid and accurate reading, or a chemically prepared paper strip.

Fever has since the earliest times been recognised as a feature of illness. Whereas then, treatment was aimed at its control as a symptom, in current medical practise, its cause (in persistent cases) must be elucidated, in order to manage the case appropriately.

How much importance is nowadays ascribed to the characteristics of a fever? Apart from malaria, with its well-recognised patterns, relatively little. It may be of interest to look at the importance accorded to fevers, in various medical text books. If we peruse some of them published over the last 300 or more years, a pattern will be seen to emerge, see table 2.1. Thus we see that since 1958, the percentage of space given to describing fever in disease as a proportion of the total number of pages in the book, has fallen considerably from 10% to 0.5–1.2%, whereas in Sydenham's book, it was 22.8%.

Plasmodium. In or around 500 BC, Hippocrates noted that some people suffered a fever which spiked twice each day (quotidian), every third day (tertian), or every fourth day (quartan). In 1880, a French army surgeon looking down the microscope at a blood film of a soldier suffering a fever, recognised the pigmented parasites within the red cells. There are 4 main species, *Pl.falciparum, vivax, ovale,* and *malariae*.

The Plasmodium is transmitted into the body of people by the bite of a female anopheline mosquito, in whose salivary glands and stomach it lives. It is only the female, because males do not take blood meals. Females do in order to produce fertile eggs. Once inside the human, it has a complicated life cycle, and the Plasmodia get back into the mosquitoes when they bite and have a blood meal.

An opportunity to study the natural history of a benign malarial infection was accorded about 50 to 60 years ago, when it was discovered that having malaria lessened the effects of neuro-syphilis. It was therefore used as a form of treatment, patients being subjected to the bites of selected mosquitoes, known to be harbouring *Pl. vivax*. About 14 days after the bite, patients exhibited the typical tertian fever. In some cases it was quotidian, which implied that they possessed 2 distinct families of the parasite, each resulting in tertian fevers but on consequent days. The fever would go through a typical 'hot', 'cold', and 'sweating', stage. Tertian fever is also found in *Pl. ovale* infection.

Pl. malariae produces a quartan fever. The outlook after infection with these is generally good, though deaths among infants are not uncommon. However, the dangerous form of the disease is that ascribed to *Pl. falciparum*. It alone does not manifest regular quotidian, tertian or quartan patterns. Alarm bells ring when delirium, convulsions or coma ensue. These are features of malaria affecting the brain, the disease being known as cerebral malaria. There may be abdominal symptoms such as diarrhoea and vomiting, with severe dehydration with blood in the stools. To confuse matters further, there may be relatively few parasites visible on a blood film, (the usual method of diagnosing malaria is by examination of thick and thin blood films, taken on several days). Thus, cerebral malaria may appear like severe gastro-enteritis. Massive bursting of red blood cells, ('haemolysis') may occur, releasing haemoglobin, the pigment of the red cell. This can clog the kidneys, which then leak the dark pigment into the urine, giving the so called 'blackwater fever'.

The treatment of malaria, is mostly by chloroquine, which is effective against most of the cases of vivax, ovale, or malariae. Falciparum unfortunately is often resistant. Quinine is an alternative, though quinine resistance has also appeared. Severe malaria in a non-immune patient with a high blood parasite count is a medical emergency, and requires urgent treatment with intravenous quinine.

Dengue fever is caused by a virus borne by an arthropod, and is therefore known as an 'Arbor' virus. The arthropod is the Aedes mosquito. It has caused epidemics since the late 18th century. Since 1920, there have been epidemics in the

Gulf of Mexico region of the USA, Greece, Australia and Japan. Between 40 and 80% of the populations of cities have been affected. It is characterised by an incubation period of 5–8 days, rapid rise in temperature, with shivering. Its most typical feature is severe pain, coining the term 'breakbone fever'. Sometimes there is a measles like rash. Occasionally, the fever after lasting 3–4 days, subsides, only to return 2 days later, giving the typical 'saddleback' appearance to the temperature chart. Despite inspiring a strong suspicion to the sufferer that he or she is about to expire, the disease is almost always non-fatal. An exception to this is 'Dengue haemorrhagic fever', which is believed to occur when there are 2 or more distinct serotypes (variants) of the virus causing sequential infection. It has only been described in S. E. Asia, in children. There is severe haemorrhage into the skin, ear, and gut. The immune system is violently over-triggered, resulting in the normal reserve of substances involved in blood clotting being used up. As might be anticipated, this is followed by massive bleeding.

Epidemic typhus fever, is caused by the body louse. Typhus was first described by Fracastorius, in 1546. The word '*typhus*' is derived from the Greek, '*typhos*', meaning smoky or hazy. Typhus and typhoid were not separated into 2 entities until 1837, when Gerhard in Philadelphia was able to draw attention to their differences. Typhus has played a major role in the outcomes of history, reducing armies to helpless patients, and having the ultimate say in the results of military campaigns. In Eastern Europe and Russia, between 1918 and 1922, it is estimated to have caused at least 3 million deaths. In 1915, in Serbia, 400 doctors were infected. 126 died.

In 1916, the organism causing this disease was named *Rickettsia prowazeki*, being found only in Man and the body louse. It was a frequent cause of illness and death amongst the inmates of the concentration camps in World War II. The lice do not like to experience cold, hence when their host dies, they leap to another individual in close proximity. Likewise, if they get too hot, i.e. their victim is running a high fever. The organism itself is very small, between the size of most bacteria, and the far smaller viruses. Its shape is both rounded (coccoid), and rod-like (bacillary). The faeces shed by the lice are rich in *R. prowazeki*, and as a consequence, when garments of louse infected individuals are shaken, or in any way moved about, rickettsia-bearing faeces spread through the air, and as a consequence of inhalation, the organisms gain direct entry to humans. This was probably what happened during the 'Black Assize', q.v. The organism has a predilection for the cells lining small blood vessels, caused endothelial cells. Damage to them is followed by thrombosis, throughout various organs depending where the infected endothelial cells are situated. These result in the typical typhus nodules. The typhus rash is of value in making the diagnosis. It starts on the trunk, and generally spares the extremities and face, unlike in Rocky Mountain Spotted fever, where the rash first affects the wrists, ankles and back.

The disease is treated with doxycycline, tetracycline or ciprofloxacin. Improved hygiene, and use of insecticides can eradicate lice and fleas.

above 39°C, shivering, headache, and a dry cough, with some chest pain. There may be crackles audible when a stethoscope is applied to the chest.

The disease usually clears up within a few weeks, but chronic cases can occur, involving the liver, heart lining (endocarditis), heart muscle (myocarditis), the eye (uveitis), and bones. Treatment is with doxycycline. In chronic cases, combination therapy with doxycycline plus rifampicin or clindamycin is tried. Total clearance of the infection in chronic cases is difficult.

Rheumatic fever affects people aged between 5 and 15 years. It used to be common in the UK, (as a medical student, the cases were seen on the wards, and many patients with the chronic aftermath of the disease, namely mitral stenosis (narrowing of the mitral valve), or mitral regurgitation (leakiness of the valve), were seen. Some patients had similar changes in their aortic valves, and some had both).

The disease would typically start with a sore throat, due to infection by a particular strain of streptococcus. (It was known as the haemolytic streptococcus because, when grown on a blood agar plate, it would produce an area of clarity around the colonies, where the red blood cells had been lysed (burst), by a substance called *haemolysin*, produced by these bacteria). A few weeks later, the child would develop a painful swollen joint, which after a few days or a week, would subside, only to be followed by a similar event in another joint. So this would go on from joint to joint. This was termed a 'flitting arthritis', and interestingly, did not result in any permanent joint damage. Together with this there would be a fever which, despite contributing to the naming of the disease, had no special features, except that whereas a fever due to any old sore throat would subside within a week or so, this would go on for weeks or months. In addition, there would be a characteristic rash, termed *erythema marginatum,* see figure 9.1 in chapter 9, and in some cases, nodules would appear under the skin. One peculiar feature in a few cases, was an apparent fidgetiness which was not an expression of boredom or naughtiness, but signalled involvement of the brain, the involuntary jerky movements being termed *rheumatic chorea,* or *Sydenham's chorea.* Not always evident was the fact that the heart and/or its surrounding membrane, the pericardium, was also affected by inflammation. This might be apparent by changes detectable on an electro-cardiogram implying a degree of slowing down of the heart's electrical conducting system between its chambers, or by murmurs detected by the stethoscope, suggesting inflammation of the mitral valve (the so-called Carey-Coombs murmur), or a scratchy murmur over the heart area of the chest, due to an inflamed pericardium, known as *pericarditis.* The treatment, traditionally, has been high dose aspirin, and still is, though the risk of Reye's syndrome (q.v.) needs to be taken into consideration. Any residual streptococcal infection would be eradicated by penicillin. If there was evidence of heart involvement during the acute rheumatic fever illness, steroids would also be given.

Eventually, children would get over the attack of rheumatic fever, though some would experience recurrences. Any heart murmurs heard would disappear. The disease would then be forgotten. Many years later however, patients might notice themselves becoming short of breath on exertion, some would notice palpitations and irregular beating of the heart, some swelling of the ankles together with shortness of breath. In some case, coughing up of blood, *haemoptysis*, would occur. On examination, the pulse might be irregularly irregular, a condition termed atrial fibrillation. Listening to the heart, the doctor might notice a low pitched rumbling murmur below the left breast extending out towards the side of the chest, especially when the patient held their breath in expiration. In such a case, the doctor would diagnose mitral stenosis. The treatment would consist of a diuretic to offload excess fluid, and attempts to regularise the heart beat by the administration of a suitable timed electrical shock. Failing this, anti-coagulants would be required to minimise the threat of a clot forming inside the heart and travelling to the brain causing a stroke. If the heart continued to fail, and especially if the heart rate was rapid, digitalis would be employed, initially prior to the 1950s as digitalis leaf in powdered form, then later as digoxin, these drugs being derived from the foxglove. Nowadays, patients would undergo an operation to widen the narrowed mitral valve orifice, or to replace it with an artificial valve.

The cause of chronic rheumatic heart disease has caused much head scratching amongst the medical fraternity. This is because try as one may, the streptococcus which we know to be the culprit can never be found within the damaged heart tissue, though examination shows certain features indicative of a chronic inflammatory process. One interesting finding has been that antibodies which act against the streptococcus, also appear to act against the patient's own heart muscle. An evolutionary wile of the streptococcus has been to resemble the host's tissue, but not everyone's immune system is taken in by this ruse. The clever immune system goes after the streptococcus, but to the patient's cost.

The disease though rare in the UK, Western Europe and North America, is still common in the Middle and Far East, Eastern Europe, and South America. With the entry into the European Community of several Eastern European countries, medical teachers and medical students can look forward to the reappearance of many interesting cases, but the cost will have to be borne by an increasingly over-stretched National Health Service.

Rift Valley Fever occurs in South and East Africa. It is caused by a virus, called flavivirus, which commonly affects livestock such as sheep, and goats. It may also affect camels. It requires an insect to spread the disease. 2–3 days after being bitten, fever develops. Typically it gets better, but then recurs before departing. In severe infections however, the course is very different. Eye, brain or liver damage may occur, and in some cases there is severe haemorrhage. Death may occur in 50% of these cases. There is no special treatment, general support is required to keep the patient alive until the disease is overcome.

Rocky Mountain Spotted Fever, like typhus, is a rickettsial disease, being caused by *R. rickettsii*. It is tick borne, and transmitted to Man from rodents. 4–10 days after the bite, a dark coloured scar (called an 'eschar') develops at the site of the bite, and the lymph nodes in the region supplied become enlarged. Thus if the arm has been bitten, it is the nodes (also known as glands) of the armpit which enlarge, whereas if the leg is the site, then the groin nodes enlarge. There is fever, muscle pain, headache, and a rash which is red and raised ('maculopapular'). These spots may bleed into the skin, when they are termed 'petechial'. Rarely, there may be involvement of the brain, bone marrow and the heart. The diagnosis may be established by finding antibodies in the blood directed against *R. rickettsii*.

Trench fever is a disease spread by the body louse, and so-called because it was prevalent during the first World War, and was one of the major medical problems. After the war it disappeared, only to reappear albeit in a smaller scale during World War II. The causative agent is a bacterium, nowadays called *Bartonella quintana*. It is again being seen in refugees and the homeless. One feature, though not in all cases, is a fever which recurs every 5 days. It appears like a form of influenza, with shivering and muscle pain, but differs in that there is a rash which comes and goes with the fever. There may also be enlargement of the spleen, which feels hard. It is never fatal, and resolves by itself, though in severe cases, recovery may be expedited by treatment with erythromycin or doxycycline.

Typhoid, or **enteric fever**, is the name given to the disease caused by *Salmonella typhi*. It is only found in Man, and is spread by infected food or water. The organisms are excreted in faeces or urine. The disease course lasts between one and eight weeks. It starts inconspicuously with feeling ill, with headache and fever which is described as remittent, climbing higher each day to 104°F or even 105°F. When patients have such a high temperature, in most other illnesses, the pulse also is rapid. Not so in all cases of typhoid fever. Whereas one might anticipate a pulse rate of well over 100 per minute, in this disease it may only be 85 or thereabouts. Constipation, a cough and abdominal distension are variable features. A fifth of patients have a nosebleed. Loss of appetite is typical. At the end of the first week, a characteristic rash may be seen in whites. The spots are called 'rose spots' and occur on the upper abdomen and lower chest typically. At this time the spleen may be slightly enlarged. Diarrhoea may occur. Complications include perforation of typhoid ulcers of the gut, and haemorrhage from the gut. Pneumonia, inflammation of the gall-bladder (in which S. typhi may reside after the acute illness is over), and infection of bones, 'osteomyelitis', may occur. Pregnant women usually abort during the course of the illness. The treatment of choice is the antibiotic ciprofloxacin, but sometimes, especially on the Indian subcontinent, the organisms are resistant. In these cases, chloramphenicol (which used to be the preferred treatment), co-trimoxazole, or amoxicillin may be tried.

Yellow fever, Benjamin Rush's nemesis, (q.v.) is now known to be caused by a type of virus called flavivirus. It is nowadays confined to Africa, South and Central America. It is spread by mosquitoes. When mild it mimics influenza, or dengue fever (q.v.) In severe cases, the liver is affected, leading to jaundice and bleeding (the liver is responsible for making several of the substances involved in blood clotting). Coma and death ensue. There is no specific treatment, more it is supportive i.e. trying by all means possible to keep the patient alive until recovery occurs. A vaccine to prevent the disease is available, but not for children under 9 months of age, or immune suppressed patients, because it is a live vaccine.

Chapter Three

THE HERBALS

In Ancient Greece there was a thriving market in plants possessing alleged medicinal value. Herbalists were also known as root diggers, and druggists as drug-sellers. Herbalists protected their trade by proclaiming all manner of superstitions centred around the assumption that herb-collecting was a dangerous process for the uninitiated. As an example, Theophrastus ridiculed their directive that Peony should only be collected at night, because if a woodpecker happened to see someone collecting the fruit in daylight, their vision would be endangered (presumably by act of said woodpecker!).

Herbals were books devoted to herbs or plants in general, describing their properties and virtues. Initially they were manuscripts, but later, with the invention of the printing press, they appeared in book form. Many were in effect printed versions of earlier manuscripts, others were printed *ab initio*.

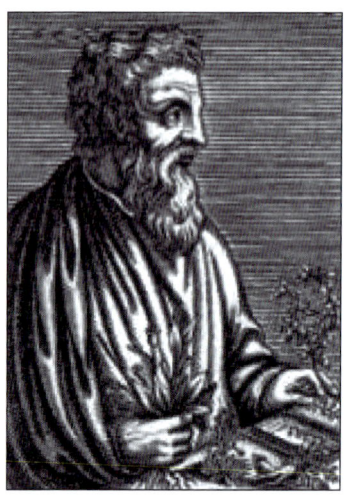

Figure 3.1. Pedanius Dioscorides.

Consequently, many books ascribed a certain print date, in fact referred to material from an earlier age. They also served to convey botanical knowledge. Before the birth of Christ, the works of note included that by **Diodes of Carystos** (c.300 BC), a work on medical botany written in Greek. However Aristotle is believed to have produced botanical writings of an abstract nature, and of which there are but few remains. In them he asks the question why a grain of corn gives rise in its turn to a grain of corn, and not to an olive. In 287 BC Theophrastus, to whom Aristotle had bequeathed his library, wrote a botanical work utilising information from Diodes, and also from folklore. Between 111–64 BC, Crateuas, personal physician to Mithridates VI, wrote an illustrated work called *Roots*. However, a major step forwards was the five-book treatise by **Dioscorides** (40–80 AD), a Greek physician, at the time of Nero and Vespasian, see figures 3.1 and 3.2. His home town was Anazarbus, then part of Roman Cilicia, but nowadays in Turkey. His work was not strictly a herbal because it also included reference to mineral and animal products as drugs. An author picture from the fol. 5 verso is shown in figure 3.3. The centre of this picture has unfortunately been damaged by the ravages of time. On the right is seen 'Pedanios Dioskurides', a book in his hand in which he is writing. The female in the centre of

Chapter Three – The Herbals

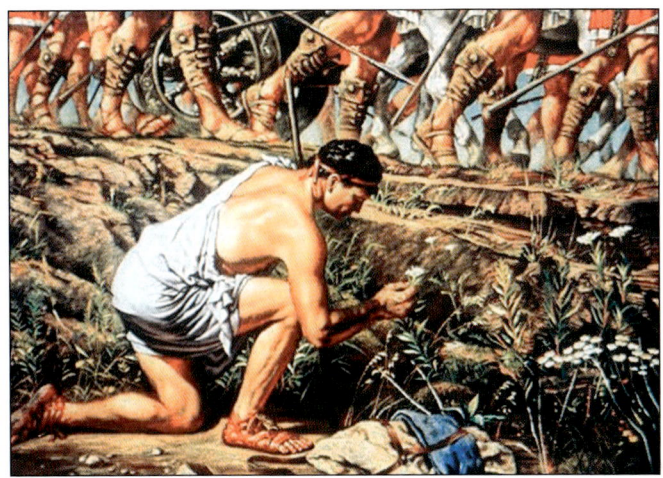

Figure 3.2. Dioscorides, a scientist looks at drugs. Painted by Robert Thom (1915–1979). (Reproduced with permission of the Pfizer Corporation).

the picture is an allegorical figure – Epinoia, or Reasoning power. She is holding a mandrake root, also possessed of medicinal value and is able to help him appreciate the scientific value of the herbs by self-education (Heuresis). On the left is seen the artist of the plant picture, and he is turning round to see the mandrake which he is drawing. Dioscorides' style included firstly a picture of the plant with its root system, fruit and flower, then the name of the plant, its habitats, followed by a botanical description, then its drug properties, its medicinal uses, side effects, quantities and doses, methods for preparation, tests for detecting adulteration, veterinary use, magical uses, and geographical location. Subsequent 'modern' herbals contain more details about growth pattern, frequency of flowering etc. The purpose of the early herbals was primarily medicine, and of the later ones, botany. These and the following remarks are based on an account by Dr. John M. Riddle Ph.D, Professor of History at the University of North Carolina, when commissioned by the editors of the Classics in Medicine series in 1986 to write some notes to accompany Hans Biedermann's *Medicina Magica*. A copy of Dioscorides' herbal, **Materia medica** – a five book series – is to be found in the National Library in Vienna. It is fantastically well preserved and was presented to the emperor's daughter, Anicia Juliana, on her birthday in 512 A.D. It probably remained in the royal library until the fall of Constantinople in 1453. Eventually, as a consequence of an ambassador of the Holy Roman Empire discovering the manuscript in the possession of a Turkish bookseller, it was procured and sent to Vienna. A similar one was found about a century later in Naples, which suggests that both originated from a common source. The work

The Fall and Rise of Aspirin

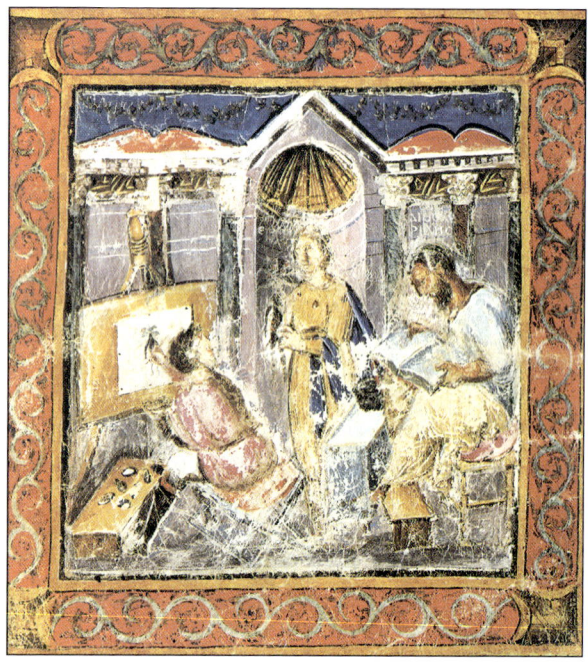

*Figure 3.3. Illustration from the Wiener Dioskurides.
(Reproduced with permission of the Classics of Medicine Library, Gryphon Editions).*

described the use of no fewer than seven hundred plants, as well as animal and mineral drugs. Thus, in a strict sense, Dioscorides' books were not purely confined to herbalism. Dioscorides was a true seeker after truth. Everywhere he went, he asked people which herbs they had found to be of value. He observed the identification, harvesting, preparation, and administration of drugs so that he could form his own opinion on their effectiveness by observing the results on patients. When plants had toxic (harmful) effects, he would quote the safe dose. Many drugs of the era were believed to possess magical effects. In these instances, Dioscorides would make this obvious by preceding the description with phrases such as: "rural people report…" or "it is said that…" At that time there were also lapidaries (accounts of the medicinal values of stones), and bestiaries (medical value of animal products). Dioscorides and other herbalists prescribed willow bark for headache, autumn crocus for gout, the Madagascan rose for cancer. Respectively, we now know these ingredients owed their effects to precursors of aspirin, colchicine and vincristine respectively.

At that time, there was a conflict between religious mysticism and clinical objectivity as developed by Hippocrates. This of course affected the herbals, lowering their scientific value. Nevertheless, Dioscorides was able to walk the narrow path

Chapter Three – The Herbals

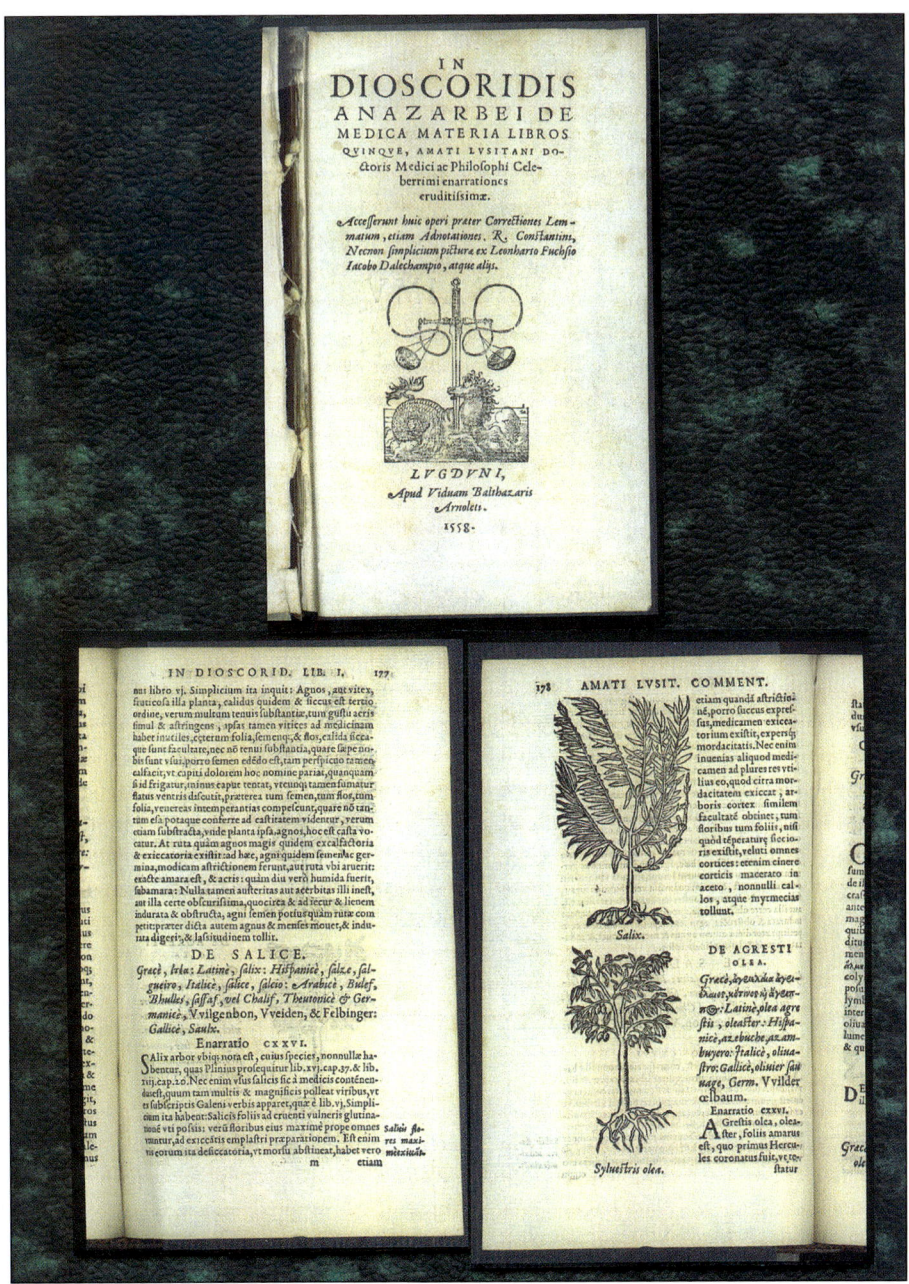

Figure 3.4. Dioscorides' Materia Medica Book 5. Title page and description of the willow (Salix). (With permission from the National Library, Vienna).

between the two, whilst illuminating what was factual. In his work, see figure 3.4, he favoured the grouping together of drugs by their uses, then stating their source as from trees, aromatics, roots, pot herbs. Others preferred an alphabetised approach. Later versions of Dioscorides' work were alphabetised by manuscript copyists, as was the case with the 6th century Juliana manuscript. It was at this time that the work was translated from Greek to Latin, which brought it within the scope of many more readers. Currently of course we have both, textbooks of pharmacology following the Dioscorides approach, in the arrangement of chapters, but with an alphabetised index.

e.g. "1.136. ITEA. Salix sp. Cynodon dactylon Pers. Willow.

Salix is a tree knowne to all whose fruit and leaues & barck & iuice have an astringent qualitie. The leaues being broken small, & dranck with a little pepper and wine doe help such as are troubled with the Iliaca Passio. Being taken of themselves with watwer they cause inconception. The fruit being dranck is good for such as spit blood, & the barck doth doe for the same. Being burnt, & macerated in vinegar, it takes away the calli and the clavi, being anointed on them. But the iuice out of ye leaues & barck, being warmed with Rosaceum in a cup of Malum Punicum, doth help ye griefs of the eares, and the decoction of them is an excellent fomentation for ye Gout. It doth also cleanse away scurfe. There is a iuice also taken of it at ye tyme of its flowring, the barck being cut, for it is found concreted within. It hath a power of cleansing away such things as darken ye Pupillae."

Around the third century AD appeared a herbal ('herbarium') attributed to **Apuleius Platonicus**. It is among the earliest to acquire the appellation 'herbal'. It was possibly the first instance of a work bringing to Britain a systematic account of plants with medicinal value. The Bodleian Library possesses a translation allegedly made for King Alfred. Most of it is about the virtues of herbs. Plants were regarded as "simples", meaning the simple ingredients of compound medicines. Plants were illustrated in a colourful and elegant manner, though in less detail than in Dioscorides. Included among medicinal virtues were spells and charms e.g. "if any propose a journey, then let him take to him in hand this wort Artemisia, – then he will not feel much toil in his journey." Subsequent to the appearance in Italy of the earliest printed editions of the Apuleius Platonicus Herbarium, came three works of great importance. These were printed in Mainz, the home of **Johann Gutenberg** (1397–1468), inventor of the moveable type printing press (c.1450). (Caxton's first printed book was in 1474). Gutenberg's first book printed using this technique was the Bible in Latin. In 1484, the Latin **Herbarius latinus** appeared. It was composed of two parts, the first containing crude illustrations of 150 German plants arranged by Latin name, with an accompanying local German name, and a discussion of the plant in Latin. The second part was not illustrated, but described 96 other plants with their properties, such as use as laxatives etc. In 1485 the German, **Herbarius zu Teutsch**, and in 1491, derived from the latter, the **Hortus Sanitatis** appeared. These

Chapter Three – The Herbals

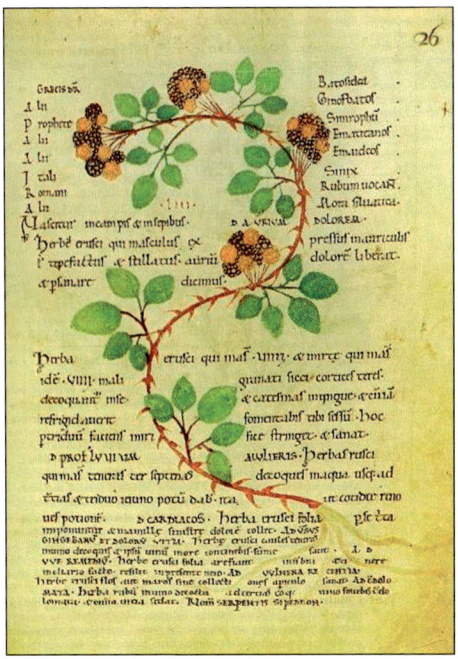

Figure 3.5. Rubus fruticosus from the Apulonius Platonicus herbal.

works are regarded as the doyens among printed herbals. Among the illustrations are several in which, where the herb is believed to possess the power of healing a particular bite or sting of an animal, that animal also is drawn on the same block. Quoting from the Herbarius Sanitatis:

"Many a time and oft have I contemplated inwardly the wondrous works of the Creator of the universe: how in the beginning He formed the heavens and adorned them with godly, shining stars, to which He gave power and might to influence everything under heaven. Also how He afterwards formed the four elements: fire, hot and dry-air, hot and moist-water, cold and moist-earth, – and gave to each a nature of its own; and how after this the same Great Master of Nature made and formed herbs of many sorts and animals of all kinds, and last of all, Man, the noblest of all created things."

The idea was that health required the correct mixture and blend of these elements. The work continues:

"While man keeps within this measure, proportion or temperament, he is strong and healthy, but as soon as he steps or falls beyond the temperament or measure of the four natures, which happens when heat takes the upper hand and strives to stifle cold, or, on the contrary, when cold begins to suppress heat, or man becomes full of cold moisture, or again is deprived of the due measure of moisture, he falls of necessity into sickness, and draws nigh unto death. – Of a truth I would as soon count thee the leaves on the trees, or the grains of sand in the sea, as the things which are the causes of a relapse from the temperament of the four natures, and a beginning of man's sickness. It is for this reason that so many thousands and thousands of perils and dangers beset man. He is not fully sure of his health or his life for one moment. While considering these matters, I also remembered how the Creator of Nature, Who has placed us amid such dangers, has mercifully provided us with a remedy, that is with all kinds of herbs, animals and other created things to which He has given power and might to restore, produce, give and temper the four natures mentioned above."

Thus was ill-heath explained, and the rationale for the use of herbs. It encompasses the most obvious features of many diseases, namely feeling hot, or cold, both characteristic of the development of a fever, and also dehydration, which could accompany fluid loss from diarrhoeal illnesses.

In England, Anglo-Saxon herbals have survived. One such is the Bury St. Edmunds herbal, an illustration from which is depicted, see figure 3.5. It shows a bramble, *Rubus fruticosus*, from Apuleius Platonicus Herbarium, c.1120 AD, and is currently in the Bodleian Library, manuscript no. 130.

Banckes' Herbal

The first true English Herbal was published in 1525. It was not illustrated. The title page states:

"Here begynneth a newe mater, the whiche sheweth and treateth of ye vertues and proprytes of herbes, the whiche is called an Herball". At the end is stated:

"Imprynted by me Rycharde Banckes, dwellynge in London, a lytel fro ye Stockes in ye Pultry". It is probably an abridgement of an English manuscript dating from mediaeval times. A quaint description of "Capillus veneris", is:

"This herbe is called Mayden here or waterworte. This herbe hath leves lyke to Ferne, but the leves be smaller, and it growth on walles and stones, and in ye myddes of ye lefe is as it were blacke heere". Several other herbals appeared under names including **Cary's** or **Copland's**, **Askham's**, and **Macer's**. All were, in reality, derived from Banckes. There is more than a quaint touch in Bancke's description of Rosemary. He advises the reader to:

"take the flowres and make powder therof and bynde it to the right arme in a lynen clothe, and it shall make the lyght and mery.... Also take the flowres and put them in a chest amonge youre clothes or amonge bokes and moughtes shall not hurt them.... Also boyle the leves in whyte wyne and wasshe thy face therwith.... thou shall have a fayre face. Also put the leves under thy beddes heed, and thou shalbe delyvered of all evyll dremes.... Also take the leves and put them into a vessel of wyne.... yf thou sell that wyne, thou shall have good lucke and spede in the sale.... Also make the a box of the wood and smell to it and it shall preserne thy youthe.

Also put therof in thy doores or in thy howse and thou shalbe without daunger of Adders and other venymous serpentes. Also make the a barell therof and drynke thou of the drynke that standeth therin and thou nedes to fere no poyson that shall hurt ye, and yf thou set it in thy garden kepe it honestly for it is moche profytable".

Banckes' Herbal was very popular and ran to several editions.

The Grete Herball
This English herbal first appeared in 1526, translated from the French ("Le Grant Herbier"). In its introduction, it referred to the uses of herbs, as well as alluding to the four elements (fire, water, air and earth).

"Consyderynge the grete goodnesse of almyghty god creatour of heven and erthe, and al thynge therin comprehended to whom be eternall laude and prays etc. Consyderynge the cours and nature of the foure elements and qualytees where to ye nature of man is inclyned, out of the whiche elementes issueth dyvers qualytees infyrmytees and dyseases in the corporate body of man, but god of his goodnesse that is creatour of all thynges hath ordeyned for mankynde (whiche he hath created to his owne lykenesse) for the grete and tender love, which he hath unto hym to whom all things erthely he hath ordeyned to be obeysant, for the sustentacyon and helthe of his lovynge creature mankynde whiche is onely made egally of the foure elementes and qualitees of the same, and whan any of these foure habounde or hath more domynacyon, the one than the other it constrayneth ye body of man to grete infyrmytees or dyseases, for the whiche ye eternall god hath gyven of his haboundante grace, vertues in all maner of herbes to cure and heale all maner of sekenesses or infyrmytees to hym befallyng thrugh the influent course of the foure elementes beforesayd, and of the corrupcyons and ye venymous ayres contrarye ye helthe of man. Also of onholsam meates or drynkes, or holsam meates or drynkes taken ontemperatly whiche be called surfetes that brengeth a man sone to grete dyseases or sekenesse, whiche dyseases ben of nombre and ompossyble to be rehersed, and fortune as well in vilages where as nother surgeons nor phisicians be dwellyng nygh by many a myle, as it dooth in good townes where they be redy at hande. Wherfore brotherly love compelleth me to wryte thrugh ye gyftes of the holy gost shewynge and enformynge how man may be holpen with grene herbes of the gardyn and wedys of ye feldys as well as by costly receptes of the potycarys prepayred".

The Grete Herball concludes:

"O ye worthy reders or practicyens to whome this noble volume is present I beseche yow to take intellygence and beholde ye workes and operacyons of almyghty god which hath endewed his symple creature mankynde with the graces of ye holy goost to have parfyte knowledge and understandynge of the vertue of all maner of herbes and trees in this booke comprehendyd".

With regard to bathing, we are told that according to Galen;
"many folke that hath bathed them in colde water have dyed or they came home".
Depression ("melancholy"):
"To make folke mery at ye table, take foure leves and foure rotes of vervayn in wyne, than sprynckle the wyne all about the hous where the eatynge is and they shall be all mery".

The Grete Herball attributes the value of Artemisia to Diana and the Centaurs, but when it comes to managing a case of mad dog bite, one is advised to entreat the Virgin Mary before proceeding with any remedy. Medical practice early in the twentieth century as then, utilised liquorice for coughs, but by the 1960s, for treatment of peptic ulcers; together with laudanum, henbane, and opium as narcotics.

The herbal also exposes methods used by the unscrupulous for the faking i.e. adulteration of drugs, "to eschew ye frawde of them that selleth it".

The illustrations used in the Grete Herball were also incorporated in another work, the translation into English by Laurence Andrew of the **"Liber de arte distillandi"** (book of the art of distillation) by **Hieronymus Braunschweig**.

Gerard's Herbal

The most notable English herbal is that of **John Gerard** (1534–1612), first published in 1597, see figure 3.6. He is the best known of all the English herbalists, but, in the opinion of Agnes Arber (see bibliography), and with the following reasons, scarcely deserves the fame. A 'Master in Chirurgerie', and hailing from Cheshire, he had a good reputation as a gardener. His garden was in Holborn, then a most fashionable area in London. In 1596, he published the first complete catalogue of the contents of a single garden (his). He may well have cringed at the mention of the name 'Dr. Priest', this being the person contracted to translate the work of the great **Rembert Dodoens** (1517–1585), the first internationally renowned Belgian botanist. Priest unfortunately died before completing his task. Gerard jumped in, and with minor rearrangement, published it as his own. He acknowledged that Dr. Priest had died whilst translating Dodoens, but then dishonestly stated that Priest's translation had perished together with Priest! The herbal is a massive volume, and includes approximately 1800 wood-cuts. Gerard made numerous mistakes in labelling these wood-cut illustrations, which required amendments by de l'Obel (later Physician to William the Silent). Gerard's reputation as a serious herbalist and observer is most poignantly called into question by his belief that barnacle geese were produced by trees! He relates that these trees bear shells which hatch into barnacle geese in the 'Orchades' (Orkney Islands). In fairness however it must be stated that earlier as well as later writers still held this belief. It was not until 1633, twenty one years after his death, that Thomas Johnson edited the work with its account of 2850 plants. He corrected numerous errors, and the repute of the work soared. Gerard however, who scarcely deserved any credit, is the name that persists.

Chapter Three – The Herbals

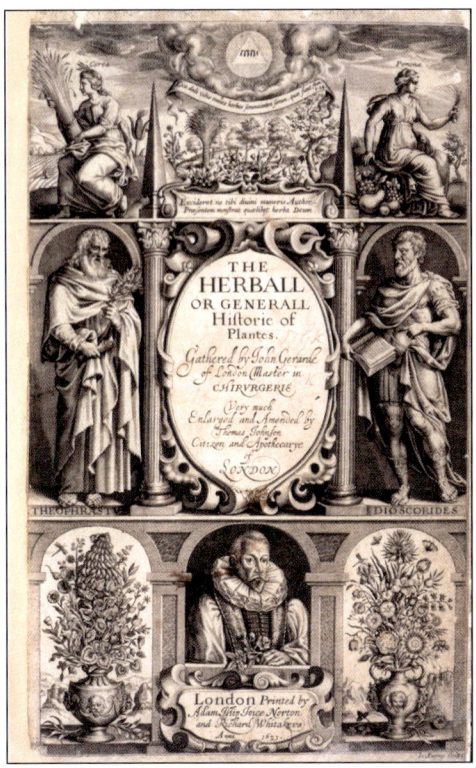

*Figure 3.6. The herbal of John Gerard (1534–1612).
Reproduced with permission of the British Library.*

**The herbal or Generall Historie of Plantes 1633
Gathered by John Gerarde of London
Master in Chirurgerie**
The Vertues (taken from page 1392).
"The leaues and bark of Withy or Willowes do stay the spitting of blood, and all other fluxes of bloud whatsoever in man or woman, if the said leaues and barke be boiled in wine and drunke. The greene boughs with the leaves may very well be brought into chambers and set about the beds of those that be sick of fevers, for they do mightily coole the heate of the aire, which thing is a wonderfull refreshing –. The barke hath like virtues: Dioscorides writeth, that this thing being burnt to ashes, and steeped in vinegar, takes away cornes and other risings in the feet and toes –. Saith Galen, doe slit the barke whilst the Withy is in flouring, and gather a certain juice, with which they vie to take away things that hinder the sight, and this is when they are constrained to use a cleansing medicine of sicke Patients thin and subtill parts –"

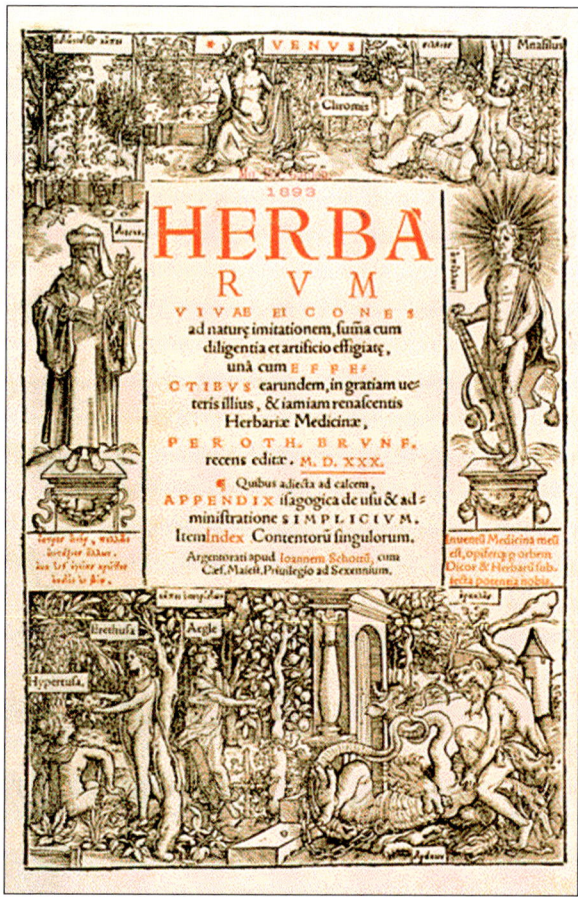

Figure 3.7. Brunfel's Herbal (1530).

The Brunfels herbal (see figure 3.7.)
Otto Brunfels (1488–1534), a physician and naturalist, was a Carthusian monk who became a Lutheran clergyman. He has been credited with publishing the first original description of a regional flora. He spent many years collecting plants around his native city of Bern, Switzerland and arranged his work according to the medicinal properties, rather than in alphabetical form. His book includes beautiful woodcuts by Hans Weiditz, considered to be some of the finest botanical illustrations of the 16th century. It marked the beginning of modern taxonomy (scientific classification). It was printed in his adopted city of Strasbourg. He became the founder of a school and concentrated his research on botany and medicine. The illustrations in his Herbarium broke with tradition in that they were more realistic and less stylized.

Chapter Three – The Herbals

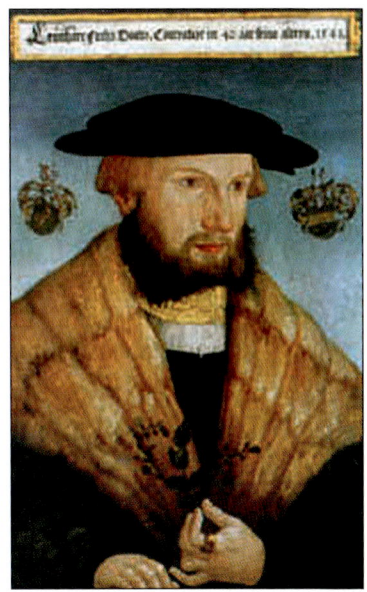
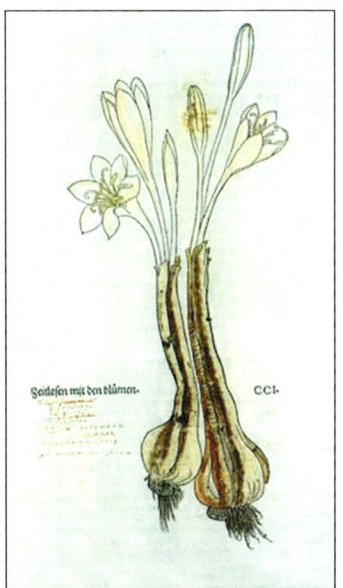
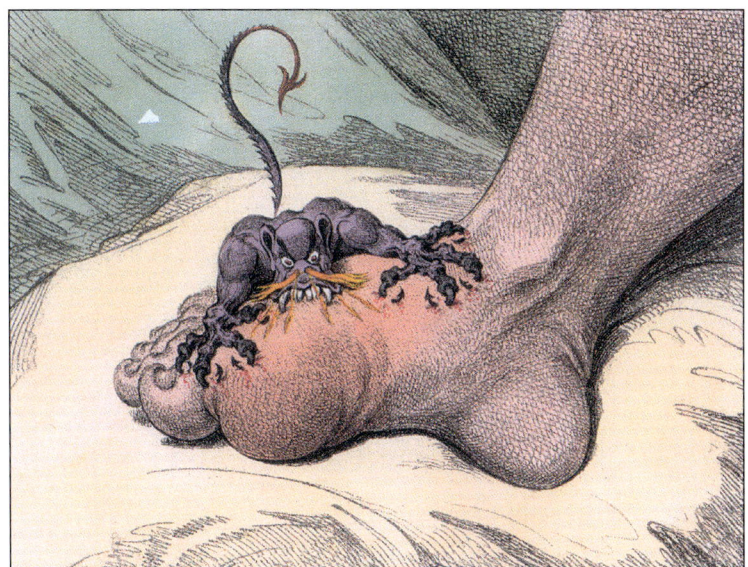

Top Left: Figure 3.8. Portrait of Leonhart Fuchsius (1501–1556).
Right: Figure 3.9. Colchicum autumnale, (1543),
from "New Kreuterbuch", by Leonhart Fuchsius (1501–1566).
Bottom: Figure 3.10. The gout, as depicted by James Gillray (1756–1816).

The Fuchsius herbal
Leonhart Fuchsius (1501–1566), see figure 3.8. was a German physician and botanist. He was influenced by the works of Dioscorides, Hippocrates and Galen, and founded one of the first German botanical gardens. In the figure 3.9, taken from his book, "New Kreuterbuch", is seen an example of Autumn crocus, from which the drug colchicine, traditionally used for the treatment of gout, see figure 3.10, was derived.

The Ryff herbal
Walter Hermann Ryff (c.1500–1548) commenced his training as an apothecary's apprentice in Gustrow, Mecklenburg before moving to Strasbourg where he was the municipal physician. In 1540 he published **"Der erste (–drit) Theyl der Kleynen Teutschen Apotek, Confect"**, see figure 3.11, 1562 edition.

In part 1, he recommends diets for invalids and sick persons, with recipes for melancholy, insanity, and plague. The work includes recipes for meat, fish, fowl, vegetables, herbs and beverages including wine (for pleasure as well as for medicinal purposes!). There is also an entire section on herbal infusions. In 1545 he published

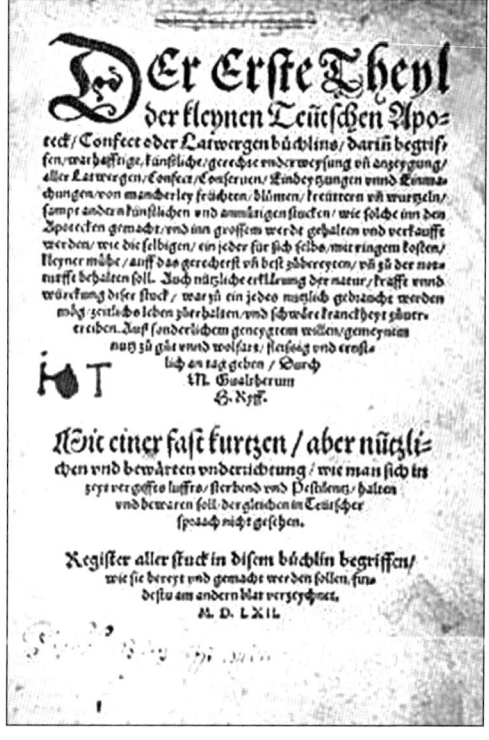

Figure 3.11. First page of the Ryff herbal, 1562.

Chapter Three – The Herbals

his valuable treatise on diets for invalids: "Neue Kochbuch, fur die Krancken". It includes woodcuts of instruments, doctors visiting patients, nurses and children around a sick bed, and hospital equipment such as the latest toilet.

In figure 3.12. is seen the title page of a later work which appeared in 1573. It promises a list of the noblest and most popular herbs together with their differences, types, nature, power, ability and effect. They will be useful and most necessary not only in illness, but also for the promotion and maintenance of bodily health. Descriptions of electuaries (medicines combined with a sweetener e.g. honey), and use of musk sachets, scented powders their mode of production and use, also the correct mixing and preparation of laxatives, together with a useful regimen for surviving and behaving in the face of death and pestilential fevers. All this by the erudite (author), Argent. Medicum, never previously issued in print. With the freedom of the Roman Kaiser's Majesty, for the past 8 years. Printed in Strasbourg by Josiam Rihel, 1573.

On the subject of wintergreen, in chapter LXI it states: (this is an approximate translation with omissions):

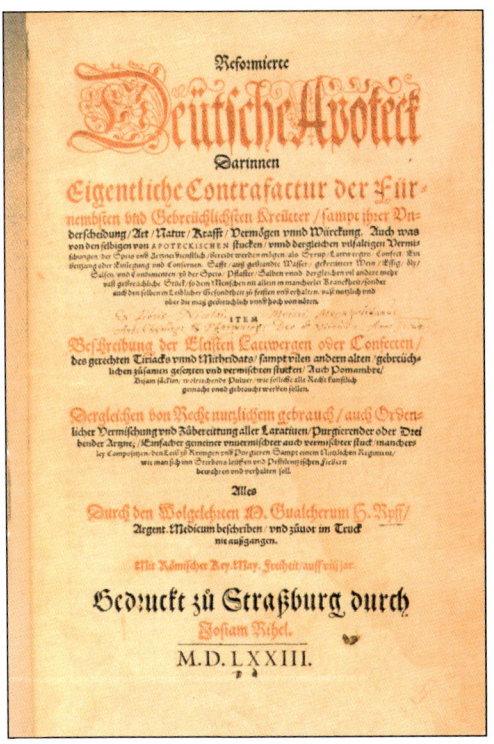

*Figure 3.12. The Ryff herbal, 1573.
(Reproduced with permission of the British Library).*

The Fall and Rise of Aspirin

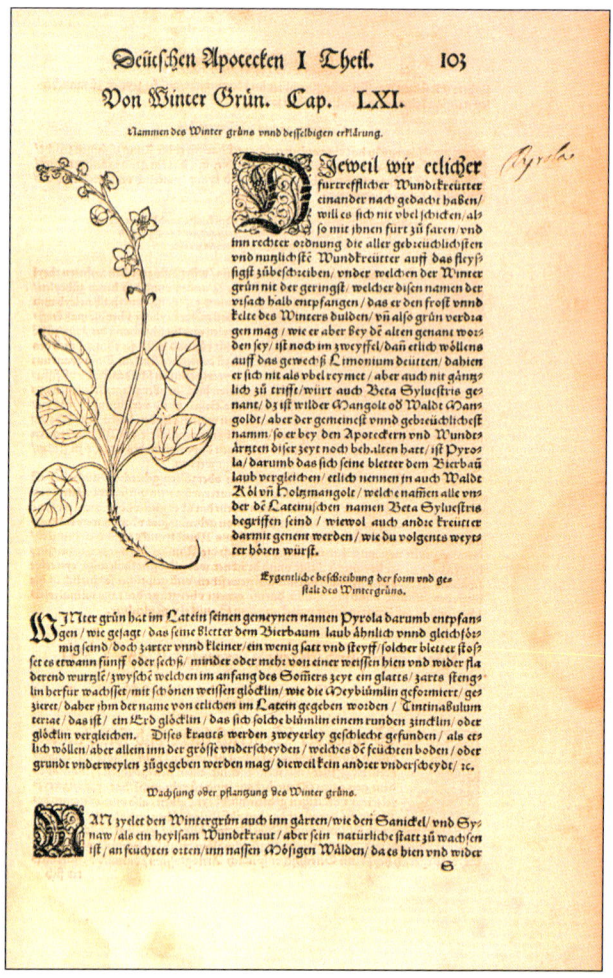

Figure 3.13. Wintergreen described in the Ryff herbal. (Reproduced with permission of the British Library).

'While we have treated a number of excellent healing (wound) herbs one after the other it would be appropriate to continue with these in similar fashion and to carefully describe in the right order the most popular and useful healing herbs, among which Wintergreen is not the least which has received the name for the reason that it stands up to the frost and cold of winter but what it was named by the Ancients is unclear – Wintergreen may also be cultivated in the garden – as a healing (wound) herb but its natural habitat is on moist places in wet mossy woods –

Wintergreen has a raw taste which squeezes the tongue –

The wholesome herb of Wintergreen is nowadays used by the majority to heal fresh wounds and the stomach – Pharmacists frequently use it – as suppositories for bowel problems – This herb, drenched in wine also cleanses the damage caused by putrid pus, cancer and fistulae. Used for washing externally and covered with linen cloth, consumed by drinking, such a potion cures all internal fractures and injury –

Out of Wintergreen one may also distil a most useful water to apply to all the mentioned ailments, thus one takes Wintergreen in its best blossom and finely chopped, pouring good strong wine over it – produces an extremely effective water in old wounds instead of drinking a daily wound potion for it heals from inside also washing the wounds externally promotes betterment, cleanses and presses all open festering pus damaged parts. Cancer and fistulae well washed therewith and sprayed particularly in the depths of the fistulae and with a cloth moistened therein, refreshed several times a day –'

The Rufinus herbal (c.1287 AD)

The Rufinus codex is a handsome illuminated folio of perhaps the early fourteenth century, comprising 118 double-columned leaves. Formerly it was in the possession of Lord Ashburnham, more recently in the Laurentian Library at Florence. It is titled, "Maestro Ruffino, Liber de virtutibus herbarum". Willow (salix) is quoted in the following folios:

21rb, 26ra, 29va, 55rb, 59ra, 66va, 75vb, 83vb. Some are given below.

59ra

"17. **Gualdula** herba est dominarum. Facit gambam rotundam altam aliquando per duo brachia vel circa. In sumitate facit acum velut acrimonia longam per duas spannas vel circa, vallatam seminibus circum circa, folia longa quasi per digitum virgulata virgules rubies desuper velut de cinabrio, folia ipsa ita stricta ut folia salicis vel catupucie. Ipsa tamen folia dispartita in stipite mirabilis ordinatione disposita circum circa. Sunt enim quinque ordines in longitudine ascendendo et quilibet ordo facit –"

75vb

"7. **Oleum de salice** fit hoc moda. *Liber graduum*, folia salicis in vere colliguntur et pistantur et pistate ponuntur in tribus partibus olei olive, et dimittitur bullire ad solem. Similiter fit oleum de semperviva, acetosa, vermiculari et stellaria vel ass – hec olea frigida valent contra calidas et eas destruent".

83vb

"14. **Persicaria** alio nomine (dicitur *mg*) salesegna; nascitur in locis pinguibus et facit arbuscullum cum mutis nodis et folium eius simile foliis salicis, et si ponatur folium ex ea super linguam, mordet eam mirabiliter".

Thorndike's introduction to Rufinus' herbal lets us have a few interesting snippets. There is only one manuscript extant. Rufinus is called various things, including a holy doctor, master in the rubric or titulus of the text, and later, as a monk, and also as "brother Rufinus, penitentiary of the lord archbishop of Genoa" and "abbot of the monastery of tyre". Rufinus informs us that he had pursued the seven liberal arts in Naples and Bologna, and that after studying astronomy and astrology, using the "Tables of Toledo" or "Alfonsine Tables – c.1270" – he turned to the study of herbs. His work consists of a careful, detailed description of the plant itself – stalk, leaves, and flower as well as the differentiation of varieties plus comparisons and contrasts to similar or related flora. His work is a compilation – he states in the preface:

"I shall collect from the sayings of the ancient sages describing the virtues of herbs and their workings in inferior bodies according to what they had experienced and the truth that they were able to discover concerning these. And first, I shall quote the words of Dioscorides; second *Circa instans*; third, Macer; fourth Alexander the philosopher; fifth, the masters of salerno; sixth, Isaac; seventh, Synonyms". He clarifies his contribution by describing additional features which he attributes to himself by the interpolation of his name.

He describes an event in Ravenna, when two boys gambled with the understanding that the loser would take hemlock. This he did, and died. The scope and variety of diseases encountered by Rufinus was somewhat limited, though mention was frequently made of fevers, fistulas, tumours, stones, cough, vomit, wounds, venomous bites, epilepsy, dropsy, jaundice, asthma, arthritis, hair loss, haemorrhoids, gout, paralysis, heart disease, rheumatism. Some case descriptions are given. Mention is made of the unwise therapeutic boast made by an old wife of Bologna, who promised to cure a boy of twelve with malaria if he would trust her, and drink wild cucumber, which he did. Unfortunately, in this case the power of suggestion proved wanting, the boy died next day, and, as for the old lady – by order of the podesta of Bologna, she was burned to death. Caveat doctor! Rufinus also taught astrology to medical students.

In the 17th century, **astrological botany** took a hold in England. Associated with the name **Paracelsus**, also noted for his unshakeable belief in the **Doctrine of Signatures**, it was based on the theory that the heavenly bodies exerted a profound influence on the vegetable world. Each plant was under the influence of a star, and it was this which drew it out of the earth. Another exponent of this belief was **Nicholas Culpeper** (1616–1654), an astrologer and "physician" in Spitalfields. He achieved notoriety by publishing his "Physicall Directory," an unauthorised translation of the Pharmacopoeia (in Latin) issued by the College of Physicians, and clearly not intended by them to convey any meaning to ordinary folk. Culpeper did little to endear himself to the medical profession by calling them, "a company of proud, insulting, domineering Doctors, whose wits were born above five hundred years before

Chapter Three – The Herbals

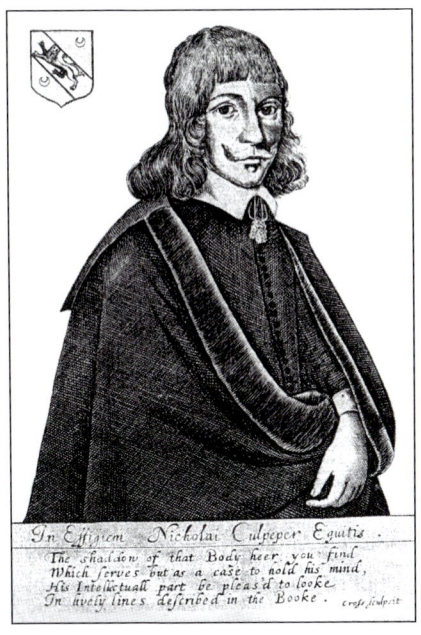

Figure 3.14. Nicholas Culpeper (1616–1654).
A Physicall Directory. Engraving by Cross.

themselves – Is it handsom and wel-beseeming a Common-wealth to see a Doctor ride in State, in Plush with a footcloath, and not a grain of Wit but what was in print before he was born?" An engraving of Culpeper is seen above, see figure 3.14.

The English Physitian or an Astrologo-Physical Discourse of the Vulgar Herbs of the Nation, Being a Compleat Method of Physick, whereby a man may preserve his Body in Health; or cure himself, being sick, for three pence charge, with such things only as grow in England, they being most fit for English Bodies.

By Nich. Culpeper, Gernt. Student in Physick and Astrologie. London. Printed by Peter Cole, at the sign of the Printing-Press in Cornhill, near the Royal Exchange, 1652

"Herein is also shewed,

The way of making Plaisters, Oyntments, Oyle, Pultisses, Syrups, Decoctions, Julips, or Waters, of all sorts of Physical Herbs, That you may have them readie for your use at all times of the year.

What Planet governeth every herb or tree (used in physick) that growth in England

The time of gathering all herbs, both vulgarly, and astrologically.
The way of drying and keeping the herbs all the yeer.
The way of keeping their Juyces ready for use at all times.
The way of making and keeping all kinds of useful Compounds made of Herbs.
The way of mixing Medicines, according to *Cause* and their *Mixture* of the *Disease* and Part of the *Body Afflicted*.

Filipendula, or Dropwort. Vertues and use
It is very effectual to open the passages of the Urine, and help the Strangury, and all other pains of the Bladder and Reins, helping mightily to expel the Stone in the Kidnies, or Bladder, and the Gravel also, and these are done by taking the in Pouder, or a Decoction of them in white Wine; whereunto a little Honey is added: The same also helpeth to expel the Afterbirth. The Roots made into Pouder and mixed with Honey into the form of an Electuary doth much help them whose Stomachs are swollen, dissolving and breaking the Wind which was the cause thereof, and also is very effectual for all diseases of the Lings, as shortness of breath, wheezings, hoarseness of the Throat, and the Cough, and to expectorate cold Flegm, or any other parts thereabouts.
It is called the *Dropwort* because it helps such as piss by drops.

Foxglove, Vertues and use
This Herb is familiarly and frequently used by the Italians to heal any fresh or green Wound, the Leavs being but bruised and bound thereon; and the Juyces thereof is also used in old Sores, to clens, dry and heal them. The Decoction hereof made up with some Sugar or Honey is available to clens, and purge the Body, both upwards and downwards sometimes of rough Flegm and clammy Humors and to open Obstructions of the Liver and Spleen: It hath been found by experience to be available for the Kings Evil, the herb bruised and applied; or an Oyntment made with the Juyce thereof and so used: And a Decoction of two handfuls thereof with four ounces of *Polipody* in Ale, hath been found by late experience to cure divers of the Falling-sickness, that have been troubled with it above twenty years". (No hint here of the profoundly significant effect on the dropsy, due to heart failure, and so elegantly to be described by Withering in 'An account of the foxglove and some of its medical uses – ' published in 1785).
"My self am confident that an Oyntment of it is one of the best Remedies for a Scabby Head that is". Thus far, no mention of willow, or meadowsweet, or anything to predict aspirin. However, in a later edition, 1824, by James Scammon, in the table of herbs and plants, we find under "The Willow-tree", on page 302:
"*Staunch bleeding, Spitting blood, Distillations on the lungs, Heat of lust, Dimness of sight, Warts, Dandriff*

Chapter Three – The Herbals

These are so well known that they need no description, I shall therefore only shew you the virtues thereof *Government and Virtues*. The Moon owns it. Both the leaves, bark, and the seed are used to staunch bleeding of wounds, and at mouth and nose, spitting of blood, and other fluxes of blood in man or woman – The leaves bruised and boiled in wine, stayeth the heat of lust in man or woman, and quite extinguisheth it, if it be long used – The flowers have an admirable faculty in drying up humours, being a medicine without any sharpness or corrosion; you may boil them in white wine, and drink as much as you will, so you do not drink yourself drunk. The bark works the same effect, if used in the same manner – the burnt ashes of the bark being mixed with vinegar, taketh away warts, corns and superfluous flesh, being applied to their place – It is a fine cool tree, the boughs of which are very convenient to be placed in the chamber of one sick of a fever".

The above is of interest, because of its many supposed uses. There is no medical evidence known to the author at the time of writing, to substantiate any of these claims, with the interesting exception of the ability to remove warts, corns and superfluous flesh. We know that salicylic acid possesses keratolytic qualities, i.e. it dissolves keratin, which is the chief substance presence in hard (horny) skin. Quite how the willow boughs placed in the room of a patient suffering from a fever would help, without first having prepared a decoction to be drunk by the patient, is tantalising. When it comes to treating agues, the good book mentions agrimony, archangel or dead nettles, barley, bilberries and whortle-berries, bucks-horn plantain, camomile, coltsfoot, dandelion, feverfew, flea-wort, and pellitory of Spain, but nothing that hints at any aspirin precursor.

In his book 'Murder, Magic and Medicine', John Mann says:

"Culpepper was especially keen on wintergreen (*Gaultheria procumbens*):

'Wintergreen is under the domination of Saturn, and is a singularly good wound herb – a salve made of the green herb stamped, or the juice boiled with hog's lard – is a sovereign salve, and highly extolled by the Germans, who use it to heal all manner of wounds and sores.' In regard to the willow, he recommended that, 'The leaves, bruised and boiled in wine, and drank stays the heat of lust in man or woman, and quite extinguishes it, if it be long used.'

Most of the herbals also mentioned extracts of willow leaves or bark as a treatment for inflammation, and these were chosen because the ancients believed that remedies were usually located in places where a disease was most prevalent. Thus, rheumatic complaints were common in damp places where the willow thrived.

To return to **Paracelsus**. His real name was Philippus Aureolus Theophrastus Bombastus, of Hohenheim. Whilst a professor at the university of Basle, in 1527, he caused an uproar by lecturing not in Latin, but in the vulgar tongue. He also burned the writings of Avicenna and Galen, preferring to interpret his own. Not surprisingly, he didn't last long and wandered about, dying in relative poverty in Salzburg in 1541.

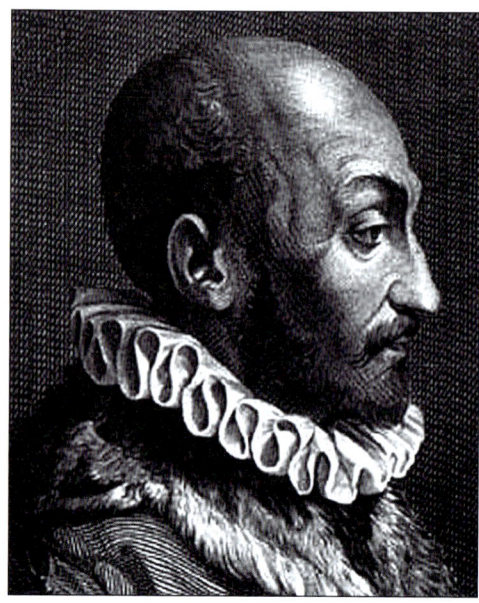

Figure 3.15. Portrait of Giambattista Della Porta.

His chemical theory led to him believing that all plants consisted of sulphur, salt and mercury. Sulphur represented ideas of change, combustibility, volatilisation, and growth. Salt stood for stability and non-inflammability, whilst mercury equated to fluidity. The virtues of plants, Paracelsus believed, depended on the relative concentrations of the aforementioned fundamental principles. And to Paracelsus is ascribed the aforesaid Doctrine of Signatures. He is quoted as saying (translated):

"I have oft-times declared, how by the outward shapes and qualities of things we may know their inward Vertues, which God hath put in them for the good of man. So in St. Johns wort, we may take notice of the form of the leaves and flowers, the porosity of the leaves, the Veins. 1. The porositie or holes in the leaves, signifie to us, that this herb helps both inward and outward holes or cuts in the skin….. 2. The flowers of Saint Johns wort, when they are putrified they are like blood; which teacheth us, that this herb is good for wounds, to close them and fill them up…"
However, there is a rival to the discovery (or fallacy) of the doctrine, and that is **Giambattista Della Porta** (1535–1615), see figure 3.15, who was born in Naples. He wrote about human physiognomony. This includes use of facial features and expression as an indication of character or ethnicity. He was perhaps attempting to produce a psychological profile of a person based on their outward appearance. From this, he reached out to the plants (herbs), believing that their healing powers would be revealed by external signs. His most famous work was the "Phytognomonica", first

Chapter Three – The Herbals

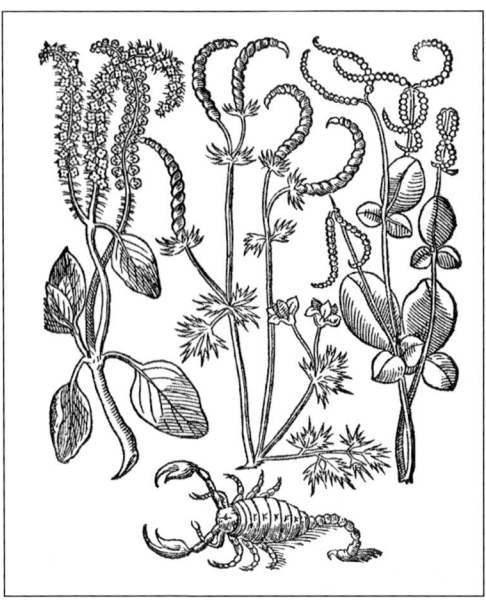

Figure 3.16. The herbs for the treatment of scorpion bite, note the articulated seed vessels.

published in Naples in 1588. The theory was fatally flawed, yet fascinating in a simplistic, even seductive way. Thus, long-lived plants would lengthen the lives of people, and the opposite for annuals. Yellow sap in a herb would perhaps therefore be assumed to cause jaundice, but in Porta's rendition, it would cure it. Butterfly shaped plants would be of value for insect bites. The Phytognomonica was illustrated, and combined the ailment to be cured with the herb which, by its appearance, and resemblance, would be of therapeutic value, see figure 3.16, as found in the Porta, Phytognomonica woodcut, 1591.

For baldness, the remedy would be found in the Maidenhair Fern, illustrated by a rear view of a head with a thick crop of hair, presumably belonging to the grateful patient.

An important name of the time, was **William Cole**, Fellow of New College, Oxford. He lived and studied botany in Putney. His version of the doctrine extended to the resemblance of the walnut to the human brain (a property which has often occurred to the author, and probably to many readers). In 1657, he wrote "Adam in Eden", thus:

"*Wall-nuts* have the perfect Signature of the Head: The outer husk or green Covering, represent the *Pericranium*, or outward skin of the skull, whereon the hair groweth, and therefore salt made of those husks or barks, are exceeding good for wounds in the head. The inner wooddy shell hath the Signature of the Skull, and the little yellow skin, or Peel, that covereth the Kernell of the hard *Meninga* and *Pia-mater*, which are the thin scarfes that envelope the brain. The *Kernel* hath the very figure of the Brain, and resists poysons; For if the Kernel be bruised, and moystned with the quintessence of Wine, and laid upon the Crown of the Head, it comforts the brain and head mightily".

The Doctrine of Signatures encompassed some confusion of thought. Whereas in the example illustrated above, the signature (scorpion) was the cause of the injury or disease, the signature might equally be the clue to the treatment e.g. the presumption that rheumatic disorders arose from exposure to damp regions, if so depicted might well include an illustration of willow trees which are commonly found in such places. One problem faced by Cole, was the fact that many plants of proven medicinal value did not readily fall into the doctrine of signatures scheme. He explained this by proposing that in these instances the plants were devoid of a signature in order to test the ingenuity of the intrepid seekers after the truth! He also bemoaned the fact that physicians tended to leave the gathering of herbs to apothecaries, who in turn relied on the words of "silly Hearb-women". Yet these women could not be all bad, as witness the experience of **William Withering**, whose discovery of the value of the foxglove in treating the dropsy, was based on a herbal remedy of an old woman in Shropshire. The doctrine was repudiated by one of the best of the 16th century herbalists, **Dodoens**. He wrote, in 1583;

" – the doctrine of the Signatures of Plants has received the authority of no ancient writer who is held in any esteem: moreover it is so changeable and uncertain that, as far as science or learning is concerned, it seems absolutely unworthy of acceptance".

Notwithstanding the doctrine of signatures, Paracelsus and Porta both deprecated the use of imported remedies, being of the opinion that nature would provide the means necessary to treat a disease in the same country where that disease occurred. Of course they were wrong, and couldn't possibly have anticipated the threats posed by air-travel as seen recently with SARS from China. But there again, perhaps they were right in regard to the discovery of salicin in the willow bark, for treating agues. Not all agues were malarial, and we didn't need to import quinine containing bark from Peru for treating fevers of which the cause was not malaria.

Chapter Four

THE BARKS

The use of willow bark dates back to ancient times. **Hippocrates** (460–377 BC), was born on the island of Cos. He was regarded as the Founder of Medicine who realised that illness generally had a physical cause, and was not due to spiritual reasons. He also realised that patients needed to be treated in a holistic manner, and not just as made up of separate parts. Many medical students upon graduation, recite the Hippocratic oath which relates to medical ethics. In addition to using lettuce juice and poppy seed oil, he used willow bark either by infusion, decoction or extract to treat pain and fever. **Aristotle** (384–322 BC), is well known for his writings on logic, physics, psychology, natural history, and philosophy. **Theophrastus** (372–287 BC), was also a Greek philosopher, and regarded as the Founder of Botany. He was taught by Aristotle, who had a botanical garden. Theophrastus was aware of the value of the Salix (willow) species. **Dioscorides** (40–90 AD), and **Pliny** (23–79 AD), who incidentally, died after inhaling toxic fumes following the eruption of Vesuvius, advised willow bark as treatment for mild to moderate pain. Subsequently it was used over the ensuing centuries by women herbalists. They would collect the bark from white willow trees (*Salix alba*) which grew along the river banks, boiling it to remove the bitter taste. Unfortunately, willow bark was much in demand for the basket trade, so they had to look elsewhere for a source of this medicine. Somehow they stumbled upon the blossoms of the meadow sweet, *Spiraea ulmaria*, which were as effective as willow bark. Interestingly, these effects were also known to the Hottentots in South Africa, and the North American Indians. But when would its effects be convincingly demonstrated in a medical setting?

Extract from 'An historical account of pharmacology to the 20th century, by Chauncey D. Leake. Published by Charles C. Thomas, Springfield, Illinois, USA 1975
"Even as late as the mid-nineteenth century of our era, the natives in the Cascade mountains of northwestern North America were found to have learned of the purgative properties of the bark of an indigenous tree, cascara sagrada (*Rhamnus purshiana*). It was only then that this safe and effective laxative was incorporated into current medical practice. It is interesting that a preparation of the crude bark, fluid extract of cascara, is preferable to the chemically pure active principle, the anthroquinone glucoside, emodin. The latter is too irritating to the bowel, but the gums, resins, and tannins in the crude preparation reduce the local irritation of the active principle, delay its effectiveness, and thus make it more gentle and satisfactory.

People everywhere found barks of trees which would help them to control diarrhoea. Barks, as we know, contain the astringent, mild antiseptic, tannin, which is effective in reducing bacterial irritation of bowels. Many such barks were later thought to be highly specific for amoebic dysentery, but their usefulness is merely due to the non-specific tannin which they contain. –

Many useful drugs came into conventional medical practice during the seventeenth century, from various places in Latin America and Africa. There the natives had long before discovered their potential medical value. Among such drugs were coca leaves and Peruvian bark from the Andes, from which in the nineteenth century such active substances as cocaine and quinine were extracted.

The ancient Greeks used willow barks and leaves crushed in olive oil to apply to rheumatic or arthritic joints or muscles. Arthritis was common in antiquity in the Near East as old Egyptian mummy bones testify. Willow (Salix) contains a glucoside called salicin; its chemical make-up led to the synthesis of salicylic acid. Its many derivatives, chief of which is aspirin (acetyl-salicylic acid), are used the world over for the relief of rheumatic and arthritic aches and pains. The Amerinds of the eastern United States used crushed leaves of wintergreen for the same purpose. We now know that oil of wintergreen is methyl salicylate and is often used in ointments to help reduce the pain of rheumatism and arthritis."

Interestingly, it would be a man of the cloth, not a physician, who would point the way. That man was the Reverend Edward Stone. And what was the active ingredient? This would not be revealed until more than a century later.

1. The Reverend Edward Stone (1702–1768)

(Much of the following is extracted from the monograph about the life of Edward Stone, written by the Reverend Ralph Mann, local historian of Chipping Norton, who kindly donated a copy to the author).

Edward Stone was born in the village of Lacey Green, Oxfordshire, on 5th November 1702, the son of Edward Stone, yeoman of Princes Risborough, and Elizabeth Reynolds of Monks Risborough. Mann described it thus:

"Edward Stone grew up in the quiet countryside around Princes Risborough. Barely touched by the turnpikes, Princes Risborough was a small country town at the foot of the Chiltern Hills in Buckinghamshire. Lacey Green itself, his birthplace, lay a few miles south east in a hollow of the hills – ", see figure 4.1. His mother died shortly after. In April 1707 his father remarried, his second wife being Elizabeth Grubb, of Horsenden. Her father was Lord of the Manor of Horsenden and Owlswick. A daughter was born in 1709.

So Edward Stone grew up, comfortably, in Princes Risborough, at the foot of the Chiltern Hills. He probably received his education at home, as there was no local grammar school. From the age of 14 years, he lived at the Manor of Owlswick, his

Chapter Four – The Barks

father having come into possession through marriage (it was bequeathed jointly to his second wife and her two sisters, who Edward Stone Senior had bought out). Owlswick was a tiny hamlet four miles north of Princes Risborough. Nearby was the village of Horsenden, of which the Manor was owned by John Grubb. It seems possible that Edward Stone junior received his education at Horsenden Manor, see figure 4.2, with his cousins. Within the grounds was the church of St. Michael, see figure 4.3. After a childhood probably spent in idyllic surroundings, at the age of 17 he went up to Wadham College in Oxford, which received about thirteen undergraduates per annum. The Admissions Register records the event as:

"– Edward Stone the son of Edward Stone of Princes Risborough, Gent". In 1724, Edward Stone was elected to a scholarship. In November 1724, he graduated BA, and in June 1727, MA. He then set about attaining Fellowship of the College. To be ordained would be of considerable advantage, and this he proceeded to do. The necessary prerequisite was to have an elementary knowledge of the bible, a desire to uphold public morality, and to pass an interview with the Bishop. This, proving no obstacle, Stone was ordained in March 1728 by the Bishop of Lincoln, to be Curate of Saunderton, Buckinghamshire, based on the church of St. Mary and St. Nicholas. It fell within the Diocese of Lincoln, see figure 4.4. However, Stone's sights were set upon Oxford, and within three months, he had once more undergone ordination, this time by the Bishop of Oxford, and consequently, as a priest, Stone took up the curateship at Charlton-on-Otmoor, at the church of St. Mary, (see figure 4.5.) a larger village than Saunderton.

Over the next two years he resided at Charlton-on-Otmoor, as Curate to the Rector, John Hill, who was a Fellow of Queens College. The arrangement was that Hill would be absent during term time, when Stone's services were required. Stone remained thus for two years only. Attendances at church were none too good. By 1740, another Curate was obtained, which resulted in considerable improvement in attendance and religious observance. One may deduce that, as a Curate, Stone did not exactly make waves. However, it would become quite clear that to be a Curate was only a stepping stone to Rectorship, a comfortable income, and the ability to rely upon one's Curate to do the work. All preceding Rectors of Charlton-on-Otmoor had been Fellows (of Queens College). By 1730, Stone had been elected to a Fellowship at Wadham College. Because he was neither a don nor a schoolteacher, he had to omit his ecclesiastical title during the seven years of his Fellowship. His subsequent responsibilities there were as follows:

1730	Fellow and Humanities Lecturer	1736	Sabbatical
1731	Librarian	1737	Librarian
1732	Bursar	1738	Bursar
1733	Bursar	1739	Sub-Warden
1734	Dean	1740	Senior Bursar
1735	Librarian		

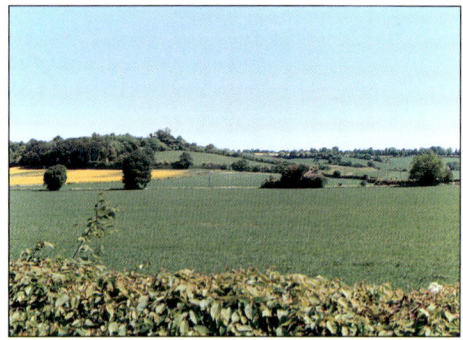 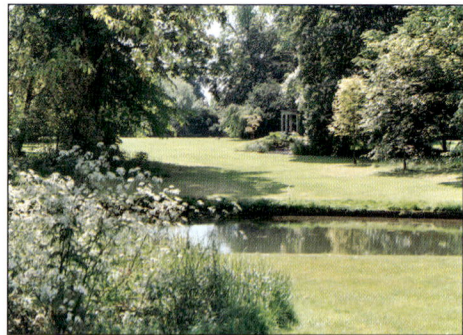
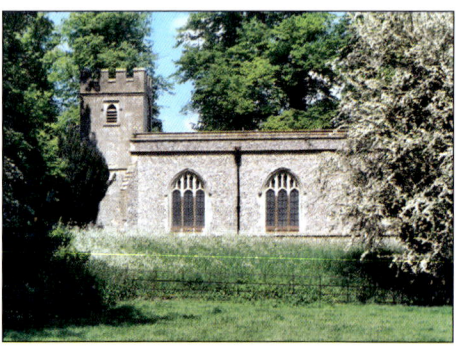 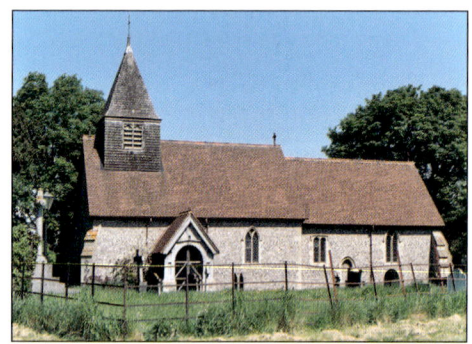

Top Left: Figure 4.1. Lacey Green – "a few miles south-east of the town (Princes Risborough) in a "hollow of the hills" (Ralph Mann). Top Right: Figure 4.2. Grounds of Horsenden Manor. Bottom Left: Figure 4.3. Parish church of St. Michael in Horsenden, Stone's first Rectorship from c.1737. Bottom Right: Figure 4.4. Church of St. Mary and St. Nicholas, at Saunderton, Stone's first Curateship, from March 1728.

In the 18th century, all was not well in academia. Incompetency among Masters was not unknown, and laziness and self-indulgence by Fellows commonplace. Class distinction was rampant, celibacy was required of the academic staff (dating back to the Middle Ages), and disaffected pro-Jacobites found sanctuary. On the other hand, there was also much that was good, including the formalisation of the tutorial system.

Another important aspect at this time was Stone's political affiliation. Wadham College was known to be pro the Whig party, whereas the university generally was militant Tory. However, the Whigs had been in power for several years, and Stone therefore might have anticipated political and ecclesiastical preferment as a consequence of his affiliation to Wadham. As a consequence, Stone's politics were to secure the patronage of influential and powerful Whig families, including the Parkers of Shirburn, the Spencer-Churchills of Blenheim, and Sir Jonathan Cope of Bruern. It should be noted, that Shirburn Castle was the seat of the Earl of Macclesfield, to whom in 1763, Stone would pen his groundbreaking communication leading to his fame, and eventually to the discovery of aspirin. And Jonathan Cope's son, Jonathan Junior, went up to Wadham in 1735, where his tutor was – Edward Stone. A friendship developed, which, as we shall see, had important consequences in 1741. In 1737, the living (i.e. Rectorship) of Horsenden fell vacant. The patron was John Grubb, brother of Edward's stepmother, who presented him. Stone was inducted as Rector of Horsenden in March 1737/8. There were not many parishioners to be cared for as there were only four houses in the parish, and the curate of nearby Little Missenden accepted responsibility for its twenty inhabitants. It would not appear that this Rectorship involved much in the way of work, though it doubtless carried a stipend.

Meanwhile, at Wadham College, certain events took place which may well have influenced Edward Stone's decision to leave for good. The first was the revelation, in 1738, that the Bursar had embezzled over £1000 of College money. The second, the following year, was the homosexual rape, by the Warden, of a young undergraduate student. Stone, in his official capacity as Sub-Warden, together with another Fellow, sought legal advice. They drew up a letter which was sent to London for the opinion of learned Counsel. Unfortunately, the matter did not come to trial, because the Warden fled the country. The third was that Stone had found a lady whom he wished to marry. Interestingly, she happened to be the daughter of his stepmother's brother, John Grubb of Horsenden. And the University in its official requirement of celibacy, ensured that marriage would require Stone's resignation. In recognition of this, the college offered him the parish of Southrop, in Gloucestershire, Wadham College being the corporate patron. After

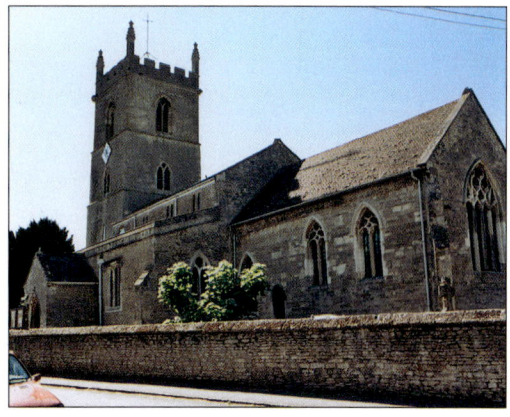

Figure 4.5. Church of St. Mary, Charlton-on-Otmoor, Stone's second Curateship, c.June 1728.

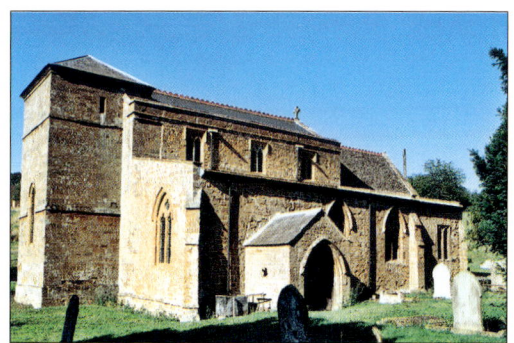

Figure 4.6. Church of St. Peter, at Drayton, near Banbury, Stone's additional Rectorship from 1741, (together with Horsenden).

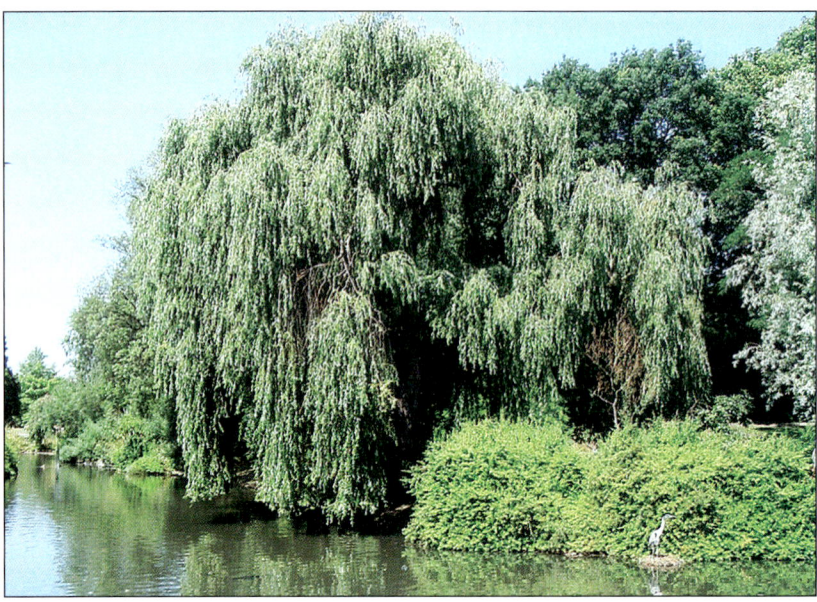

Figure 4.7. Willow tree, in typically damp surroundings. Regent's Park, London.

initially accepting, Stone turned it down, for reasons that are not clear. Exemption from celibacy was granted to some Heads of Colleges, the precise reason for which remains obscure. It would immediately be apparent therefore, that for a Fellow to resign in order to marry would entail a fall in income, no doubt to be compensated by a marriage that came with some clear cut pecuniary and other advantages. Stone chose well, perhaps repaying the favour granted him in 1737, the Rectorship of Horsenden. They married in 1741. At this time, Stone's attachment to the Copes bore fruit. Stone accepted Sir Jonathan Cope's presentation, to become Rector of Drayton, in the parish of St. Peter, (Sir Jonathan had inherited the advowson (under Anglican Ecclesiastical law, the right to recommend or appoint to a vacant benefice) of Drayton, the benefice having fallen vacant in 1741), see figure 4.6. In 1741, Edward Stone's father died.

Stone would thus, for the remainder of his life, officially remain as Rector to Horsenden and Drayton. For the next three years, Stone actually carried out the full-time pastoral work of an Anglican priest. Initially he and his wife lived in the old Parsonage House at Drayton, which was situated at the top of a hill, looking down on the church of St. Peter. A son, Edward, was born in May 1744, and baptised in St. Peter's church. However, by 1745, having obtained a permanent Curate, the Stones moved to Chipping Norton. He apparently never returned to the parish, but instead became personal Chaplain to Sir Jonathan Cope at Bruern Abbey. As there was no

Chapter Four – The Barks

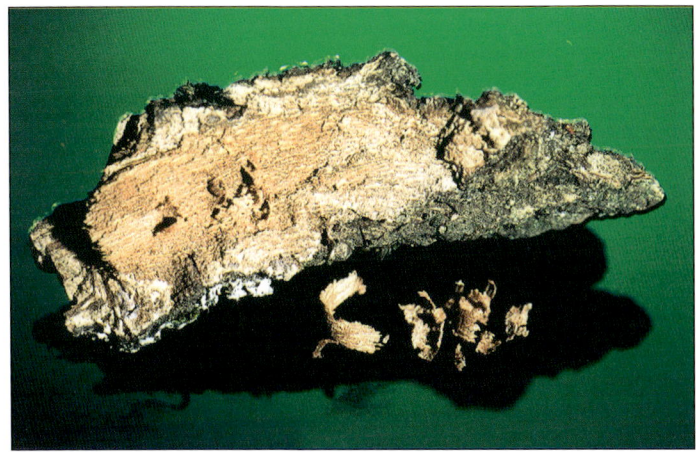

Figure 4.8. Sample of willow bark.

suitable accommodation at Bruern, the Stones lived at Chipping Norton. In 1745, their daughter, Elizabeth, was born and baptised.

It may be asked why Stone appeared to align himself with the Copes, and distance himself from his official church responsibilities. One answer may be political. The bulk of the local clergy were Tory, whereas Stone's sympathies lay with the Whigs, for whom Sir Jonathan Cope was the prospective candidate for the non-parliamentary borough of Chipping Norton in the election of 1754. Stone acted as his political agent. Eventually, it was decreed that the Whigs had won, after recounts, and some serious disturbances. The Whigs stood for the developing entrepreneurial outlook, nurtured by the nascent Industrial Revolution, whilst the Tories stood for the Crown, Parliament, the Church and the pre-existing paternal squirarchy.

Stone's service as political agent was rewarded in September 1755, when he was made a Justice of the Peace. His qualifications for this post included the fact that he possessed land in Princes and Monks Risborough, together with the Rectory and Glebe (land) of his parish at Drayton. He possessed a house in Back Lane, described in Jackson's Oxford Journal on 15th July 1775 as:

"A most commodious house, late the residence of the Rev. Mr. Stone; consisting of two handsome parlours, store-room, kitchen, excellent vaulted cellars, four bed-chambers, and four good garrets, with convenient offices, brewhouses, coal-house, a stable for five horses, and dairy, with apartments over them; a garden, and two acres of pasture adjoining, and with or without twelve acres of rich meadow land, at a small distance."

It is likely that whilst living in Chipping Norton, with his ecclesiastical title, and serving as a Justice of the Peace, he turned his mind to the treatment of agues. Quite

[195]

XXXII. *An Account of the Success of the Bark of the Willow in the Cure of Agues. In a Letter to the Right Honourable* George *Earl of* Macclesfield, *President of R. S. from the Rev. Mr.* Edmund Stone, *of* Chipping-Norton *in* Oxfordshire.

My Lord,

Read June 2d, 1763.

Among the many useful discoveries, which this age hath made, there are very few which, better deserve the attention of the public than what I am going to lay before your Lordship.

There is a bark of an English tree, which I have found by experience to be a powerful astringent, and very efficacious in curing aguish and intermitting disorders.

About six years ago, I accidentally tasted it, and was surprised at its extraordinary bitterness; which immediately raised me a suspicion of its having the properties of the Peruvian bark. As this tree delights in a moist or wet soil, where agues chiefly abound, the general maxim, that many natural maladies carry their cures along with them, or that their remedies lie not far from their causes, was so very apposite to this particular case, that I could not help applying it; and that this might be the intention of Providence here, I must own had some little weight with me.

The excessive plenty of this bark furnished me, in my speculative disquisitions upon it, with an

D d 2   argument

[196]

argument both for and against these imaginary qualities of it; for, on one hand, as intermittents are very common, it was reasonable to suppose, that what was designed for their cure, should be as common and as easy to be procured. But then, on the other hand, it seemed probable, that, if there was any considerable virtue in this bark, it must have been discovered from its plenty. My curiosity prompted me to look into into the dispensatories and books of botany, and examine what they said concerning it; but there it existed only by name. I could not find, that it hath, or ever had, any place in pharmacy, or any such qualities, as I suspected ascribed to it by the botanists.

However, I determined to make some experiments with it; and, for this purpose, I gathered that summer near a pound weight of it, which I dryed in a bag, upon the outside of a baker's oven, for more than three months, at which time it was to be reduced to a powder, by pounding and sifting after the manner that other barks are pulverized.

It was not long before I had an opportunity of making a trial of it; but, being an entire stranger to its nature, I gave it in very small quantities, I think it was about twenty grains of the powder at a dose, and repeated it every four hours between the fits; but with great caution and the strictest attention to its effects: the fits were considerably abated, but did not entirely cease. Not perceiving the least ill consequences, I grew bolder with it, and in a few days encreased the dose to two scruples, and the ague was soon removed.

It was then given to several others with the same success; but I found it better answered the intention, when a dram of it was taken every four hours in the intervals of the paroxisms.

I have

[197]

I have continued to use it as a remedy for agues and intermitting disorders for five years successively and successfully. It hath been given I believe to fifty persons, and never failed in the cure, except in a few autumnal and quartan agues, with which the patients had been long and severely afflicted; these it reduced in a great degree, but did not wholly take them off; the patient, at the usual time for the return of his fit, felt some smattering of his distemper, which the incessant repetition of these powders could not conquer: it seemed as if their power could reach thus far and no farther, and I did suppose that it would not have long continued to reach so far, and that the distemper would have soon returned with its pristine violence; but I did not stay to see the issue: I added one fifth part of the Peruvian bark to it, and with this small auxiliary it totally routed its adversary. It was found necessary likewise, in one or two obstinate cases, at other times of the year, to mix the same quantity of that bark with it; but these were cases where the patient went abroad imprudently, and caught cold, as a post-chaise boy did, who, being almost recovered from an inveterate tertian ague, would follow his business, by which means he not only neglected his powders, but, meeting with bad weather, renewed his distemper.

One fifth part was the largest and indeed the only proportion of the quinquina made use of in this composition, and this only upon extraordinary occasions: the patient was never prepared, either by vomiting, bleeding, purging, or any medicines of a similar intention, for the reception of this bark, but he entered upon it abruptly and immediately, and it

was

[188]

was always given in powders, with any common vehicle, as water, tea, small beer and such like. This was done purely to ascertain its effects; and that I might be assured the changes wrought in the patient could not be attributed to any other thing: though, had there been a due preparation, the most obstinate intermittents would probably have yielded to this bark without any foreign assistance: And, by all I can judge from five years experience of it upon a number of persons, it appears to be a powerful absorbent, astringent, and febrifuge in intermitting cases, of the same nature and kind with the Peruvian bark, and to have all its properties, though perhaps not always in in the same degree. It seems likewise to have this additional quality, viz. to be a safe medicine; for I never could perceive the least ill effect from it, though it had been always given without any preparation of the patient.

The tree, from which this bark is taken, is stiled by Ray, in his Synopsis, Salix, alba, vulgaris, the common white Willow. Hæc omnium nobis cognitarum maxima est, et in satis crassam et proceram Arborem adolescit.

It is called in these parts, by the common people, the willow, and sometimes the Dutch willow; but, if it be of a foreign extraction, it hath been so long naturalized to this climate, that it thrives as well in it as if it was in its original soil. It is easily distinguished by the notable bitterness and the free running of its bark, which may be readily separated from it all the summer months whilst the sap is up. I took it from the shoots of three or four years growth, that sprung from Pollard trees, the diameters of which

shoots,

[189]

shoots, at their biggest end, were from one to four or five inches: it is possible, and indeed not improbable, that this cortex, taken from larger or older shoots, or from the trunk of the tree itself, may be stronger; but I have not had time nor opportunities to make the experiments, which ought to be made upon it. The bark, I had, was gathered in the northern parts of Oxfordshire, which are chiefly of dry and gravelly nature, affording few moist or moory places for this tree to grow in; and therefore, I suspect that its bark is not so good here as in some other parts of the kingdom. Few vegetables are equal in every place; all have their peculiar soils, where they arrive to a greater perfection than in any other place: the best and strongest Mustard-seed is gathered in the county of Durham; the finest Saffron-Flowers are produced in some particular spots of Essex and Cambridgeshire; the best Cyder-apples grow in Herefordshire, Devonshire and the adjacent counties; the roots of Valerian are esteemed most medicinal, which are dug up in Oxfordshire and Glocestershire: And therefore why may not the Cortex Salignus, or Cortex Anglicanus, have its favourite soil, where it may flourish most, and attain to its highest perfection? It is very probable that it hath; and perhaps it may be in the fens of Lincolnshire, Cambridgeshire, Essex, Kent, or some such like situations; and, though the bark, which grew in the county of Oxford, may seem in some particular cases to be a little inferior to the quinquina, yet, in other places, it may equal, if not exceed it.

The powders made from this bark are at first of a light brown, tinged with a dusky yellow, and the longer they are kept, the more they incline to a cinnamon

[200]

cinnamon or lateritious colour, which I believe is the case with the Peruvian bark and powders.

I have no other motives for publishing this valuable specific, than that it may have a fair and full trial in all its variety of circumstances and situations, and that the world may reap the benefits accruing from it. For these purposes I have given this long and minute account of it, and which I would not have troubled your Lordship with, was I not fully persuaded of the wonderful efficacy of this Cortex Salignus in agues and intermitting cases, and did I not think, that this persuasion was sufficiently supported by the manifold experience, which I have had of it.

I am, my Lord,

with the profoundest submission and respect,

Chipping-Norton, Oxfordshire, April 25, 1763.

your Lordship's most obedient humble Servant

Edward Stone.

XXXIII. An

Figure 4.9. Edward Stone's letter to the Royal Society.

what inspired this can only be guessed. From his publication, figure 4.9, we gather that "by accident" he happened to taste some willow bark. How this came about he did not say. Imagine perhaps a small stack of Cinchona bark lying on a table beneath a willow tree. A piece of bark by chance somehow was scraped off, and fell among the Cinchona. Stone was collecting some Peruvian bark to treat a friend, when he noticed to his anger and surprise, that there was a small piece of contaminating willow bark in the goods. Cheating on Peruvian bark was well known, usually by contamination, and for this reason pure Cinchona was scarce, and very expensive. Out of mild curiosity, and in order to convince the seller that the goods were contaminated, he tasted the willow bark with the intention of proving to the vendor that it was not the genuine article because it didn't taste bitter. But, amazingly, it did taste bitter! There being nothing to lose, he decided to try it on his friend. His discovery might well have been ignored, but it was his great good fortune by this time to have befriended his tutee, Lord Parker, whose father was the Earl of Macclesfield, President of the Royal Society. Thus his letter to the Earl had a much improved chance of publication, and, as a consequence, the world had its first detailed description of the use of the willow bark in the treatment of agues (fevers, often accompanied with shivering bouts). However, the world took little notice at the time.

An example of the type of tree from which he removed the bark is shown below, see figure 4.7, together with a sample of the bark itself, see figure 4.8.

Edward Stone's letter to the Royal Society, claiming the discovery of the use of the willow bark is reproduced on the following pages, figure 4.9.

Little notice of Edward Stone's paper appears to have been taken, until the paper written by **Samuel James**, a surgeon, in 1792, see figure 4.10.

2. Samuel James, on the willow

In the preface, the author states with great modesty that he is a young provincial (Hoddesdon) practitioner, and that what he has to say may well be consigned to neglect and oblivion. He is of the opinion that he has, if not discovered, at least improved upon a medicine that is beneficial to mankind, and particularly for the poorer classes (the reader will recall that Peruvian bark was very expensive).

"That every climate possesses antidotes for the different disorders with which its inhabitants are afflicted, is an old, I believe, a just observation: but it seems to be the lot of human nature to overlook the merits of what is easily procured and costs but little, and to be captivated with a commodity which can only be acquired with difficulty and expense. Thus we go to the Western extremity of South America for a remedy of disorders, for which we have a better at home; and send annually out of the kingdom a considerable sum of money to purchase a bark, when we have a tree in our fields which offers us one of equal, if not superior virtue, and which may be cultivated almost without trouble or cost".

He goes on to allude to the Reverend Edward Stone's discovery nearly thirty years previously, and deplores the fact that so little notice appears to have been taken of it. Though included in Materia Medica, it was not to be found in the chemists' ("Druggists") shops. He observed that there were eleven species of willow, and announced that he had discovered the best. These were the leaves of Salix Latifolia (the broad leaved Willow). They were described in William Withering's Botanical Arrangement thus:

"The leaves of the Salix Latifolia are egg-shaped, downy on the undersurface, waved at the edge, with little teeth towards the end." Withering went on to mention use of the wood as a source of charcoal for gunpowder and pencils. In Lapland, the bark would be used to make a sort of leather for gloves, a decoction of the leaves for heartburn. The flowers were of interest to bees, and the leaves would be eaten by horses, cows, goats, and sheep.

Like others, James compared the different species of willow with reference to their relative astringency. One test was to boil two ounces of bark in water, then study the effect of vitriolated iron which led to a black discolouration of the bark. Using a comparative discolouration test he concluded the relative strengths were as follows:

8oz. Of the decoction of the bark of the oak were as strong as
9oz. Of that of the broad-leaved Willow, as
12oz. Of that of the dwarf Willow, as
20oz. Of the Peruvian bark, as
24oz. Of the bark of the white willow.

He lamented the fact that the eminent Dr. Cullen did not experiment on the various different bark species, because if he had, and found the special merit of the broad leaved willow, then it would surely have by now been in more general use.

He went on to describe 10 cases based on three year's experience.

Case I
J.B. aged 40. Male. Quartan fever 1789. Treatment with the Peruvian bark failed. Next James tried the white willow bark, but without benefit. He did however respond to the decoction made from the broad-leaved willow. *(Author's comment – if this was malaria, and it well could have been, then its failure to resolve after taking the Peruvian bark may have been a sign that it was of inferior quality. Why it should respond to one species of Salix and not another is a mystery. One would question the quality of the white willow bark used. Or perhaps, broad leaved bark is in some way superior. Possibly a field to research, especially as resistant strains of malaria are becoming an increasing problem).*

Case II
J.G, aged 16, gender not stated, quotidian fever 1789. Equal success to case I. Many other similar cases. For agues and intermittent fevers.

Case III
Mrs. S. Aged 45. This patient had all the appearances of scrofula (tuberculosis involving the lymph glands). With knee pain and swelling. She was unable to walk without the use of crutches. She developed shivering attacks (rigors), and swelling appeared in the inner aspects of both thighs, plus severe pain in the loins. After incising and draining about two pints of pus, the patient became very ill, with a high temperature. Peruvian bark was given, but the discharge continued and the patient became weaker. However, administration of decoction of broad-leaved willow bark made the patient feel better and the discharge lessened. *(Author's comment – this was in all likelihood what in medical terminology is called a psoas abscess. In this condition, TB of the spine causes pus to track down the front of the spine and along the path of the psoas muscle, which links the spine to the thigh bone (femur) and is brought into use when the hip joint is flexed. It can appear ('point') over the upper inner thigh, and in this case was probably bilateral. The same remarks concerning efficacy as were made in regard to case I apply).* In chapter 5, we will see that synthesized salicylic acid was found to possess antiseptic properties.

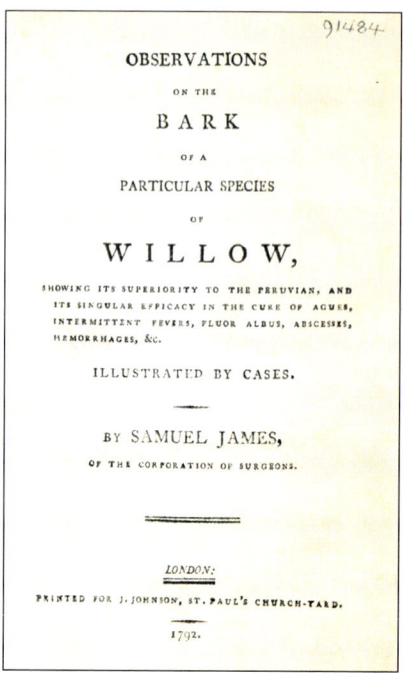

Figure 4.10. James' book on willow bark 1792. (Reproduced with permission of the Wellcome Library).

Case IV

G.V, male, aged 10. Severe pain in middle of thigh bone. Also, an abscess of the thigh, which responded, after incision and drainage, to administration of decoction of broad-leaved willow bark.

Case V

W.F, male, aged 7. Similar case to case IV. Effectiveness of the treatment deduced by Mr. James (the author of the paper), because the discharge lessened. *(Author's comment – in current thinking, this would be ascribed simply to the act of surgically draining the abscess, and not to any intrinsic quality of the willow bark itself).*

Case VI

W.B. aged 40, male. Violent pains in loins and hips. Rigors. Swelling in the loin on the right side. Again a psoas abscess, with the gradual appearance of swelling in the right thigh. Eventually, after surgical drainage, pain relief was achieved by the administration of decoction of broad-leaved willow bark. After apparently improving over a six weeks period the patient developed severe right sided pain and cough. He coughed a lot of purulent material, then died. Mr. James sought permission from his wife to carry out an autopsy. This was given, and, in the company of a surgeon and a clergyman, was duly performed. They found that the psoas abscess had also tracked upwards, to the right lung, and the membrane around it (the pleura), attaching these tissues to the ribs. He concluded that these kinds of abscess are best treated by a combination of drainage and willow bark. *(Author's comment – whilst almost certainly tuberculous, the unfortunate patient may in addition have suffered a pulmonary embolus whilst apparently improving over the 6 week period, especially if he had been advised to keep to his bed. Coughing purulent material would suggest super-added pyogenic infection (i.e. another bacterial infection, in addition to the tuberculosis).*

Case VII
E.R, aged 33, male. Chest pain and cough. Four pints of pus were drained from the left side of the chest, between the fifth and sixth ribs. Ten months later, he suffered a recurrence of symptom together with fever and night sweats. This was obviously due to TB. Again, drainage was performed. He had night sweats, and fevers, which responded to willow bark. He took 12 pints of decoction and never once had any side effects. *(Author's comment – Whilst TB was certainly on the cards, the empyema (pus within the pleural space) could have been due to pyogenic bacteria. In either case, the fever, though not the underlying disease, could have responded to the willow bark extract – the same train of thought which must have exasperated Jurgen Lehmann, see chapter 8).*

Case VIII
J.S. aged 6. Male. Swollen knee, plus pain and signs of inflammation. Drainage from two inches above the ankle yielded a quantity of pus. The greater part of the tibia was destroyed by tuberculosis. He took a considerable amount of the decoction, and in general improved. Later, he developed swollen glands in his groins. These improved with the willow bark decoction.

Case IX
H.L, aged 39, female. Back pain and miscarriage at 5 months gestation. Troubled by vaginal haemorrhage, and persistent discharge, which improved with the willow bark treatment. *(Author's comment – probably coincidental, however claims to reduce vaginal discharge by willow bark have been made by herbalists).*

Case X
H.M, aged 41, female. Severe white discharge 10 days post-partum. Continued for 16 weeks. Failed to respond to various treatments, but did to willow bark.

"I shall conclude with a single observation. I have found the oak bark a very efficacious remedy where it agreed with the patient, but that was seldom the case. Of the bark of the broad-leaved willow, I can however say with truth, that I have never known it to disagree, whether the dose has been small or large, and have never been forced to leave it off on such account, a single instance excepted; and that was in a very weakly constitution."

The author is clearly convinced of the superiority of the goat broad–leaved willow bark. His selected cases reflect a majority of post-partum and tuberculosis sufferers. These were the days before the advent of any antibiotics, or the chemotherapeutic agents (sulphonamides) which preceded them. Infections left to their own resources frequently lead to abscess formation, with eventual bursting. This is Nature's way, but in the meantime and subsequently, there is enormous suffering. The place of the willow bark was clearly to give some symptomatic relief from pain and suffering.

3. W. White on the willow

Another writer convinced of the value of the willow bark was **W. White**, a surgeon in Bath, see figure 4.11. He began thus:

"To the Physicians and Committee of Managers of the Bath City Infirmary and Dispensary;
This work
IS MOST RESPECTFULLY INSCRIBED, BY THEIR MOST OBEDIENT, AND FAITHFUL SERVANT,
The author
Member of the Corporation of Surgeons, and Apothecary to the Bath City Infirmary and Dispensary Bath: Printed and Sold by S. Hazard Sold also by Vernor and Hood, Poultry, London, 1798."

Then, like James, he described a series of similar experiments as a means to describing the chemical properties of the willow bark. Unlike James however, he drew no conclusions, before diving into his case descriptions. In all, 24 cases were described.

Case the First

February 22nd Jof. Pernell, aged 30. Tertian agues. Four times daily he was given a decoction of Salix latifolia and his fevers ceased The total period of observation however was only 9 days.

Case the Second

Ann Milsom, aged 4. Quotidian ague for the past 7 weeks. The fever left her within 2 hours of taking the decoction. 1 week later, it returned. Upon resumption of the decoction, the fever abated as did the cough, over a two week period.

Chapter Four – The Barks

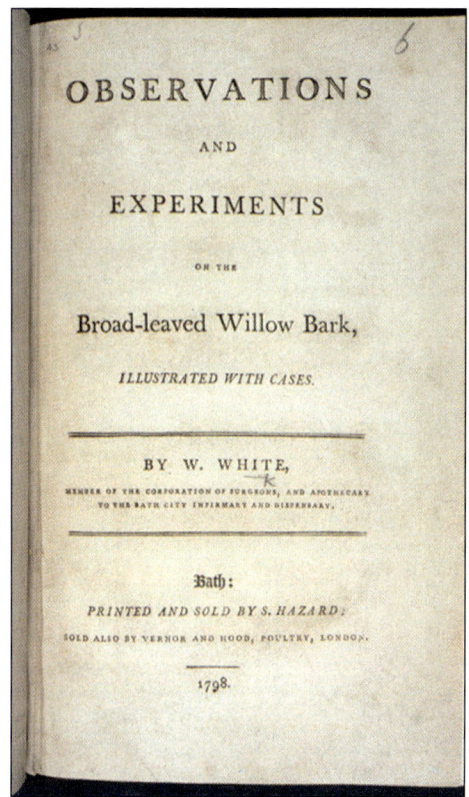

*Figure 4.11. Title of White's book 1798.
(Reproduced with permission of the British Library).*

Case the Third
Frances Heath, aged 20. Hot flushes for several days. Resolved after taking the decoction.

Case the Fourth
Geofrrey Longford, aged 14. Headache, vomiting and diarrhoea. Chills abated within one week of taking the decoction.

Case the Fifth
William Pike, 40 years or more. Fever, cough, chest pain, cough and shortness of breath. Initially treated with yellow (Peruvian) bark, but no response. Responded to decoction of broad-leaved willow bark. *(Author's comment – probably symptomatic relief of a viral or bacterial respiratory tract infection).*

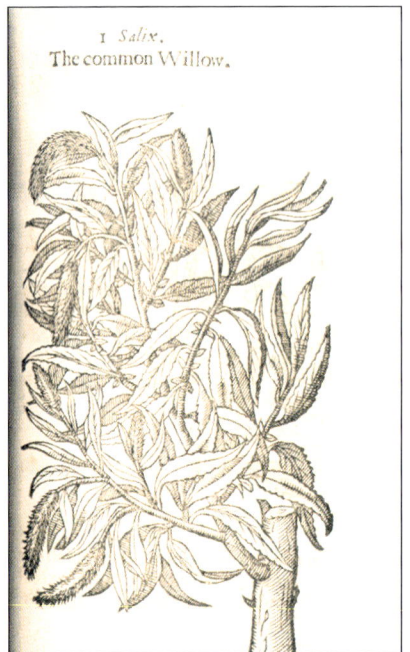 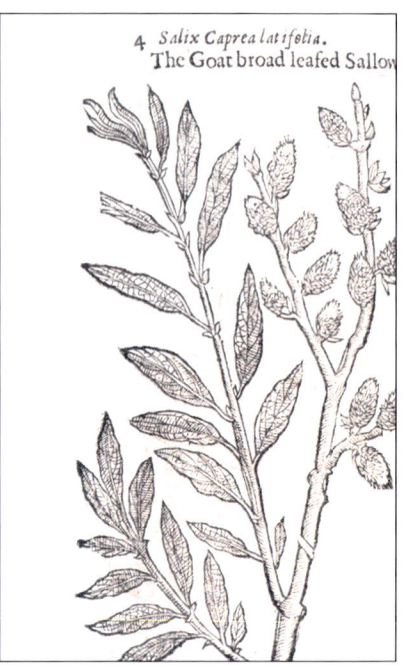

Left: Figure 4.12. The common willow, from W. White's book.
Right: Figure 4.13. Goat broad-leaved willow, from White's book.
(Both reproduced with permission of the British Library).

Case the Sixth
John Eades, upwards of 40 years. Sense of heat at night, with considerable thirst and passing urine whenever he drinks. Symptoms present for about 4 months. Improved with treatment. Recurrence in April, after working in gardens in severe weather. No urinary symptoms on this occasion. Didn't improve with salix decoction, but eventually got better anyway. *(Author's comment – one wonders whether this man was developing diabetes. Salicylates can have a mild sugar lowering effect. It is unlikely that he would have had long-lasting relief).*

Case the Seventh
A. Nott, female, head pain, deafness and debility. Fever every day with perspiration, initially 3 weeks ago, also had diarrhoea and vomiting. Cured within a week on treatment. *(Author's comment – 3 week's history of an infection. Could have been otitis media. We aren't told what remedies had previously been tried, but they may have been responsible for the diarrhoea and vomiting. The willow bark extract probably helped the fever, and the patient got better anyway).*

Case the Eighth
J. Debank aged 6, female. 2 weeks history of headache, backache, sickness, thirst, furred tongue. Gradually improved after taking emetics, but evening fevers at about 6 o'clock persisted. Responded to the decoction.

Case the Ninth
William Golesney, aged about 30. 10 weeks ago, shivering, vomiting and diarrhoea. Occasional blood in the stools. Diarrhoea ceased a week ago, but still experiencing a fever at ten o'clock each evening. Responded and was cured after 2 weeks treatment with the decoction. *(Author's comment – many possible causes. 9 weeks of diarrhoea and occasional blood in the stools might suggest chronic inflammatory bowel disease, either Crohn's or ulcerative colitis. In those days, other causes such as typhoid, salmonella, shigella or amoebic dysentery would also be possibilities).*

Case the Tenth
Sarah Fudge, aged 36. 5 day history of head and back pain. Flushes, perspiration, frequently feels chilly. Decoction resulted in considerable improvement in the head and back pain, cured within 3 weeks. *(Author's comment – a viral infection, treated much as it might be today).*

Case the Eleventh
Martha Comber, aged about 40, 'chilly fits' (presumed fevers) for several weeks. Decoction accompanied by resolution of illness within a week. *(Author's comment – nowadays, one would suspect urinary tract infection, which doesn't necessarily declare itself by urinary symptoms. Alternatively, gall bladder infection could be the cause).*

Case the Twelfth
A. Lane, aged 30, female. Backpain, weakness, giddiness, diarrhoea. Ill for 3 weeks. At onset, had fever, less febrile when first seen. Cured within 2 weeks of the treatment.

Case the Thirteenth
Marsh. Male 35 years old. For the past week had suffered headache and shivering attacks. The patient received powdered willow bark and had less pain. 2 weeks later, the fever returned, but eventually resolved.

Case the Fourteenth
Mary Mason, aged 30 years. Chills, and hot flushes. Had recently recovered from 'low fevers.' Received the decoction. Within a week the chills ceased and by 2 weeks was recovered.

'I have to say in favour of the willow, that except in a single instance (which may be noticed in the case of Collins), I have never found it to disagree with the stomach or bowels.' He went on to state that he felt it to be inferior to the Peruvian bark as an antiseptic, but was a greatly superior tonic. The antiseptic property was ascribed to its bitterness, rather than to its astringency (this being measured at the time by the ability to tan leather). He concluded that willow was particularly useful in cases of general debility – accompanied by appetite loss, also for intermittent or remittent fever, mild typhus, convalescent states such as after giving birth, and for uterine prolapse. These properties were regarded as evidence of its usefulness as a tonic. When tried for irregular intermittents, he felt it to be superior to the Cinchona, but admitted that he had not seen sufficient numbers of cases to be sure of this.

In France, **Germain Sée** (1818–1896) used salicylate for the treatment of rheumatic fever, including chorea (a neurological complication of rheumatic fever characterised by involuntary movements), and for rheumatoid arthritis. He also used it to treat gout, though the definition and differentiation of gout and rheumatoid arthritis at the time was imprecise.

4. G. Wilkinson on the willow

In 1803, **G. Wilkinson** a corresponding member of the medical society of London, Licentiate of the Royal College of Surgeons and Honorary member of the Chirurgo-Physical Society Of Edinburgh, and of the literary and philosophical society of Newcastle upon Tyne published his paper titled:
"Experiments and observations on the cortex *salicis latifolia*". Dedicated to:
Professor John Sheldon FRS, professor of anatomy in the Royal Academy of Arts.

The contents consist of preliminary observations on medical science, a general history of the cinchona and reasons why it fell short of its original reputation. Next a general history of the Salix latifolia. Previous findings are described, including those of Dr. James, Mr. White, Dr. Beddoes and others. A botanical description follows, then its sensible qualities. Finally, its preparation and mode of exhibition.

Introduction
"Although medicine is a science, or art, which, when compared with various other learned studies, seems pretty generally allowed to be far distant from a state of perfection, yet the rapid improvements and truly valuable discoveries which it has acquired within the last century, must be acknowledged abundantly to transcend those of our predecessors –"

" – the Cinchona ruber – having excited general attention, the labours of the ingenious Dr. Saunders made us not only better acquainted with the general history of

Chapter Four – The Barks

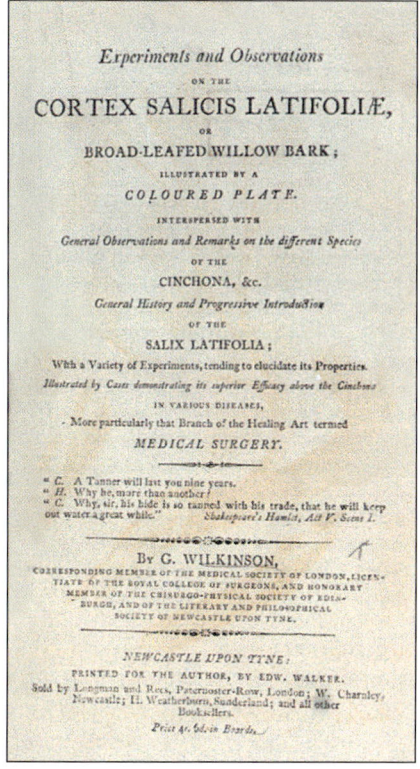 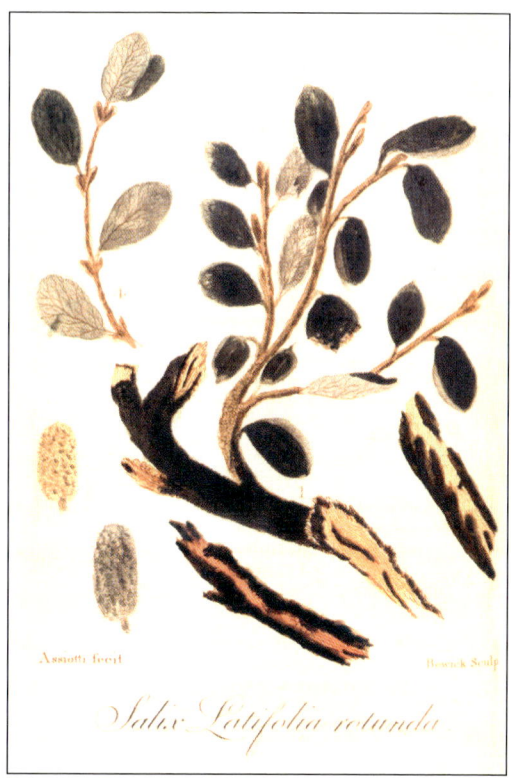

Left: Figure 4.14. Wilkinson's book on willow bark, 1803.
Right: Figure 4.15. Goat broad leafed willow Salix latifolia. (Wilkinson).
(Both reproduced with permission of the British Library).

that in common use – He says he had long suspected that the Peruvian bark in common use was very inferior in power and efficacy to that recommended by the early writers on the subject, more especially by our countrymen Sydenham and Morton –"

General history of the Salix Latifolia

To the modest and candid Mr. James, Surgeon, of Hoddesden, in Hertfordshire, we were indebted ten years ago, for the introduction into practice of the Salix Latifolia, and as he has hinted, excepting himself, "no Englishman has written at large on its virtues." More than three years experience in many remarkable cases, has enabled this gentleman to prove its decisive superiority over the Cinchona: nor has this useful vegetable escaped the notice of the indefatigable and humane friend to the human race, the illustrious Dr. Beddoes – the testimony of Mr. White, apothecary to the Bath City Infirmary and Dispensary, published in the year 1798 – puts it beyond a doubt that we possess at our doors, a vegetable bark as much superior to the Peruvian, as the vaccine disease is superior to the variolous –

It is true that Mr. Stone, an English clergyman, communicated to the Royal Society a paper, in 1763, on the beneficial effects of the willow in agues and intermittent fevers, but this appears to be a quite different species from that of which I am now treating. – It must however, be recollected, that the plant he was then speaking of was the Salix vulgaris alba arborescens of C. Bauhin, or what is usually termed the white willow, which Mr. James found by repeated trials, much inferior to that which he has recommended.

From the favourable account given by Mr. Stone of the Salix Alba, Dr. Cullen has strongly recommended it as a substitute for the Cort. Peruv in agues and intermittents. The author goes on to lament the failure to take up the new treatment instead of the traditional Peruvian bark:

"– not only on its being more easily procured, but also from its being far less expensive than the Cinchona, yet when we reflect on the rooted unwillingness, perverse obstinacy and tenaciousness, that mankind in general have ever shewn to adhere to early impressions habitually fixed, it can be no wonder that it has met the fate of almost every thing newly offered –"

Salix caprea

"It grows to a tolerable large tree, covered with a greyish bark, a little bitter – This species of willow varies very much in the shape of its leaves. It grows in damp woods, by the sides of rivers, and ditches –

The most proper time of gathering the bark is in May, June, and until the middle of July, as after this period, it is found to adhere too firmly to the tree, as not easily to be peeled off – It should be cut into pieces, not more than five inches in length, and the large thick bark to be one or two inches in breadth. This must be done while green, and then it should be dried in the house, in a place where no sun or fire comes. This renders it convenient and neat, for stowage, or packing for carriage, dries it more regularly, and fits it for the mortar, either for decoction or infusion –

Perhaps what I have further to remark on this subject, and which has been entirely passed over by Messrs White and James, will be another matter of no small importance to its preparation, which is this, – that taking it for granted, that whenever this bark is prescribed, it must be understood to be more or less in a dried state –"

The author goes on to describe several experiments he carried out comparing the tanning properties of salix with tormentil, oak, yellow, red (Cinchona), and angostura barks. The purpose was to determine the most effective antisepsis mediated by tanned tissue.

Chapter Four – The Barks

Finally, he describes 16 cases treated with willow bark. Cases 1–4 were female with mainly gynaecological complaints, and who, for whatever reason, appeared to improve subsequent to treatment. Case 5 was a man aged 32 with scrophulous (i.e tuberculous), lymph glands. He also suffered from a quartan ague (a fever every fourth day. This could have been due to malaria. However, it had not responded to Peruvian bark treatment. He was given twelve ounces of strong decoction, and he recovered perfectly i.e. he had suffered fevers for three months, but no more.

The cases were summarised.

"Summary Remarks and General Observations on the Medical Properties and Effects of the Salix Latifolia, compared with the Cinchona; with some reflections on Tonics and Antiseptics, &c.

From the foregoing experiments and cases, I trust it is proved that the salix is greatly superior to the cinchona, and that very little doubt will remain in the minds of the candid and liberal part of the profession, of its deserving much more notice and attention than it has hitherto received.

Being much less expensive than the cinchona, I found many favourable opportunities of dispensing it among the poor, labouring under almost every variety of disease, in which the use of the Peruvian bark was indicated. The further I extended it, the more I was convinced of the pre-eminence over the barks in common use, and except when prescribed by physicians, have now adopted it as a substitute for the cinchona.

It very seldom disagrees with the stomach or bowels; but it ought not to be administered without being preceded by an emetic, or gentle laxative, in cases where such preparatives are clearly indicated.

With cold stomachs, or such as appear to be morbidly affected by the powerful stimulus of ardent spirits, or excessive use of port wine, it has been sometimes found to disagree, and requires to be combined with aromatics, – Like good port wine, which often proves disagreeable to those unused to it, it becomes more and more agreeable by perseverance. It does not produce such a degree of constipation as need be considered dangerous –

Like the cinchona, it does not purge, nor is it likely to produce any such effect in decoction, whatever it may do in powder, in which state I have never yet employed it.

– If we reason from analogy, by comparing their effects on the dead, with the living animal fibre, those vegetables possessing the largest share of tanning principle, ought certainly to be esteemed the most powerful tonics. –

How far bitterness may be essentially necessary for the perfection of vegetable tonics, as febrifuges, is not for me to determine. In the case of intermittents and typhus, in which I have administered the salix, it did not appear defective from want of this property.

– In thus noticing the failure of the cinchona in some of the fevers of the West Indies, and I may add, in the yellow fever of Philadelphia, where from the testimony of Drs. Chisholm and Rush, it proved hurtful, I shall not attempt to assign the true causes of its failure –

I should have remarked, that exclusive of the singular efficacy I experienced from the salix in the variety of diseases assuming an intermitting, or a periodical type, I have found it superior to the cinchona in what may be termed that species of pulmonary hectic so often the constant attendant of long continued catarrhs, and acute pneumonic inflammations, and which may be justly esteemed among the leading causes of phthisis pulmonalis. –

I urge this more strongly, from the unexpected success I have experienced in four cases of this sort, in three of which the patients were indebted for their recovery to the free use of the salix decoction, even after having used the digitalis, and the cinchona, without any manifest benefit. In the first of these instances, though continued for some time, the digitalis proved on the whole injurious by debilitating the system. –

And here I think it is not improper to observe that it may be thought by many, that I have expressed myself in terms too sanguine in favour of the salix to the prejudice of the cinchona, as may have been the case with others respecting the digitalis, in dropsies, phthisis pulmonalis, & co. but this, whether true or not, must be left to time and experience to determine. It has proved in my practice abundantly more efficacious than the cinchona; and when it is considered that it is a much less dangerous remedy than the digitalis, the risqué attendant on its exhibition as a substitute for the cinchona, cannot be esteemed of that importance as to deter any one from giving it fair trials. Mr. White says "Since the introduction of this bark into practice, at the Bath City Infirmary and Dispensary, as a substitute for the cinchona, not less than twenty pounds a year have been saved to the charity, which circumstances will render it a very valuable article to all hospitals where much bark is used.

What opposition may probably arise to the introduction of the salix, from dealers and speculators in the cinchona, as an article of commerce, I cannot say. But if once this domestic vegetable gets fairly introduced into general use, those very persons, and our good friends, the Spaniards will be enabled (if not compelled) to furnish us with cinchona more genuine than, from its extensive consumption, they have hitherto done, and it will be less liable to be adulterated at home with barks of an inferior quality."

Summary of Wilkinsons 16 cases

Case 1
Name: Jane Drew   *Age:* c.40   *Sex:* F
Complaints: Nervous, dyspeptic, irregular periods, vaginal discharge, constipated and at other times, diarrhoea. Painful legs and ankles, legs sometimes oedematous.

Chapter Four – The Barks

2 months after treatment with salix, anxious. But found to be pregnant. Safely delivered at term. *(Author's comment – unlikely to have had any beneficial effect on the vaginal discharge, but may have reduced the pain in her lower limbs. Could this have facilitated her pregnancy?!!).*

Case 2
Name: Mrs. E.H.   *Age:* 38   *Sex:* F
Complaints: Nervous, dyspeptic, debility, vaginal discharge, back and loin pain. Treated by another (person) with mercurials. Developed signs of mercury poisoning. Other remedies sufficed, but persistent vaginal discharge. Cured by willow bark decoctions. *(Author's comment – unaware of any evidence of its efficacy for relieving vaginal discharge although herbal remedies including willow bark do make this claim).*

Case 3
Name: Mrs. A.P.   *Age:* 48   *Sex:* F
Complaints: Uterine prolapse and discharge. Took willow bark decoction. Discharge went. Appetite and strength returned.

Case 4
Name: ?   *Age:* 30   *Sex:* F
Complaints: Violent loin and thigh pain. Uterine prolapse and discharge. Previously treated with Peruvian bark. All symptoms nearly totally disappeared. 8 and a half pints of decoction of willow bark taken. Shortly afterwards became pregnant. *(Author's comment – uterine prolapse at age 30. Perhaps a reflection of the inferior obstetric service of the time. High infant mortality. Violent pain extending from the loin to the groin is the classical description of a kidney stone travelling down the ureter (renal colic).*

Case 5
Name: W. Hoggitt   *Age:* 32   *Sex:* M
Complaints: Scrophula of lymph glands with discharges over hands, neck, ankle, angle of jaws and back of head. Quartan ague (i.e. a fever every 1st and 4th day). Treated for the past 3 months with Peruvian bark. He received 12 ounces of strong willow bark decoction, 2 pints. Recovered perfectly. *(Author's comment – perhaps an example of the ability to relieve fever even when due to tuberculosis, though not to cure it).*

Case 6
Name: Thomas Williamson   *Age:* 18   *Sex:* M
Complains: Tertian ague (fever every 1st and 3rd day). Temporary response to willow bark. Fever returned. Responded to 8 half pints. *(Author's comment – a case of malaria? in which case the willow bark would have been of little value).*

Case 7

Name: William Crank   *Age:* 18   *Sex:* M

Complaints: Fever after exposure to cold and wet. Shivering, headache, sickness, loin and limb pain. Treated with willow bark, but returned to sea too soon. Relapsed, but eventually responded, 5 half pints.

Case 8

Name: William Grozier   *Age:* 43   *Sex:* M

Complaints: Seaman Fever, shivering, limb pain, headache, nausea, vomiting. Took Peruvian bark. Improved, then relapsed. 7 half pints. Cured within 9 days. *(Author's comment – possibly viral gastritis).*

Case 9

Name: W. Walker   *Age:* 18   *Sex:* M

Complaints: Chills, headache, limb pain. Eventually cured after 8 half pints. *(Author's comment – influenza?).*

Case 10

Name: Mrs. B.   *Age:* 75   *Sex:* F

Complaints: Pyrexia, inflamed and painful eyes, cough, shivering. Patient stated she would not take any bark (Peruvian). Took willow bark decoction every 2 hours. Relapsed, but refused any more. Got better any way. *(Author's comment – slow to respond upper respiratory tract infection).*

Case 11

Name: M.W.   *Age:* 52   *Sex:* F

Complaints: Obese, intemperate. Several months previously, abscess of right side of abdominal wall. Fistulae formed. Had received great quantities of powdered cinchona and some of it as a decoction. No benefit. Treated with 10 ounces of willow bark decoction, and on 4 further occasions over the next fortnight, continued for 8 weeks. Much improved by August. *(Author's comment – Crohn's disease? well known to predispose to fistula formation. Often accompanied by fever, though not mentioned here. Willow bark unlikely to have had any effect on the fistula).*

Case 12

Name: Wife of Peter Burn   *Age:* 46   *Sex:* F

Complaints: Pyrexia, rib pain, rigors, sweats. Hard swelling appeared on right side (presumed abdomen). Yellow skin, brightly tinged urine, white stools. Large hard tumour in right hypochondrium. Tender, with pain felt at the right shoulder. Abscess drained. She improved, but still had paroxysms of fever. Treated with decoction of willow bark. Feverish symptoms very soon left her. Took 2 pints. *(Author's comment – interesting. Obviously a case of obstructive jaundice, possibly secondary to an abscess of the gall bladder extending under the diaphragm, known as a subphrenic abscess. Diaphragmatic pain, as any medical student knows, is referred to the shoulder).*

Case 13

Name: A soldier's wife   *Age:* 25   *Sex:* F

Complaints: Dull pain left kidney which occurred 6 weeks post partum. Kidney enlarged. Swelling extended over the spinal muscles. Abscess drained – several hydatid cysts emerged. Subsequently developed a fever, which resolved after 6 half pints. *(Author's comment – hydatid cysts uncommon nowadays. Possibly reflected living in contact with dogs, pigs or sheep. Usual site of cysts is within the liver, from which the abscess probably originated).*

Case 14

Name: Thomas Smith   *Age:* 52   *Sex:* M

Complaints: Violent pain in right thumb, hand, wrist, and rigors, fever and delirium. Deep seated suppuration among the hand tendons. Inflammation extended up the forearm. Previous medical attendant had mentioned possible amputation. Had already been treated with Peruvian bark. Then received decoction of cortex salicis every 3 to 4 hours. The abscess was drained. The ulnar bone protruded, the radius was loose. Then pain in the right hip, with another abscess. 2 quarts of pus were drained. "Of all the medicines prescribed for him, the decoction of salix pleased him most." *(Author's comment – Of course it would, as it would have been effective at relieving the severe pain of osteomyelits, which the Peruvian bark had no hope of doing).*

Case 15

Name: William Swales   *Age:* 17   *Sex:* M

Complaints: Back pain and lower limb weakness. Projecting 4th and 5th dorsal vertebrae. Discharging. No response to prior cinchona. Treated with salix decoction for 1 month. Successful. Took 40 pints. The spine did not recover its form. Now no longer going to sea, instead employed as a weaver. (2 other cases of incurved spine treated successfully). *(Author's comment – Probably a case of tuberculous osteomyelits, also known as Pott's disease. Symptomatic relief to be expected, though no benefit against the infection itself).*

Case 16

Name: Benjamin Johnson   *Age:* 26   *Sex:* M

Complaints: Swelling of calf of left leg. Local applications. Discharged, with spread to heel and instep. Nearly 2 years later, similar symptoms on right side. Amputation of left leg advised. Heel bone exfoliated. He gradually improved with 40 pints of willow bark decoction. *(Author's comment – may have had a deep vein thrombosis. Superficial meddling may have resulted in secondary infection. The willow bark would have had an effect on blood clotting, which surreptitiously proved beneficial. Alternatively, the patient may have had a ruptured cyst at the back of his knee, also known as a popliteal or Baker's cyst. Fluid can then track down the calf muscle as far as the ankle).*

5. Dr. Thomas John Maclagan (1838–1903) on the willow

(An excellent review of his life is to be found in the Scottish Medical Journal, 1987; 32: 141–146, by Stewart & Fleming). Maclagan attended school in Perth, and entered Edinburgh medical school in 1855. He became Resident Medical Superintendent at Dundee Royal Infirmary in 1864, various prominent medical and nursing staff having died of typhus or typhoid immediately prior to his appointment. It was therefore a brave and dedicated man who chose to take up the post. Medical admissions at the time totalled about 50 per week, far fewer than nowadays. Between 1858 and 1866 there were 2492 cases of typhus. In 1867 he published a paper on "Thermometrical observations" which included detailed studies using a clinical thermometer (Casella's straight self-registering). A photograph taken at the time of his marriage is seen opposite, figure 4.16.

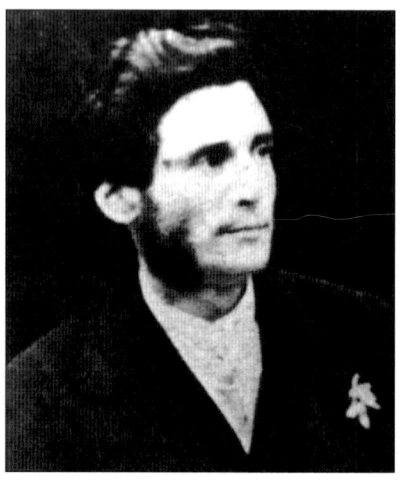

Figure 4.16. Thomas Maclagan (1838–1903). (Reproduced courtesy of Tayside Medical History Museum, University of Dundee; copyright the Maclagan family).

He published an important paper in two parts in the Lancet on March 4th and March 11th 1876, see figures 4.17, and 4.18, titled "The treatment of acute rheumatism by Salicin". In the introductory section, he states:

"In reference to the action of quinine on the various forms of intermittent and remittent fever, and, indeed, with reference to the action of the Chinchonaceae generally on the disease of tropical climates (ipecacuanha in dysentery, for instance), there is one fact which has always strongly impressed me – namely, that the maladies on whose course they exercise the most beneficial action are most prevalent in those countries in which the Chinchonaceae grow most readily; nature seeming to produce the remedy under climatic conditions similar to those which give rise to the disease.

Impressed with this fact, and believing in the miasmatic origin of rheumatic fever, it seemed to me that a remedy for that disease would most hopefully be looked for among those plants and trees whose favourite habitat presented

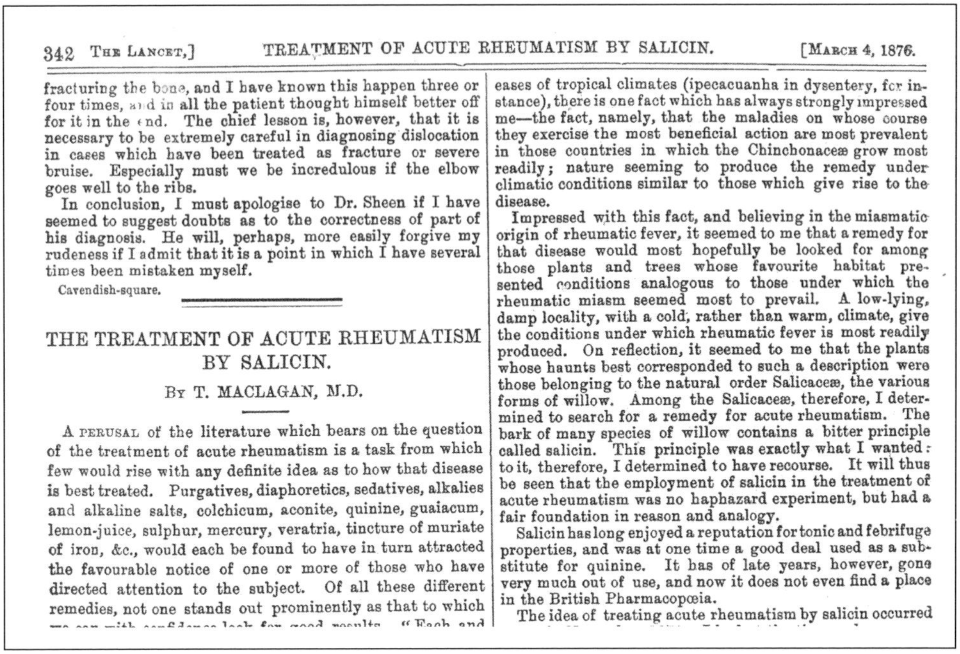

Chapter Four – The Barks

> 342 THE LANCET,] TREATMENT OF ACUTE RHEUMATISM BY SALICIN. [MARCH 4, 1876.
>
> fracturing the bone, and I have known this happen three or four times, and in all the patient thought himself better off for it in the end. The chief lesson is, however, that it is necessary to be extremely careful in diagnosing dislocation in cases which have been treated as fracture or severe bruise. Especially must we be incredulous if the elbow goes well to the ribs.
>
> In conclusion, I must apologise to Dr. Sheen if I have seemed to suggest doubts as to the correctness of part of his diagnosis. He will, perhaps, more easily forgive my rudeness if I admit that it is a point in which I have several times been mistaken myself.
>
> Cavendish-square.
>
> ### THE TREATMENT OF ACUTE RHEUMATISM BY SALICIN.
>
> BY T. MACLAGAN, M.D.
>
> A PERUSAL of the literature which bears on the question of the treatment of acute rheumatism is a task from which few would rise with any definite idea as to how that disease is best treated. Purgatives, diaphoretics, sedatives, alkalies and alkaline salts, colchicum, aconite, quinine, guaiacum, lemon-juice, sulphur, mercury, veratria, tincture of muriate of iron, &c., would each be found to have in turn attracted the favourable notice of one or more of those who have directed attention to the subject. Of all these different remedies, not one stands out prominently as that to which
>
> eases of tropical climates (ipecacuanha in dysentery, for instance), there is one fact which has always strongly impressed me—the fact, namely, that the maladies on whose course they exercise the most beneficial action are most prevalent in those countries in which the Chinchonaceæ grow most readily; nature seeming to produce the remedy under climatic conditions similar to those which give rise to the disease.
>
> Impressed with this fact, and believing in the miasmatic origin of rheumatic fever, it seemed to me that a remedy for that disease would most hopefully be looked for among those plants and trees whose favourite habitat presented conditions analogous to those under which the rheumatic miasm seemed most to prevail. A low-lying, damp locality, with a cold, rather than warm, climate, give the conditions under which rheumatic fever is most readily produced. On reflection, it seemed to me that the plants whose haunts best corresponded to such a description were those belonging to the natural order Salicaceæ, the various forms of willow. Among the Salicaceæ, therefore, I determined to search for a remedy for acute rheumatism. The bark of many species of willow contains a bitter principle called salicin. This principle was exactly what I wanted: to it, therefore, I determined to have recourse. It will thus be seen that the employment of salicin in the treatment of acute rheumatism was no haphazard experiment, but had a fair foundation in reason and analogy.
>
> Salicin has long enjoyed a reputation for tonic and febrifuge properties, and was at one time a good deal used as a substitute for quinine. It has of late years, however, gone very much out of use, and now it does not even find a place in the British Pharmacopœia.
>
> The idea of treating acute rheumatism by salicin occurred

Figure 4.17. Maclagan's paper on treatment of acute rheumatism. (Lancet March 4th 1876. Reproduced with permission of Elsevier).

conditions analogous to those under which the rheumatic miasm seemed most to prevail. A low-lying damp locality, with a cold, rather than warm, climate, give the conditions under which rheumatic fever is most readily produced. On reflection, it seemed to me that the plants whose haunts best corresponded to such a description were those belonging to the natural order Salicaceae, the various forms of willow. Among the salicaceae, therefore, I determined to search for a remedy for acute rheumatism. The bark of many species of willow contains a bitter principle called salicin. This principle was exactly what I wanted: to it, therefore, I determined to have recourse. It will thus be seen that the employment of salicin in the treatment of acute rheumatism was no haphazard experiment, but had a fair foundation in reason and analogy".

The above is an example of the **Doctrine of signatures** previously described. In accordance with this idea, remedies will be found either by locality, or by some other physical or mystical property, to exert a beneficial effect. Paracelsus (1493–1541) said:

"I have oft-times declared, how by the outward shapes and qualities of things we may know their inward Vertues, which God hath put in them for the good of man.

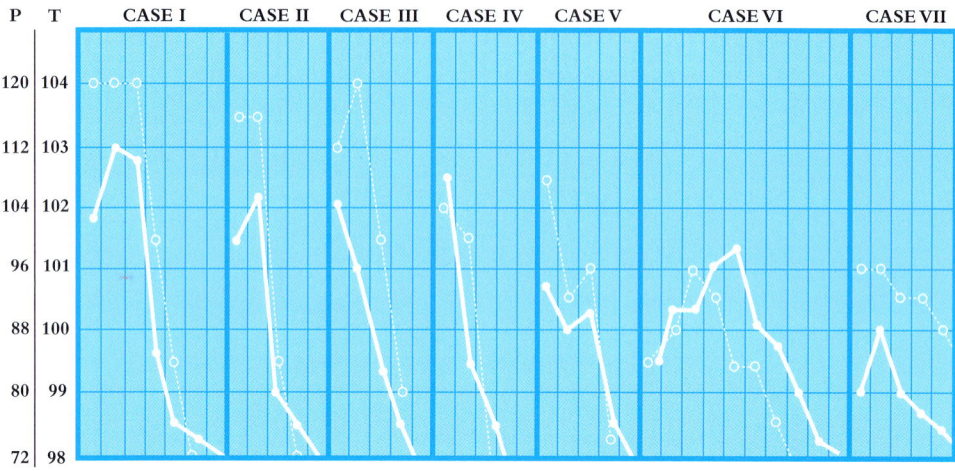

Figure 4.18. 7 cases of acute rheumatism treated with salicin by Maclagan.

So in St. John's wort, we may take notice of the form of the leaves and flowers, the porosity of the leaves, the Veins. 1. The porositie or holes in the leaves, signifie to us, that this herb helps both inward and outward holes or cuts in the skin 2. The flowers of St. John's wort, when they are putrified they are like blood; which teacheth us, that this herb is good for wounds, to close them and fill them up –"

As an example of the doctrine of signatures, consider the discomfort arising from a nettle sting. As every child knows, the application of a dock leaf is symptomatically beneficial. The Rev. Edward Stone, in 1763, and Dr. Thomas Maclagan in 1876 applied the same principle. And eventually, as will be described later, aspirin was discovered. What would the currently trained scientific mind make of this? To the author, the answer is simple – it is a form of natural, albeit pharmacological, selection. In the same manner that naturally occurring genetic mutations are tried out in Nature, and those offering benefit lead to survival, whilst those that give no benefit, or are positively harmful, die out, so, by trial (not necessarily of a scientifically robust nature), Nature will select out those that are beneficial from those that are not. Had the "signaturists" permitted their searches to have taken place in other locations, it is quite possible they would have come up with some similarly efficacious remedies. The Old Lady of Shropshire, whose herbal tea remedy was used to cure the dropsy, did not know that dropsy was due to heart failure, nor that foxglove leaf was the active ingredient in her remedy. William Withering discerned that it was the likely active ingredient, and put it to the test. The doctrine was there – namely that Nature could provide the "cure" – but in this case the "signature" was missing. People possessed of the dropsy do not have more foxgloves growing in their areas than others.

Chapter Four – The Barks

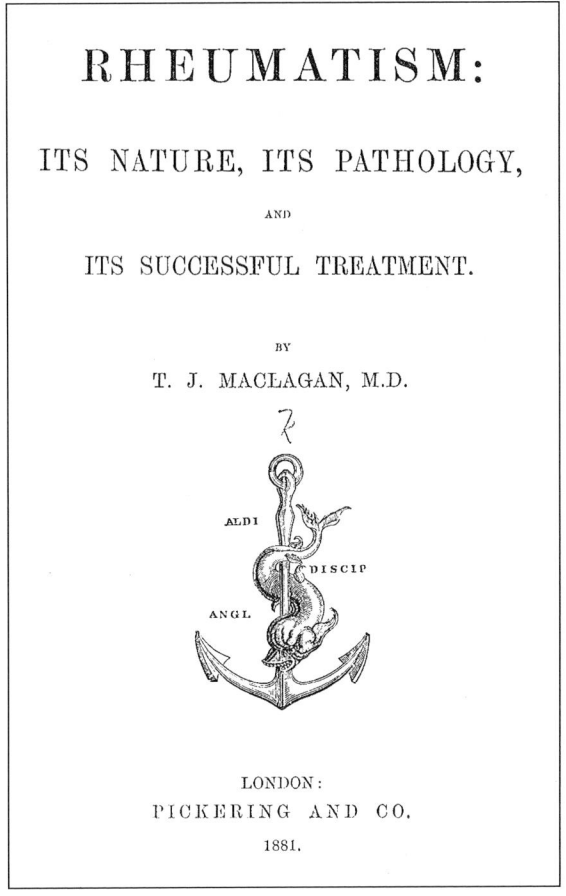

Figure 4.19. Title page of Maclagan's book on Rheumatism, 1881.

Next, as was the custom, Maclagan went into general practice. He was Attending Physician on the staff of Dundee Infirmary from 1877, but in 1879 left for London, where he lived in Cadogan Place, Belgrave Square. He built up a fashionable practice. In 1882, he succeeded in obtaining membership of the Royal College of Physicians of London, but was never made a Fellow. Perhaps this was because he arrived late in London, and did not obtain the equivalent of a consultant post. Despite this he published widely.

In 1881 he published his book, see figure 4.19.

Rheumatism: Its nature, its pathology, and successful treatment. By T.J. Maclagan M.D. London: Pickering & Co. 1881

In the preface he states:

"A PERUSAL of the literature which bears on the question of the treatment of acute rheumatism (rheumatic fever) is a task from which few would rise with any definite idea as to how that disease is best treated. Purgatives, diaphoretics, sedatives, alkalies and alkaline salts, colchicum, aconite, quinine, guaicum, lemon juice, sulphur, mercury, veratria, tincture of muriate of iron etc would each be found to have in turn directed attention to the subject. Of all these different remedies not one stands out prominently, as to that which we can with confidence look for good results. We have, indeed, no remedy for acute rheumatism – a malady which not infrequently proves fatal, which is always accompanied by great pain, and is a fruitful source of heart disease.

Under these circumstances I need make no apology for bringing under the notice of the profession a remedy which, so far as my observations have gone, has given better results than any which I have hitherto tried – and I have tried all the usual remedies over and over again.

In the course of an investigation into the causation and pathology of acute febrile ailments which has for some time engaged my attention, I was led to give some consideration to intermittent and to acute rheumatic fever. The more I studied these ailments, the more I was struck with the points of analogy which existed between them. On a detailed consideration of these I shall not now enter. Suffice it to say that they were sufficiently marked to lead me to regard rheumatic fever as being, in its pathology, more closely allied to intermittent fever than to any other disease, an opinion which further reflection and extended experience have served only to strengthen. Such are the opening sentences of the paper in which, in March 1876, I introduced salicin to the notice of the profession, as a remedy in acute rheumatism –" 9, Cadogan Place, London SW, May 6, 1881.

"Febrile symptoms are marked. The pulse and respirations are increased in frequency. The temperature varies from 100° to 104° Fahr., but has no distinctive range. The general course of the fever is remittent rather than continued – In some cases, fortunately in very few, the temperature runs up to 106°, 108°, or even 110°. –

Acute rheumatoid arthritis resembles subacute rather than acute rheumatism – It comes on more gradually than rheumatism. It attacks the small joints as frequently as the large. It shows no tendency to shift from joint to joint."

In the 4th chapter, on the nature of rheumatism, he states:

"Rheumatic inflammation has been regarded by some as differing from ordinary inflammation, not essentially, but only in the peculiarity of its seat. By others it is looked upon as specific in nature, as resulting from the action on the fibrous and serous tissues, of a special poison, which does not operate in the production of other than rheumatic inflammation.

The former is the view taken by those who regard the disease as the direct result of exposure to cold and damp; the latter that held by those who look upon it as due to the action of a *materies morbi* circulating in the blood.

That exposure to cold and damp suffices to produce acute rheumatism, is an old view which finds its chief support in the fact that the disease often occurs after such an exposure. But so frequent is such exposure in this country, that it would be difficult to point out any disease which might not be attributed to this agency, –

It is common to find patients attributing an attack of typhus or typhoid fever to that cause; but no medical man would endorse such a view, though the sequence of events may be clear enough to the patient."

He then describes his experiences of typhus and typhoid, both of which attacked him within a four year period. The former occurred whilst angling in Scotland, up to his knees in water. His friends had no hesitation in blaming the disease as being due to his exposure to cold and wet environments. He however was confident he had caught it from the typhus wards at the Edinburgh Infirmary, where he had been working up to three days previously. Similar exposure was blamed by his friends when he contracted typhoid fever, but he blamed the drains of the hospital which were being repaired at the time.

Maclagan then goes on to discuss the nature of the presumed 'rheumatic poison.' Based on the acidity of the perspiration, the urine and even the saliva, there was a theory that rheumatism was due to excessive lactic acid. This had led its followers to treat the condition with alkalis. The results were poor, and clearly lent no support to this theory. He then considered the miasmatic theory of rheumatism, comparing it to malaria:

"In studying malarial disease, the facts which force themselves most prominently on our attention are as follows:

1. They are specially apt to occur in low-lying damp localities, in certain climates, and at certain seasons of the year.
2. Some people are more likely to be attacked than others.
3. They have no definite period of duration.
4. They are not communicable from the sick to the healthy.

Now we cannot fail to see that these are quite the attributes of acute rheumatism. It is most common in temperate climates, at certain seasons, and in damp, low-lying localities. It has no fixed period of duration. It is not communicable from the sick to the healthy. Some people are more liable to it than others; and the poison, we have reason to believe, enters the system from without –

It is evident that the rheumatic poison, both in its history, and in its effects on the system, bears a close analogy to the poison of malarial fevers than to any other morbis agency –

Indeed, like the common malarial fevers, rheumatic fever may be divided into two kinds, *remittent* and *intermittent*."

Only in the second edition of his book, published in 1896, by Adam and Charles Black of London, does he mention the malarial parasite by name, –

"It is with the plasmodium malariae as it is with the relapsing fever; it is present in the blood during the pyrexia and absent during the apyrexia – " (Incidentally, the title page of the second edition mentions the fact that he is 'Physician in ordinary to their Royal Highnesses Prince and Princess Christian of Schleswig-Holstein').

To return to the first edition, he then gives an excellent resume of previous treatments for acute rheumatic fever and their advocates. Being regarded as a phlegmasia i.e. an inflammation dependent on exposure to cold, its remedy was by many, felt to be blood letting. Sydenham, the father of English medicine, in 1666, wrote that the cure of rheumatism was by blood letting, 10 oz on days 1, 2, 3 or 4, 6 or 7. Interestingly, and demonstrating commendable clinical honesty, 10 years before his death, Sydenham writing to a colleague (Dr. Brady), said:

"I, like yourself, have lamented that rheumatism cannot be cured without great and repeated losses of blood. This weakens the patient at the time; and if he have been previously weak, makes him more liable to other diseases for some years – Reflecting upon this, I judged it likely that diet, simple, cool and nutritious, might do the work of repeated bleedings, and saving the discomforts arising therefrom. Hence I gave my patients whey instead of bleeding them."

Around 1840, the name of Bouillaud was synonymous with the ordered regular practise of blood letting, and he espoused the concept of repeating a bleed before the (assumedly beneficial) effect wore off. Other remedies included purgatives, diaphoretics (i.e. perspiration inducing drugs) especially ipececuanha and antimony in combination with opium, and Dover's powder, cinchona and its alkaloid, quinine. Morton was the first to use cinchona in acute rheumatism, Cullen advised against it. Colchicum also had its proponents, though Garrod, whilst acknowledging its efficacy in gout, said that:

" – It possesses no influence in checking the progress of rheumatic fever."

With so many instances of failed medical treatment, some more enlightened physicians gave up all medicinal treatment and simply kept the patient warm in bed, with a light diet and the administration of a placebo. A Dr. Flint in 1863 published an account of 13 cases treated this way with good results. (American Journal of the Medical Sciences, 1863, July). In 1865, Dr. Sutton reported 41 cases treated at Guy's Hospital with mint water (Guy's Hospital Reports, 1865).

"Early in 1876, Stricker and Riess published a most favourable account of their experience of its" (salicylic acid) "employment in that disease". (Stricker. Berliner Klinische Wochenschrift 1876, no's 1 and 2). Riess Ibid. 1876, no. 7.

"The conclusions at which he had arrived are thus formulated by Stricker:

Chapter Four – The Barks

1. Salicylic acid appears to be a rapid and radical remedy in recent cases of genuine acute rheumatism of the joints.
2. It is not injurious to the human organism, when administered every hour in doses varying from 7½ to 15 grains.
3. It can be given in these doses for a longer time to young and strong individuals than to the old and feeble.
4. In the latter, it produces toxic symptoms more readily than in the former.
5. The toxic symptoms vary in degree.
6. Those most commonly met with are noises in the ears, difficulty of hearing and diaphoresis; when these occur, the administration of the medicine should be discontinued.
7. If salicylic acid be found to fully answer the expectations entertained regarding it, the internal administration of a certain quantity may be expected to prevent the occurrence of fresh attacks in hitherto unaffected joints, and also secondary inflammation of serous membranes, especially the endocardium.
8. To prevent relapse, the medicine must be continued in smaller doses for some days after the termination of the main treatment.
9. Salicylic acid is of doubtful value in chronic articular disease.
10. It is not likely to be of use in gonorrhoeal or diarrhoeal rheumatism, or in the polyarthritis attending septicaemia."

Maclagan goes on to make the interesting observation:

"Previous to the publication of the German reports, I had myself, while making my observations on salicin, tried salicylic acid in a case of subacute rheumatism. It did good to the rheumatism, but caused so much irritation of the throat and stomach that it was omitted and salicin given instead –

Results so striking as those got by the German observers from salicylic acid, and by myself from salicin, could not fail to attract general attention. Observations were made on all hands. The journals in England, France, Germany and America contained numerous reports of cases of rheumatism treated by these drugs.

– The favourable experience of Stricker and Riess is endorsed by German physicians generally. In France, it has been equally successfully – In America, Dr. Brown – " (Boston Medical and Surgical Journal 1877, Feb 8th).

Dr. Maclagan was also a contributor to a book titled:

"Twentieth Century Practice. An International Encyclopedia of Modern Medical Science by Leading Authorities of Europe and Asia. Edited by Thomas L. Stedman M. D. New York City. In 20 volumes. Volume II. Nutritive Disorders Published in London by Sampson Low, Marston and Company Limited, St. Dunstan's House, Fetter Lane, Fleet Street, E.C.1895. Dr. Maclagan is described as follows:

RANGE OF TEMPERATURE IN A FATAL CASE OF ACUTE RHEUMATISM COMPLICATED WITH PERICARDITIS. (SYDNEY RINGER).

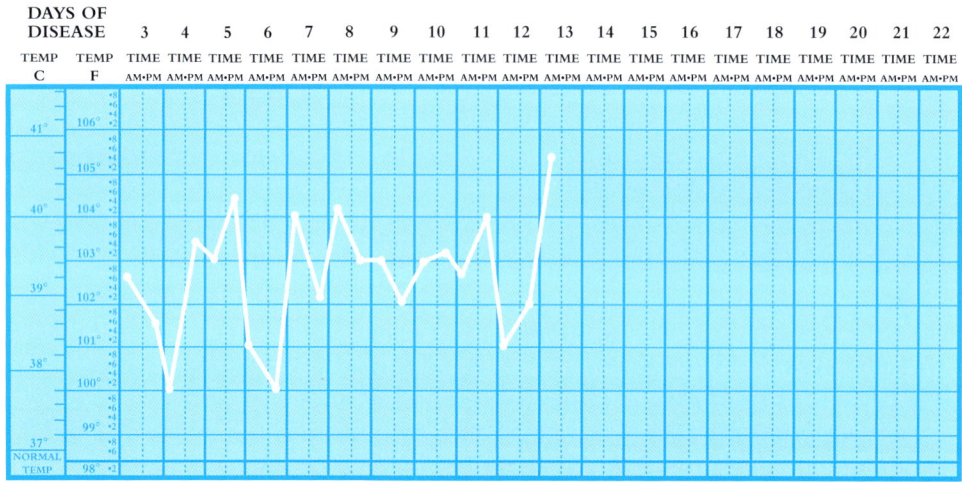

Figure 4.20. Fatal case of acute rheumatism – temperature chart.

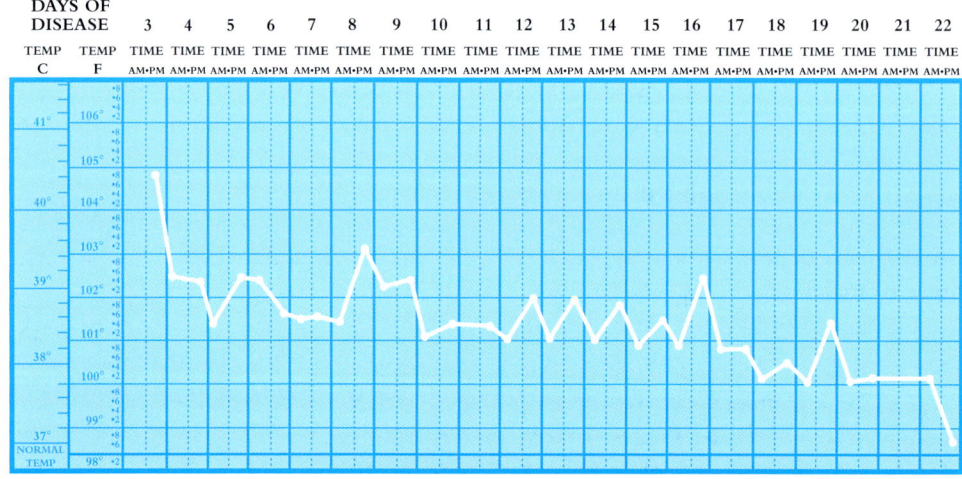

Figure 4.21. Range of temperature in a case of acute rheumatism affecting many joints simultaneously.

Chapter Four – The Barks

Left: Figure 4.22. Chemical formula of quinine.
Top: Figure 4.23. Chemical formulae of aspirin and its sodium salt.

Thomas J. Maclagan, M. D. M. R. C. P. London. Physician-in-Ordinary to Prince and Princess Christian of Schlëswig-Holstein; Formerly Physician to the Dundee Royal Infirmary and Examiner in Medicine and Pathology, University of Aberdeen.

Distinguished co-authors included Sir Dyce Duckworth, Physician at St. Bartholomew's Hospital, as well as Physician to the Prince of Wales, and Archibald E. Garrod, Assistant Physician to the Hospital for Sick Children, Great Ormond Street and who, interestingly wrote the section on "Arthritis deformans." (One might have anticipated him writing on the subject of gout, as it is a metabolic disease, in which field Garrod is regarded as supreme).

In this book Maclagan gives a description of 9 cases of rheumatism, which are summarised. He discusses the mode of action of salicyl compounds in rheumatism, see figures 4.20 and 4.21. He reviews the use of cinchona (Peruvian bark) in the treatment of intermittent fevers, pointing out that the mechanism by which it works has never been explained. He states that he has tried quinine in all types of ague, but has only found it of value in intermittents and remittents. However, the fact remains that whilst quinine could cure cases of malaria, it could not cure other forms of fever. Likewise, salicylates could cure rheumatic fever but not the fever of malaria.

Having described the principal clinical publications on the use of willow bark extract in the 18th and 19th centuries, a word or two on the bark it supplanted – Jesuit's bark, derived from the Cinchona trees found in South America.

Cinchona belongs to the family Rubiaceae, and is found from Bolivia to Venezuela on the eastern slopes of the Andes. It grows at altitudes up to 10,000 feet. It was a useful source of quinine, the formula of which is seen in figure 4.22. Also shown are the formulae of sodium salicylate and acetylsalicylic acid (aspirin). They are trees or shrubs, and can reach a height of as much as 100 feet. The bark is corky, fissured and bitter. Around 1630 Spanish Jesuits learned about the beneficial effect of its bark. It was first used for the treatment of fever by a Jesuit priest in Peru, and in all likelihood, he gained this knowledge from native Indians. The priests employed the natives to harvest the bark, and interestingly, for each tree cut down, five had to be planted in the shape of a cross. Subsequently it became known as **'Jesuit's bark'** see figure 4.23, and was greatly in demand in Europe particularly in Italy and Spain. By 1645, the bark had reached Rome for use in the Vatican. Protestants refused to use it on principle, considering it an evil papal plot. Thus poor Oliver Cromwell, suffering from malaria, was denied a cure, and died of it in 1658. Notwithstanding quinine's suspicious reputation, it was used to treat Charles II of England, and Louis XIV of France.

In 1655, the Jesuit's bark reached England, and is mentioned in the London Pharmacopoeia of 1677. In 1663 appeared a paper by **Sebastiano Bado**, describing the miraculous fever bark from Peru, see figure 4.24. This was the original source of the legend of the cure of the Countess of Chinchon, wife of the Viceroy of Lima, of her fever. The subsequent mis-spelling of the word 'Chinchona' was the error of Linnaeus, and this error has been perpetuated. It was chiefly used for 'ague' (malaria), but in reality, ague probably referred simply to 'fever' which in some, but not all cases was due to malaria. Thus, the effectiveness of willow bark in agues shows that, in at least some cases, the fever was not due to malaria, because aspirin is not effective in malaria. Prominent physicians of the time, included **Prujean**, **Sydenham** and **Sloane** (who had invested heavily in it during his sojourn in Jamaica in 1687–89).

Quinine was isolated from the bark of cinchona in 1820 by Pelletier and Caventou of Paris, but unfortunately for them they failed to patent it. In 1865, seeds of quinine plants were smuggled out of South America by Charles Ledger for about 20 dollars, which was equivalent at the time to the price paid for Manhattan Island. These seeds were used to produce plantations in Java, and led to a Dutch monopoly replacing the South American one.

Sir Hans Sloane (see above), founded the Chelsea Physic Garden in London, from where the example of the leaves of the Cincona tree, see figure 4.25, are seen below.

Quinine was subsequently manufactured in London, Amsterdam, Philadelphia and Germany. The Peruvian government had a monopoly on the bark, and the price demanded reflected this. The Dutch established large plantations of high quality in Java which captured 95% of the market. The availability of quinine no doubt facilitated the colonisation and exploration of the 19th century, especially in the tropics.

In the book titled 'Henry Wellcome', by Robert Rhodes James, there is a graphic description of Wellcome's 1878 expedition to Ecuador.

"Words are inadequate to picture the terribly broken and precipitous character of these Andean ranges; on every side traces of ruptured violence is distinctly visible; every rock shows the marks of a tremendous crushing force; the irregular masses of rock and earth heaped together form tortuous ridges and bold craggy spurs, with numerous intersecting fissures, ravines and vast chasms; every physical feature is

Chapter Four – The Barks

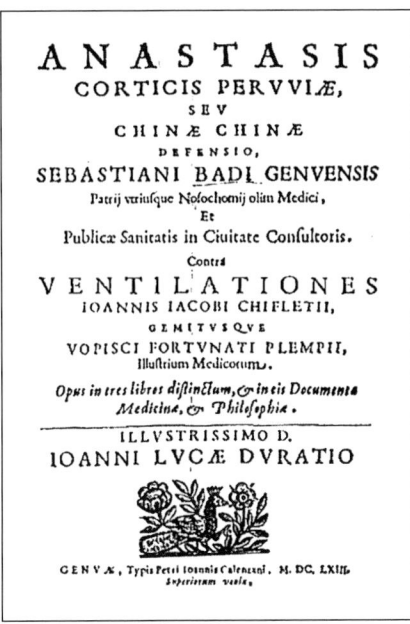

Figure 4.24. Sebastiano Bado's 1663 opus on the fever bark.

modelled on magnificence and grandeur – In many places while penetrating the forests, we were obliged to dismount and climb, while our mules were lifted almost bodily up the jagged steeps by the peons; finally we reached a point beyond which it was impossible to take the animals. Leaving them – we gained a point on one of the great spurs, where we saw spread out before us a boundless undulating sea of wilderness, as far as the eye could reach, a gorgeous expanse of matted verdure, illumined by showy blossoms of glowing colours. –

The surpassing grandeur of this view was enrapturing beyond expression. On every hand the manifold and varied beauties unfolded themselves with almost bewildering rapidity; but suddenly a huge bank of clouds drifted upon us like a Newfoundland fog, curtailing the scene for a few moments and then quickly passing on.

Our guide soon described some Cinchonas in the distance with glistening leaves, which reflected brightly the vertical rays of the sun.

This characteristic reflex of the foliage, together with the bright roseate tints of the flowers, afford the means of discovering the Cinchonas amongst the mass of forest giants. In prospecting by the appearance of the leaves alone, a novice is easily misled by the India Rubber tree, which has a glossy leaf very like the magnolias of our southern states and when seen in the distance in the bright sunlight is easily mistaken for the Cinchona. –

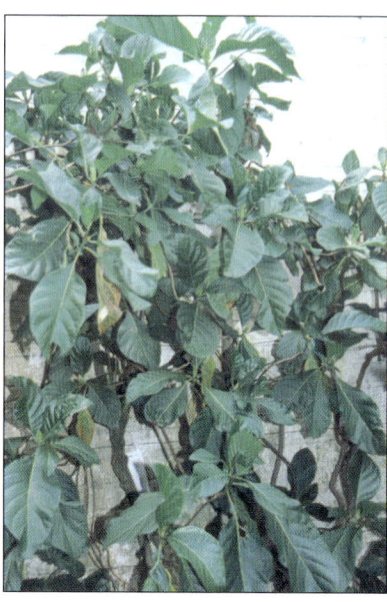

Figure 4.25. Cinchona officinale in the tropical hothouse at the Chelsea Physic Garden. Taken from an article by Dr. Tim Cutler, the College Representative of the Royal College of Physicians of London at the Chelsea Physic Garden, which appeared in the College Commentary, September/October 2003. (With permission of the Royal College of Physicians of London).

The older Cinchona trees as found, in the virgin forest, are really very grand and handsome. They appear to seek the most secluded and inaccessible depths of the forest for their habitation. They are rarely grouped in large numbers or close together, but are distinguished in more or less irregular, scattering patches; sometimes single trees are found widely separated from any others of its family, variety and diversity are notable features of tropical forests.

The Cinchona Succiruba ranges from forty to eighty feet in height, trunks straight and branches regular; leaves opposite, evergreen, broadly oval; six to ten inches in length, of a rich, dark green colour, sometimes tinged with crimson – The bark of the tree is usually completely covered and fringed with mosses of the most delicate, lace-like texture." Wellcome went on to describe the techniques for stripping the bark and conveying it to ports. He was appalled at the low rates of pay received by the local work force, and the dangers they faced. The Indians regarded malaria with terror.

"As regards the prospects of further supplies of Cinchona barks from the native forests of South America, the outlook is exceedingly discouraging, the greatly increased use of Cinchona alkaloids during the past few years, with the consequent demand for larger supplies of bark, has caused a very thorough working of the old forests and energetic seeking for new ones. The discoveries of paying forests are becoming more and more rare every year, and the new forests are found at greater distances from the shipping ports and more difficult of access.

The track of country yielding the Cinchona is not so unlimited as some writers would give us to believe, nor is the supply inexhaustible; it is a fact recognised by natives and dealers, who are well informed about the extent and resources of the Cinchona bearing districts, that if the present ruinous system of destroying the trees is continued, and no effort made to propagate new growths, they will before many years be exterminated from their native soil."

How pertinent are these remarks even today, as we witness the mindless destruction of so much of the planet's forests as a consequence of financial opportunism, with the short term risks of flooding, and in the long term, global warming with dire consequences for the whole of mankind.

In the 6th edition of 'An arrangement of British Plants' by William Withering, published in London in 1818, (the book though ascribed to William Withering was edited by his son William, Withering Senior having died in 1799), there is a detailed description of all the known willows of the time. Under the White or Common Willow, found in woods, hedge-rows, and wet meadow and pasture land, appears the following:

"T. April★

★It loves a moist and open situation; grows quickly, and bears lopping. The wood is very white, and is therefore preferred for making milk pails and butter firkins. It is also used for flooring, for chests and for boxes. It is light, tough, and pliable. The Rev. Mr. Stone, in the *Phil. Trans.* liii. p. 195, gives us an account of the great efficacy of the bark of this tree in curing intermittent fevers. He gathers the bark in summer, when it is full of sap, dries it by a gentle heat, and gives a dram of it powdered every four hours between the fits. In a few obstinate cases he mixed it with one fifth part of Peruvian bark. It is remarkable that intermittents are most prevalent in wet countries; and this tree grows naturally in such situations. Whilst the Peruvian bark remained at its usual moderate price, it was hardly worth while to seek for a substitute! But now its price is more than and the supply from South America hardly equal to the consumption, we may expect to find it dearer and more adulterated every year. The WHITE WILLOW bark is, therefore, likely to become an object worth the attention of physicians, and if its success upon a more enlarged scale of practice prove equal to Mr. Stone's experiments, the world will be much indebted to that gentleman for his communication. The bark of *S. triandria* and *fragilis* have the same properties. A set of experiments should, therefore, be instituted to ascertain which of the species ought to be preferred. – "

The Fall and Rise of Aspirin

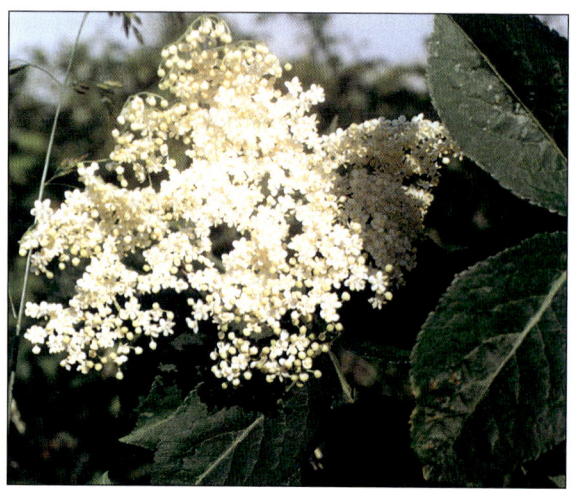 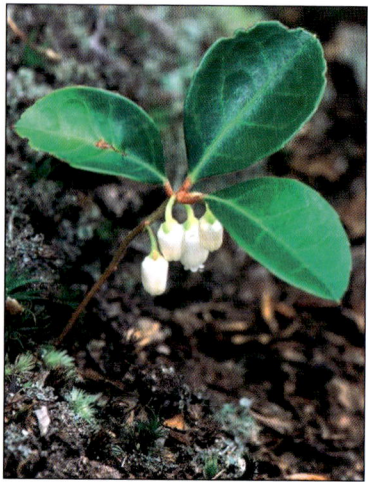

Left: Figure 5.2. Meadowsweet. (Filendipula ulmaria, previously Spiraea ulmaria).
Right: Figure 5.3. Wintergreen. (Gaultheria procumbens).
(Reproduced with kind permission of University of Kentucky.
From 'Wild flowers and ferns of Kentucky,' Thomas G. Barnes and S.W. Francis, 2004).

Chronological sequence of events leading to the production of aspirin
Isolation from natural sources

Fontana (1826) and Brugnatelli (1829) isolated small quantities of salicin.

Buchner (1828) in Munich isolated salicin.

Leroux (1829) in Paris, isolated salicin from willow bark, and demonstrated its anti-fever value.

Pagenstecher (1831), in Switzerland, distilled salicylaldehyde obtained from the meadowsweet or queen of the meadow plant (*Filendipula ulmaria*), then known as *Spiraea ulmaria*, the "Spiraea" contributing to the eventual naming of aspirin, see figure 2.

Merck (1833), in Darmstadt, isolated salicin from willow bark.

Lowig (1835), a Swiss chemist, starting from meadowsweet, was the first to prepare salicylic acid from salicylaldehyde, which he called "Spirsaure", the "Spir" coming from the genus Spiraea, and the "saure" being the German word for acid. Acetylation of spirsaure led to the term "acetylspiraure" which was then shortened to aspirin. An alternative explanation was that it was named after St. Aspirinus, an early Neapolitan Bishop, who was the patron saint against headaches.

Piria (1838), in Paris, isolated salicin from willow bark, decoctions of which were used from antiquity for the relief of pains and inflammation associated with arthritis and rheumatism. From salicin, salicylic acid was prepared.

132

Chapter Five – The Laboratory Chemists and Aspirin Manufacture

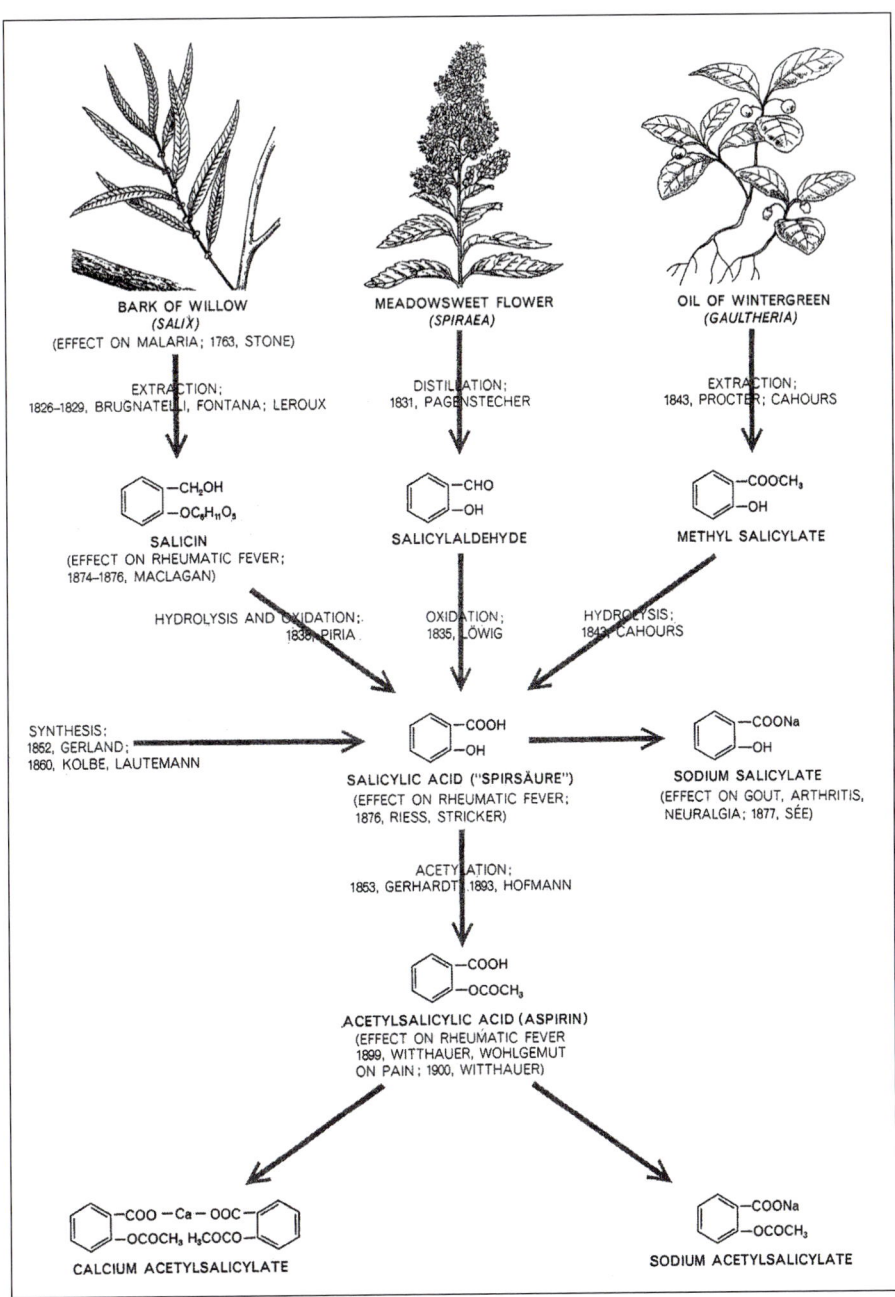

Figure 5.4. Historical overview of production of aspirin from natural sources. (From Scientific American, 1963, with permission of Donald G. Garber).

Dumas (1839), showed that Lowig's and Piria's compounds were identical, both having prepared salicylic acid, one starting with salicin from willow bark, the other with salicylaldehyde from meadowsweet.

William Procter (1843), an American, and the Frenchman **Auguste Cahours** isolated methyl salicylate from oil of wintergreen, (*Gaultheria procumbens*, or *Gaultheria hispidula*), which was an English folk remedy for treatment of "agues" i.e. fevers, see figure 5.3.

Cahours (1844), hydrolysed methyl salicylate to salicylic acid. Up to this point advances were being made in the isolation and purification of salicylates from natural sources, but it would require synthesis from other chemicals to allow economical mass production to develop.

A summary of the various paths taken in various laboratories to extract salicylic acid, and then acetylate it, producing acetylsalicylic acid (aspirin), is shown in figure 5.4, reproduced with thanks, from Scientific American, 1961.

(ii) Synthetic production

In 1852 **Henri Gerland** synthesised salicylic acid by reacting nitrous acid with anthranilic acid – this was the first example of its synthesis starting from basic chemicals as apart from a natural source. Clues as to its eventual synthesis came as a result of **Charles Gerhardt** in 1853, professor of chemistry at Montpellier. He found that by heating salicylic acid, it decomposed into phenol and carbon dioxide. The reverse reaction i.e. the production of salicylic acid from phenol by joint action of carbon dioxide and sodium, was seized upon by **Herman Kolbe** in 1860, and by 1874, together with **Lautemann** he introduced the commercial process which enabled **Friedrich von Heyden** to establish his large factory for the commercial production of salicylic acid. (Incidentally, Gerhardt had been trying to find a general expression for the molecular construction of organic acids. He later reacted sodium salicylate with acetylchloride and obtained acetylsalicylic acid (aspirin). The reaction had been very difficult to perform, and Gerhardt considered the new compound to be "of no further significance." An example of being so wrapped up in the science, that the commercial spin-off went unnoticed). Kolbe was instrumental in proving that organic (i.e. carbon containing) chemicals could be made from inorganic ones, and did not require the presence of living matter, which was the previously held belief. His seminal work, in 1843–5, was to convert carbon disulphide (regarded as an inorganic substance) to acetic acid (organic). Together with **Schmitt**, he jointly developed the reaction which bears their names: the **Kolbe-Schmitt** reaction, which consisted of heating sodium phenolate with pressurised carbon dioxide at 125°C, and 125 atmospheres, then adding sulphuric acid, and obtaining salicylic acid. In 1879, **Stricker** noted the beneficial effect of acetylsalicylic acid in acute rheumatic disorders and that the sodium salt was effective in acute rheumatic fever.

Chapter Five – The Laboratory Chemists and Aspirin Manufacture

The Bayer story

The history of aspirin cannot be told without referring to the history of the Bayer company. The founder **Friedrich Bayer**, senior, (1825–1880), see figure 5.5, was born in the Barmen-Wichlinghausen district of what is today Wuppertal. His father was a silk-worker, the textile industry being predominant at the time. When he was 14 years old, he got a job as an apprentice with Wesenfeld & Co. in Barmen. There he gained invaluable experience in the dyeing industry. Initially, he worked with natural dyes, extracted from wood. However, the field of inorganic chemistry was proceeding apace, and had enormous potential. Aniline and fuchsine literally outshone natural dyes. These dyes were extracted from tar, and when developed by Bayer and **Johann Friedrich Weskcott**, (1820–1876), a future business partner of Bayer, were of superior quality to the first generation synthetic dyestuffs. Only later would it come to light that many of the workers who came into contact with these chemicals would develop bladder cancer. By August 1863, their partnership was commercially registered as 'Friedr. Bayer et comp'. By 1867, the company employed 50 people. Bayer, senior, died in 1880, aged 55 years, leaving behind a flourishing family business. The early premises at Barmen are seen in the next figure, see figure 5.6.

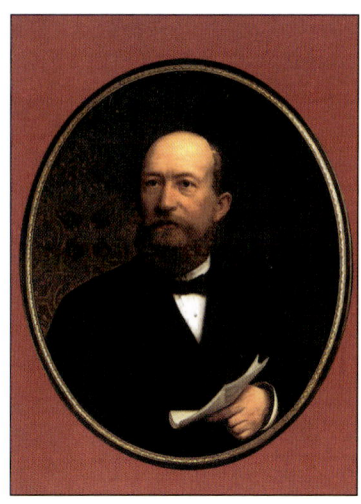

Figure 5.5. The founder, Friedrich Bayer (1825–1880). (Reproduced with permission of Bayer A.G).

In 1874, **Kolbe** and **Lautemann** formulated a feasible organic synthesis of salicylic acid from phenol and carbon dioxide. In 1876, two other German physicians, **Stricker** and **Reiss** independently reported on the value of salicylic acid in the treatment of rheumatic fever, thereby preceding **Maclagan's** book, published in 1881. By 1880, sodium salicylate was being used to treat chronic rheumatoid arthritis, and gout. In 1874, one of Kolbe's students, **Friedrich von Heyden**, formed a company, the **Heyden Chemical Company** which devoted itself to the commercial synthesis and marketing of salicylic acid. However, they inappropriately promoted it as an antiseptic, lacking the irritation of phenol, as well as any smell. Unfortunately, it never proved to be particularly effective as an antiseptic. It had been hoped that it would also be used as a food preservative for this reason.

It will be remembered that 1874 was the year Maclagan of Dundee published his case reports of the use of salicin. However, commercial pressures determined that salicin, (produced by tedious and expensive extraction from willow bark), would not

The Fall and Rise of Aspirin

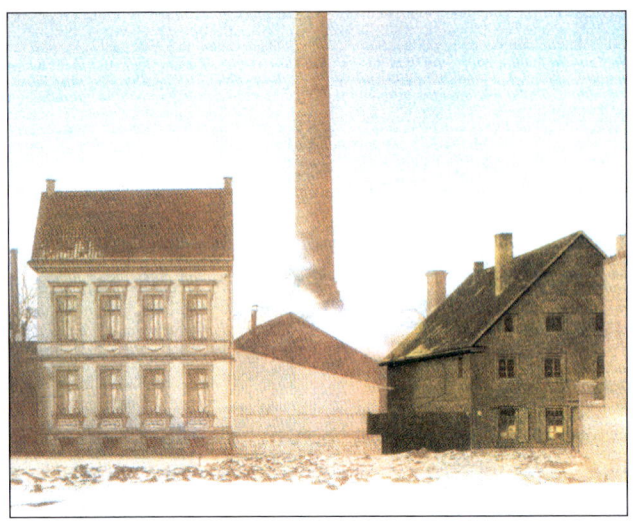
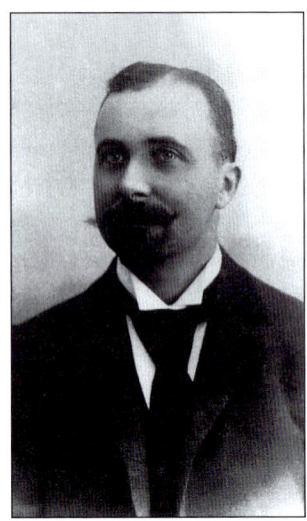

Left: Figure 5.6. Premises of Friedrich Bayer & Company in Heckinghauser Strasse, in the Rittershausen section of Barmen. (Reproduced with permission of Bayer A.G).
Right: Figure 5.7. Felix Hoffmann (1868–1946).

prove the preparation of choice because it was ten times more expensive than synthesised salicylic acid.

The name of the Bayer company is inextricably linked to that of **Felix Hoffmann**, (1868–1946), see figure 5.7.

He studied under a future Nobel prize winner, Professor Adolf von Baeyer, who recommended him to the company which he joined in 1894 as a laboratory chemist. Hoffmann's father suffered from rheumatic pains and not un-naturally encouraged his son to produce a pain-killing drug which did not taste as sickening as sodium salicylate. Hoffmann reported his synthesis of pure acetylsalicylic acid in 1897, see figures 5.8.

Its final sentence states:

"Durch ihre physikalischen Eigenschaften wie eine sauren Geschmack ohne jede Atzwirkung unterscheidet sich die Acetylsalicylsaure vorteilhaft von der Salicylsaure und wird dieselbe in diesem Sinne auf ihre Verwendbarkeit gepruft."

Translated this means:

"Due to its physical properties, such as an acid taste without any corrosive action, acetylsalicylic acid differs advantageously from salicylic acid and is being examined for its usefulness with just this in mind."

In 1899, the head of the experimental pharmacology department was **Heinrich Dreser**, see figure 5.9. According to **Arthur Eichengrun**, see figure 5.10, a colleague

Chapter Five – The Laboratory Chemists and Aspirin Manufacture

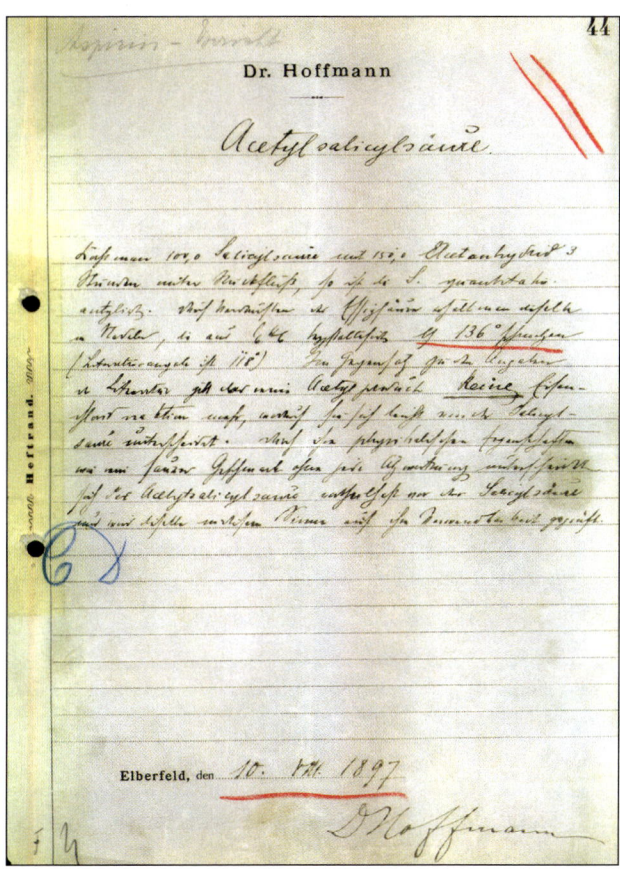

Figure 5.8. Hoffmann's description of the preparation of acetylsalicylic acid, 1897. (Reproduced with permission of Bayer A.G).

of Hoffmann, Dreser showed little interest in acetylsalicylic acid for about 18 months. In fact he feared that it might prove toxic to the heart, and vetoed the commencement of clinical studies as called for by Eichengrun. Not to be deterred, Eichengrun tested aspirin on himself and other physician volunteers. They confirmed its remarkable anti-rheumatic effects, not least on toothache. Dreser's comment – "This is the usual loud mouthing of Berlin – the product has no value." Sadly Eichengrun was later taken to Theresienstadt which was a staging post for unfortunates later to be transported East to the death camps.

Whether the development of aspirin was actually due to Hoffmann's desire to help his father, or to Eichengrun's determination to circumvent Dreser's negative opinion of its usefulness is a matter for debate, as has been put forth in Walter

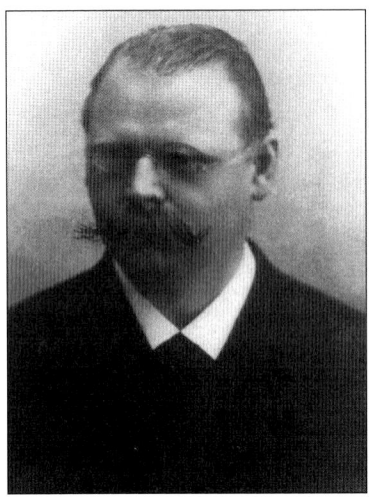 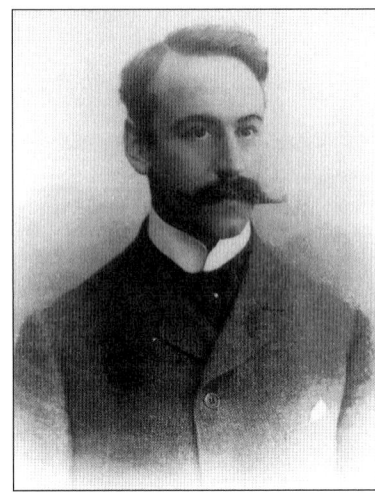

Left: Figure 5.9. Heinrich Dreser, Head of the Experimental Pharmacology Department.
Right: Figure 5.10. Arthur Eichengrun, colleague of Hoffmann.
(Reproduced with permission of Bayer A.G).

Sneader's paper in the British Medical Journal, December 23rd 2000. Dreser then reinvestigated the drug in 1898 and in 1899 published a pre-launch paper in which the history of the drug's development and properties attracted the gaze of both physicians and pharmacists. Strangely, he omitted to mention the contributions of Eichengrun and Hoffmann. And to make matters worse, only Dreser would ultimately benefit financially, because he had an agreement whereby he received payment for all drugs tested in his laboratory. Although Eichengrun and Hoffmann had patent rights for drugs developed in Germany, this only applied to the processes whereby these drugs were produced, not to the drugs themselves. Thus did Dreser become a rich man. A bitter pill indeed – for Eichengrun and Hoffmann!

Internal company communications are shown in the ensuing figures. Figures 5.11 and 5.12 are the first and second pages respectively of a circular to all the big wigs.

Translated it states:

"It is proposed to name the body (i.e. substance) of the drug -" (chemical formula drawn) – "which has the chemical name acetylsalicylic acid under the name aspirin, to protect (it) at the Imperial Patent Office. The substance is supposed to serve as an anti-rheumatic and replace salicylic acid. Are any similar (patent protected) words or similar words known in literature or in the trade? Is it a pure fantasy name or does it give evidence of its composition or effect on the body for which this name is given?

Are there any concerns which would argue against the word, or can you make other proposals?"

Chapter Five – The Laboratory Chemists and Aspirin Manufacture

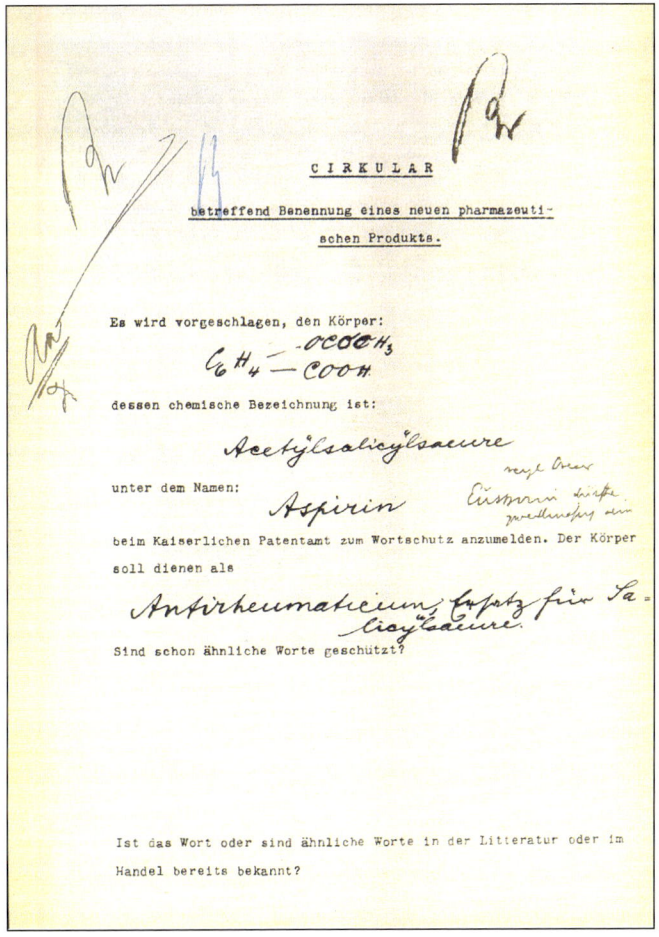

Figure 5.11. First page of company circular 23rd January 1899. The baptism of aspirin.

As publicity, Bayer, now named "Farbenfabriken" (dye fabricators) previously Bayer & Co. of Elberfeld, distributed hundreds of packages containing aspirin powder, inviting the recipients (doctors, hospitals, pharmacists) to give it a try. These days of course one cannot legally do that, because the various control agencies will not issue a product licence until it has been extensively tested, and proved itself from the standpoint of effectiveness, tolerability and safety. And even then, years after the licence has been issued, nasty side effects may become apparent only as a consequence of the drug by now having been used on hundreds of thousands, or millions of people. Such a case has recently come to light with the drug **Vioxx**. Despite being markedly less likely to cause internal bleeding than other anti-

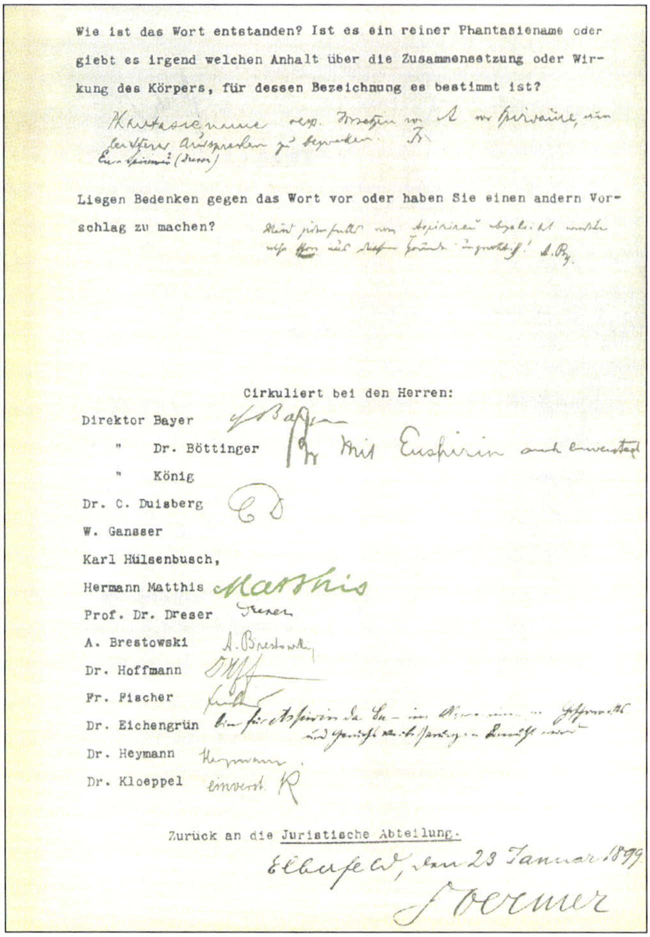
Wie ist das Wort entstanden? Ist es ein reiner Phantasiename oder giebt es irgend welchen Anhalt über die Zusammensetzung oder Wirkung des Körpers, für dessen Bezeichnung es bestimmt ist?

Liegen Bedenken gegen das Wort vor oder haben Sie einen andern Vorschlag zu machen?

Cirkuliert bei den Herren:

Direktor Bayer
" Dr. Böttinger — Mit Euspirin auch einverstanden
" König
Dr. C. Duisberg
W. Gansser
Karl Hülsenbusch,
Hermann Matthis — Matthis
Prof. Dr. Dreser — Dreser
A. Brestowski — A. Brestowski
Dr. Hoffmann
Fr. Fischer
Dr. Eichengrün
Dr. Heymann
Dr. Kloeppel — einverst. K

Zurück an die Juristische Abteilung.

Elberfeld, den 23 Januar 1899

Figure 5.12. Second page of company circular, Elberfeld, 23rd January 1899. (Reproduced with permission of Bayer A.G).

inflammatory agents, including aspirin, it was discovered to be increasing the incidence of heart attacks and strokes. Having to withdraw such a drug is the manufacturer's nightmare. Being threatened with thousands of liability suits could technically drive a company to the wall. However, in those halcyon days, there was no such threat to this commercial venture. It was even proclaimed to be a drug with few side effects – wrong again! The drug was also tried by **Kurt Witthauer** at the Deaconess Hospital in Halle, and he published his findings in April 1899. He stated that after hesitating for a long time, the Bayer factory was finally convinced by his experiences to market aspirin.

Chapter Five – The Laboratory Chemists and Aspirin Manufacture

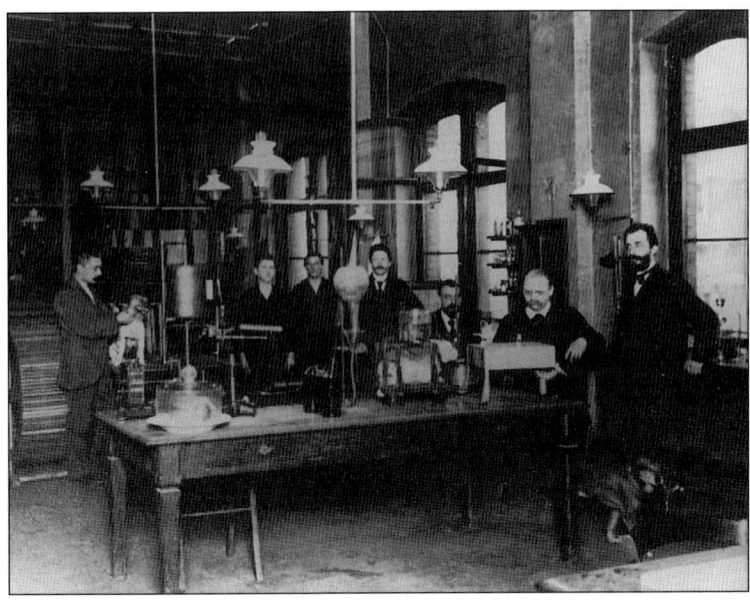

Figure 5.17. Where it all happened, Bayer's aspirin research laboratory, c.1900. (Reproduced with permission of Bayer A.G).

the same. The question of the crystalline character is apparently of no importance, and Professor Smith's conclusion is that acetylsalicylic acid may be obtained without difficulty, chemically pure, from more than one source, but that, as with other chemicals, indifferent and impure makes are on the market, and therefore the same discrimination should be used in buying it as with other drugs." This led the British Board of Trade to announce (as recorded in The Lancet, in the same issue:)

"The Aspirin Trade Mark,

The Board of Trade has made an order regarding the aspirin trade marks. The effect of which is to make the word 'aspirin' public property. As is well known, this is the trade name under which the Bayer Company introduced acetylsalicylic acid and the name under which the drug is best known. It is now open to anyone to sell acetylsalicylic acid as aspirin and it is to be hoped that this will not lead to any deterioration in the standard of the drug... there are now several makers of acetylsalicylic acid in this country, and an examination of various samples has shown that chemically most are identical with the original aspirin."

Nowadays, the professors carrying out and publishing their results would be expected to declare their interests. For instance, what if, heaven forbid, Professor Smith had been in cahoots with some shady manufacturer of inferior grade acetylsalicylic acid. And there were several inferior products, despite the published reassurances.

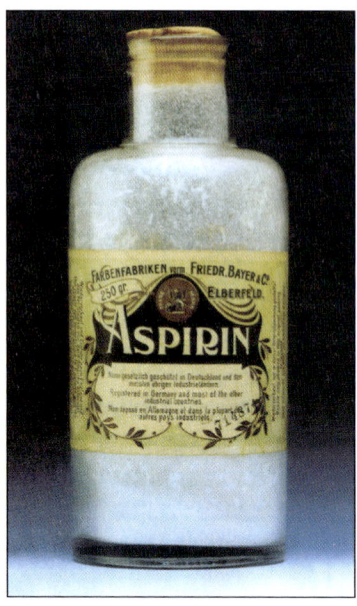

*Figure 5.18. Early example of Bayer aspirin in powder form.
(Reproduced with permission of Bayer A.G).*

The British Pharmaceutical Codex
Published by direction of the Council of the Pharmaceutical Society of Great Britain, 1911.

ACIDUM ACETYL-SALICYLICUM. ACETYL-SALICYLIC ACID
Related entry: Salicylic acid – Methyl salicylate Other tomes $C_9H_8O_4 = 180.064$.
Synonyms. – Acidum Acetosalicum; Acetosalic Acid; Acetosalin; Acidum Salaceticum; Salacetin.

Acetyl-salicylic acid, $C_6H_4(COOH)OCOCH3$, is prepared by the action of acetic anhydride or acetyl chloride on salicylic acid. It was originally introduced into medicine under the trade-name Aspirin. It is also known, in a simple or compounded form, under the trade-names Acetysal, Aletodin, Saletin, Xaxa, etc. It occurs in colourless acicular crystals, or as a white, crystalline powder, melting-point (when dry), 135°. The acid should be free from chlorides and sulphates, and leave no residue on ignition. If 1 decigram (10 gram) be dissolved in 5 mils of alcohol, 20 mils of water added, and then 1 drop of dilute ferric chloride solution, a violet colour should not be produced immediately (absence of free salicylic acid). The acid should be preserved in well-closed bottles, and kept in a dry place.

Soluble in water (1 in 300), alcohol (1 in 5), ether, or chloroform.

Chapter Five – The Laboratory Chemists and Aspirin Manufacture

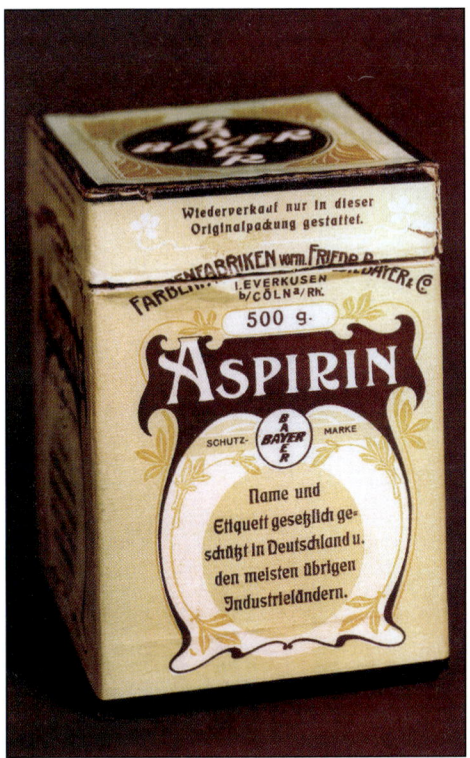 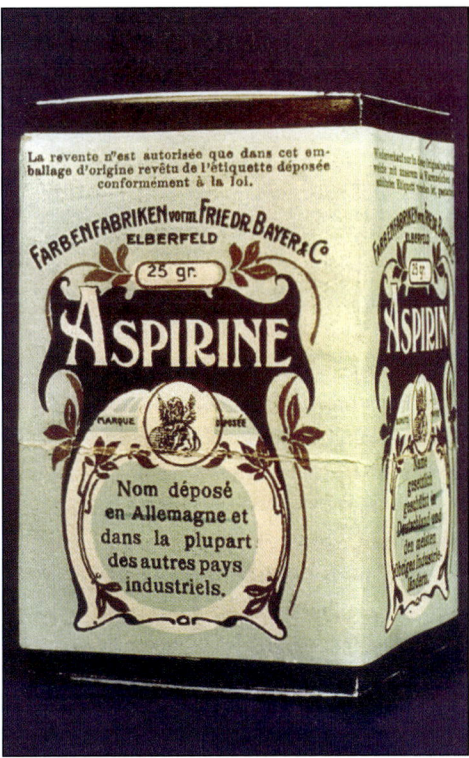

*Left: Figure 5.19. 500 grams, presumably powder, Bayer Leverkusen. Note new Bayer logo.
Right: Figure 5.20. 25 grams Aspirin powder for the French market.
(Reproduced with permission of Bayer A.G).*

Action and Uses. – Acetyl-salicylic acid passes through the stomach unchanged, but is slowly decomposed by the alkali of the duodenum, salicylic acid being liberated. It has therefore the same action as salicylic acid (see Acidum Salicylicum), but is less liable to produce objectionable secondary effects such as gastric disturbance. The powder is applied locally at frequent intervals in the early stages of tonsillitis. It is best **administered** in cachets, powders, or tablets, and should not be prescribed with alkaline substances. The aqueous and alcoholic solutions decompose on standing, salicylic and acetic acids being formed; the reaction takes place very rapidly in alkaline solutions. For administration to children the powder may be mixed with cold milk. Compressed tablets of acetyl-salicylic acid sometimes contain some free salicylic acid, produced by contact with water during manipulation; this may be avoided by the use of ethereal solution of wax or theobroma for granulation. *Dose.* – ½ to 1 gramme (8 to 15 grains).

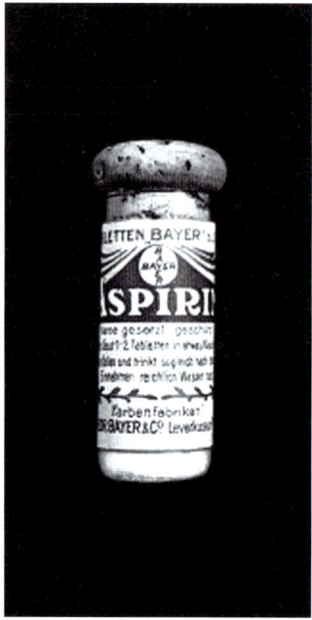 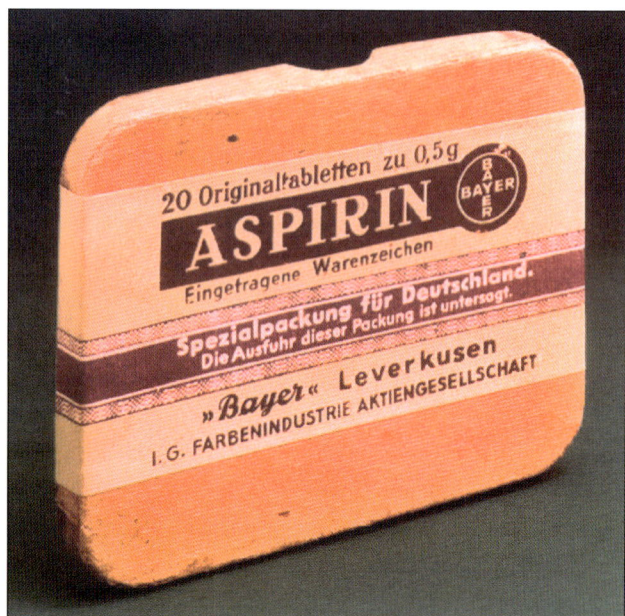

*Left: Figure 5.21. Early aspirin tablets in tubed glass container, from Bayer Leverkusen.
Right: Figure 5.22. Tin of Aspirin tablets from Bayer Leverkusen.
(Reproduced with permission of Bayer A.G).*

PREPARATION
Tablettae Acidi Acetyl-salicylici, B.P.C. – ACETYL-SALICYLIC
ACID TABLETS. 5 grains. Given for all forms of rheumatism. *Dose.* – 1 to 3 tablets.

Aspirin was now being taken in large amounts by the general public. Its pristine reputation not unexpectedly therefore began to tarnish a little. An article in the Lancet in 1917, vol.2, page 659:

"A.H. a lady of 30 years, recently consulted me on account of curious sensations in her head – she had suffered from headache for a long time for which she had taken aspirin freely –

I have no doubt that the reckless way in which aspirin is frequently prescribed would account for some obscure nervous conditions. Sisters and nurses in nursing homes are much given to doping patients with aspirin entirely on their own account, a practice which cannot be too strongly deprecated.
I am, Sir, yours faithfully,

Charles W. Chapman
Harley St, W., October 17th, 1917"

Chapter Five – The Laboratory Chemists and Aspirin Manufacture

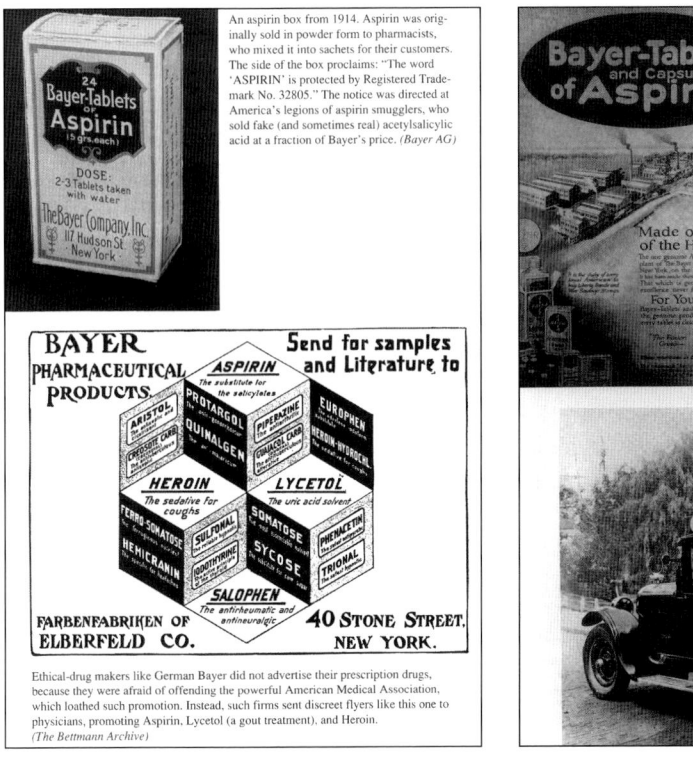
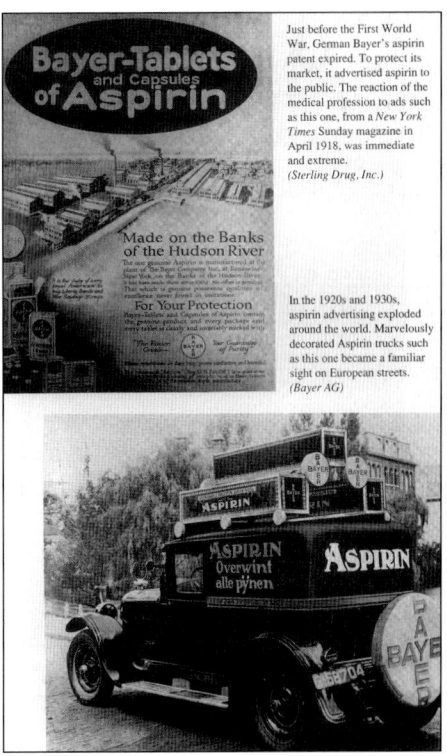

Left: Figure 5.23. Some other Bayer products of the time.
Right: Figure 5.24. Bayer advertising.
(Reproduced with permission of Bayer A.G).

Supply couldn't keep up with demand. Another big player in the aspirin stakes was emerging from, of all places, Australia. His name was **George Nicholas**, a chemist from Melbourne. Through a lot of hard work and gritty experimentation, he succeeded in producing acetylsalicylic acid of sufficient quality to satisfy the authorities there to give him a product licence, as was announced in the Melbourne Herald on 17th September 1915. In fact the claim was made that his product was even purer than that of Bayer. Nicholas, with encouragement from the local authorities, then had the temerity to claim that because their product was superior to Bayer's, only theirs should be known as aspirin! But anti-German feelings were running high, and because the name aspirin was inextricably linked to the German Bayer product, another name was needed. The name they came up with was **Aspro**. Contrast that with the frenetic desire in America to be associated with the name aspirin. But we must not forget there was a powerful pro-German feeling at the time amongst many Americans, which was literally blown

The Fall and Rise of Aspirin

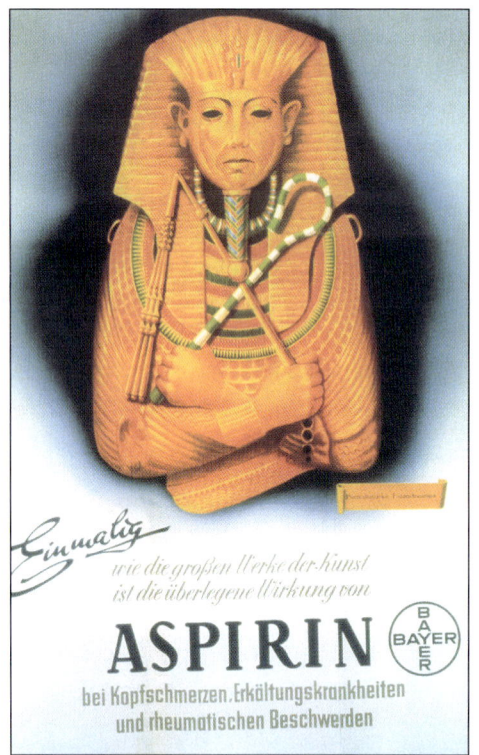 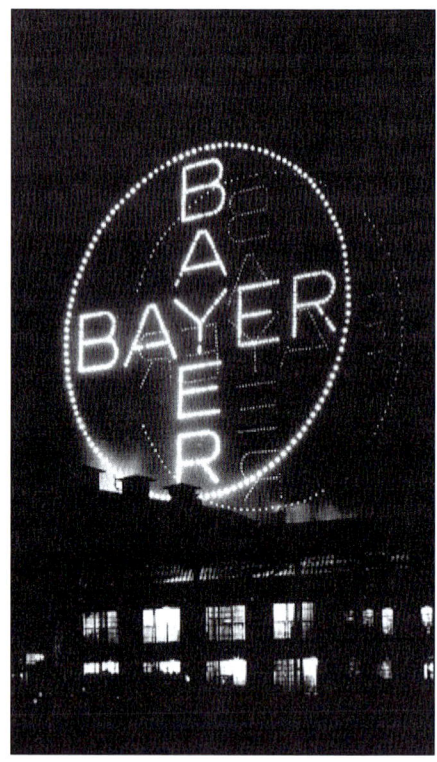

Left: Figure 5.25. Like the greatest works of art, so is Aspirin for headaches, colds and rheumatism. (Presumably Tutanchamon found them useful too!)
Right: Figure 5.26. The Bayer cross, 1933, Leverkusen headquarters. (Reproduced with permission of Bayer A.G).

out of the water when many lives were lost as a result of torpedoes fired by U-boats on their ships, however that didn't stop the attraction of the name – dollars counted.

Came the end of World War I, and the world was struck by the great flu pandemic. Aspirin being in great demand, its manufacture boomed. But anti-German feeling gained sway in America, and the Office of the Alien Property Custodian sold off the Bayer factory at Rensselaer, see figure 5.15. to Sterling Products, later Sterling-Winthrop. They then assumed the same posture as Bayer, claiming that only their product could be termed aspirin, and fought a case with the United Drug Company. They lost. The judge decided that, to the man in the street, the stuff was aspirin, and therefore could be marketed as such by anyone. This led to an explosion in competition, with rival products claiming increased speed, or safety, or the (dubious) benefits of additives which variously included phenacetin, caffeine, and codeine.

Chapter Five – The Laboratory Chemists and Aspirin Manufacture

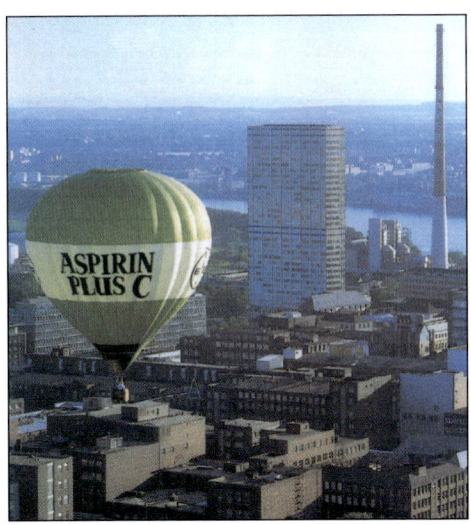 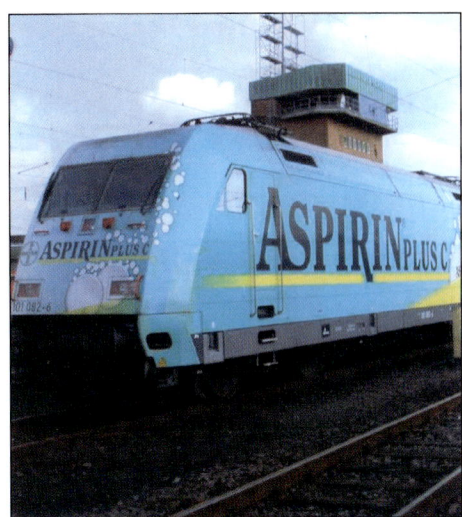

Left: Figure 5.27. Hot air balloon hovering over the Leverkusen factory.
Right: Figure 5.28. Locomotive advertising aspirin plus vitamin C.
(Reproduced with permission of Bayer A.G).

Meanwhile, back in England, several companies were in competition. (see British Pharmacopoeia 1906–1930). Amongst them were:

Manufacturer:	*Product:*
Reckitt & Colman, Hull	Disprin
Thomas Kerfoot Ltd, Lancashire	Salasprin
Genatosan Ltd, Loughborough	Genasprin
Aspro-Nicholas, Slough	Aspro

In the 1870s, Thomas Kerfoot set up a small pill and lozenge factory in Manchester. It was successful, and in 1896 relocated to Ashton-under-Lyne. During the First World War, it was one of several companies selected to manufacture its version of aspirin, which of course could no longer be imported from Germany, and which it marketed as Salasprin. It was subsequently taken over by Medeva Pharm Ltd.

With the start of World War II, Bayer (Leverkusen), was a behemoth of industry, a brilliant company, which had used the best scientific brains, and aggressive marketing strategies (not always successful, as has been shown). Nevertheless, it was a veritable *tour de force* and formed a cartel with other German manufacturers, calling themselves IG Farben. Unfortunately their strength made them a most attractive

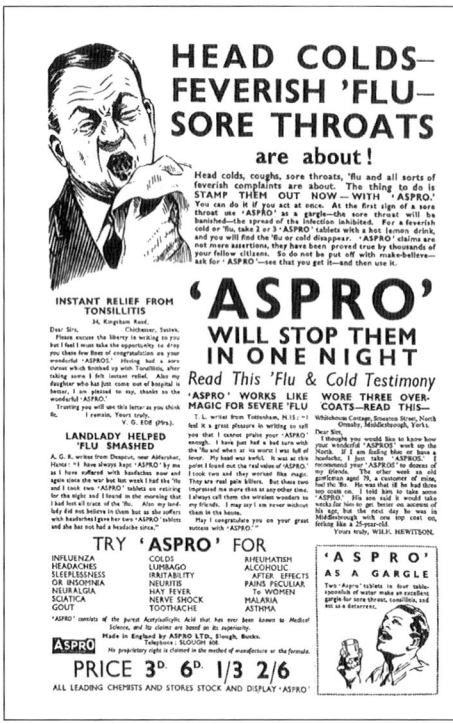
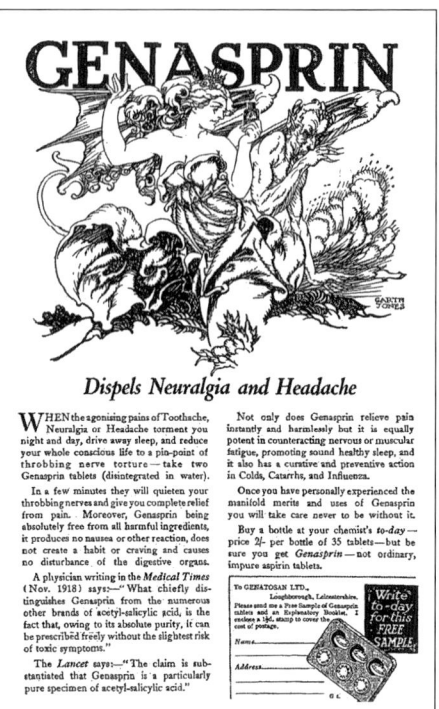

*Left: Figure 5.29. ASPRO advertisement, The Times, Saturday March 11th, 1939.
Right: Figure 5.30. Genasprin advertisement, from Genatosan of Loughborough.
From The Times, Tuesday, November 13th, 1923.*

prize for the emerging Nazi party. They were blackmailed into providing vast sums of money for the cause, but eventually became uncomfortably cooperative. IG Farben would use Jewish slave labour, and one of its subsidiaries, **Degesch** would manufacture **Zyklon B**, the poisonous gas used in the gas chambers at Auschwitz-Birkenau, and elsewhere to murder millions of Jews, and others.

In 1923, confusion over the product reigned in Britain. 'Bayer Aspirin' was available, made both by Bayer (Germany), and their lost subsidiary, now rival, Sterling Products. Into the arena stepped **Aspro**, see figure 5.29. the new boy on the block, the Nicholas product. This company adopted a highly dubious, but very successful advertising trick. Their adverts purported to show that all sorts of personages, many of whom may never have used or even heard of the drug, were espousing its qualities. Aspro and **Genasprin**, see figure 5.30, began rivalling aspirin (Bayer, and Sterling), for sales. Reckitt & Colman in Hull were very successful in marketing **Disprin**, launched in November 1948, see figures 5.31 to 5.34, emphasising its lesser risk of

Chapter Five – The Laboratory Chemists and Aspirin Manufacture

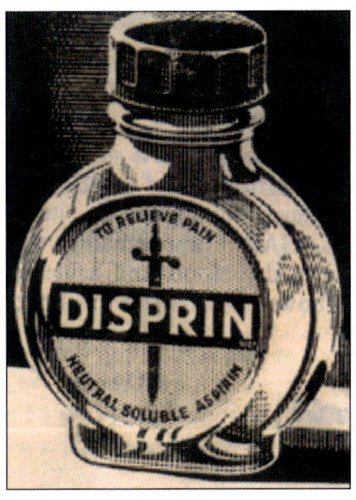 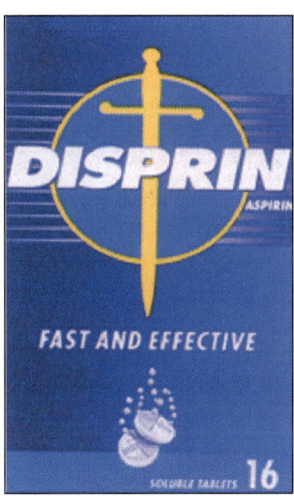

*Figure 5.31. Disprin from Reckitt of Hull.
(Reproduced with the kind permission of Reckitt Benckiser Plc).*

provoking indigestion, and its greater solubility than plain aspirin. It quickly became popular with the medical profession, and had a famous advertising slogan – "Why not take an aspirin – I mean a Disprin".

The industrial procedure for the manufacture of aspirin today differs from those of the industrial giants of the late 19th century. Those initially involved were working in small experimental laboratories, and were only interested in producing a few grams of (often impure) aspirin. Hofman, of Bayer, produced aspirin by reacting salicin (salicylic acid – obtained from willow bark), with acetyl chloride. Industry requires kilograms of reactants in mixing tanks and storage containers containing hundreds of gallons of reactants. Control of the temperature at which the reactions proceed is of paramount importance, as well as the cost of the chemicals used in the initiation, maintenance and purification of the process. In addition there are ecological concerns. Not all manufacturers use the same process. To be described is one process, as outlined in the Pharmaceutical Manufacturing Encylopaedia and U.S. patent 2,731,492.

Acetylsalicylic acid is produced by reacting acetic anhydride with salicylic acid in the presence of sulphuric acid, see figure 5.35. Acetic acid is also produced as a by-product. Nowadays, the acetic anhydride itself is produced by allowing ethylene (from natural gas), to be oxidised to acetic anhydride simply by exposure to air. In earlier days, it was produced by allowing ethanol (alcohol) to be exposed to air, in the presence of a catalyst. This resulted in acetic acid being formed (as anyone who has kept wine for too long will testify). By removing water from acetic acid (vinegar), acetic anhydride resulted.

The Fall and Rise of Aspirin

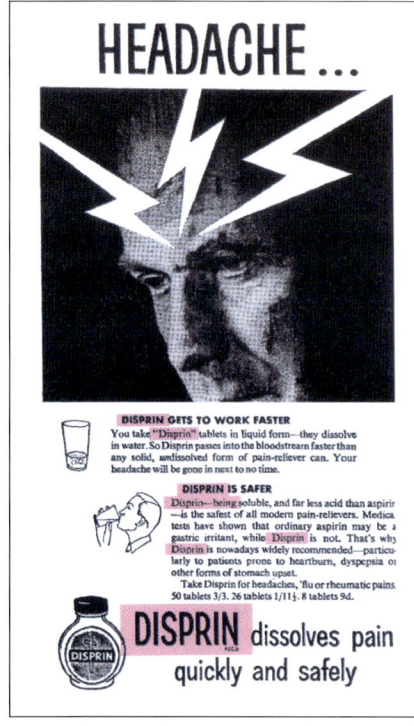 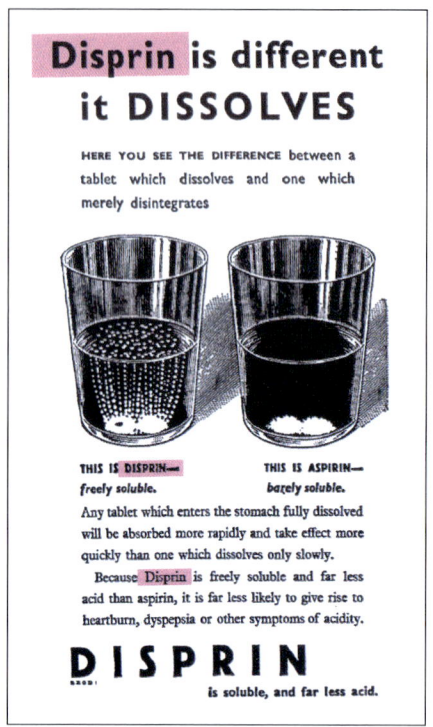

Left: Figure 5.32. Disprin for headache, from The Times, Friday November 25th, 1955. (Reproduced with the kind permission of Reckitt Benckiser Plc)
Right: Figure 5.33. From The Times, Friday September 10th, 1954. (Reproduced with the kind permission of Reckitt Benckiser Plc).

More complicated is the production of salicylic acid (having given up on willow trees!). Here goes (super simplification!).

Sodium hydroxide + phenol → sodium phenolate + water
Sodium phenolate + carbon dioxide → sodium salicylate
Sodium salicylate + sulphuric acid → salicylic acid + sodium sulphate

The main reaction takes place in a glass-lined 1500 gallon tank fitted with a water-cooled reflux condenser, automatically controlled thermometers to maintain the reaction at the desired temperature, and an efficient agitator. The process commences with the dissolving of 1532 kilos of **acetic anhydride** in 1200 kilos of toluene (a solvent which does not participate in the actual reaction that is to follow, and which will later be recovered for re-use). This is known as the mother liquor.

Chapter Five – The Laboratory Chemists and Aspirin Manufacture

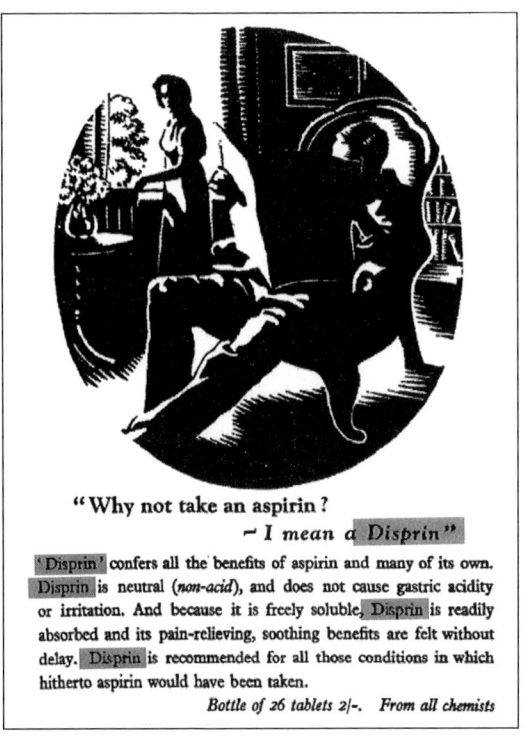

*Figure 5.34. From The Times, Friday October 21st, 1949.
(Reproduced with the kind permission of Reckitt Benckiser Plc).*

1382 kilos of **salicylic acid** is then added to the tank. The reaction is maintained at 88–92 degrees Celsius for 20 hours, then the reactants are transferred to aluminium cooling tanks and cooling takes place over a 3–4 day period. This results in the formation of large crystals of **acetylsalicylic acid (aspirin)** – the main product. The crystallised acetylsalicylic acid is washed with distilled water until all contaminating acetic acid is removed, followed by centrifugation and drying by warm air. This yields about 1790 kilos of aspirin. However, the mother liquor needs to be removed for re-processing.

This is achieved by filtration or centrifugation. The mother liquor after the above process, contains some dissolved acetylsalicylic acid, acetic anhydride, acetic acid (vinegar), and toluene. Next, ketene gas is passed through the filtrate at approximately 20 degrees Celsius, and agitated in the reactor. By the time there has been a weight increase of 420.5 kilos, the liquor will contain 180–270 kilos of dissolved acetylsalicylic acid, and 1532 kilos of acetic anhydride, in 1200 kilos of toluene. Now, by the addition of 1382 kilos of salicylic acid, the whole process is repeated.

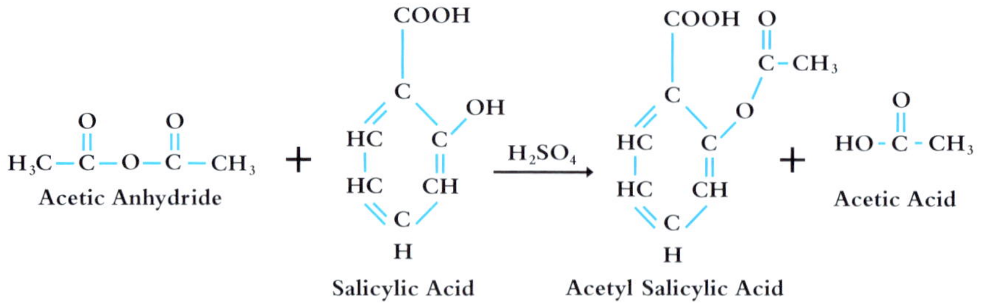

Figure 5.35. Chemical reaction for producing acetylsalicylic acid.

The production, and identification of aspirin, is commonly carried out in school laboratories, using the above shown ingredients, plus sulphuric acid. Its purpose is not simply to produce a commonly taken drug, but to illustrate the chemical principles of recycling of by-products, purification testing (very important in the pharmaceutical industry, particularly among generic products manufactured in remote places), as well as ecological considerations applied to industrial manufacturing processes.

A description of aspirin and aspirin-containing products available either on prescription or over the counter at chemist shops is shown at the end of chapter 11.

Chapter Six

THE FALL OF ASPIRIN

Aspirin, since its manufacture in the late 19th century, took the world by storm. It will be recalled that salicin and salicylic acid, though undoubtedly effective at pain relief, and symptomatically improving fevers, nevertheless were frequently accompanied by abdominal discomfort. Dr. Maclagan of Dundee noticed that many of his patients treated with salicylic acid developed a sore throat, and for a while he returned to salicin, which he found to be less irritating. Towards the end of the 19th century, there appeared reports of gastro-intestinal haemorrhages and indigestion in patients taking salicylic acid or sodium salicylate. An opportunity to study the effect of aspirin in a huge example of 'Nature's experiment' was after the end of the First World War. The notorious pandemic of 1918 killed more people than both World Wars combined. Hundreds of thousands of people took aspirin, and this was followed by an enormous number of cases of gastro-intestinal haemorrhage and in some cases this was severe, culminating in death. Many patients became constipated, some had rashes, some found their asthma was provoked. Patients who tended to take higher doses noticed ringing in their ears (tinnitus).

Reports of the direct irritant effect of aspirin on the gastric mucosa were made by Douthwaite and Lintott, who in the Lancet in 1938 published their observations in the form of coloured drawings from what they observed looking down a rigid tube equipped with a source of illumination. This rigid endoscope had been successfully passed down the oesophagus and into the stomach of a stoical patient, see figure 6.1. Controversy regarding the risk posed by aspirin has continued to rage. It must be remembered that patients with rheumatoid arthritis were, until the 1970s, among the most loyal aspirin takers, but they were not representative of the general population. They suffered chronic inflammation, their body's repair processes were often compromised, they were frequently also taking steroids, which themselves could cause gastro-intestinal bleeding. There were conflicting schools of thought, some claiming that aspirin ingestion was causally related to chronic gastric ulcer (Piper et al 1982), whereas Rees and Turnberg (1980) were of the opinion that aspirin ingestion rarely caused significant gastric pathology in normal subjects. Nevertheless, the perceived wisdom among GPs and junior hospital doctors in the 60s and early 70s, (of which the author was an example of the earlier period), was that aspirin was more likely than other non-steroidal anti-inflammatory drugs (NSAIDs) to cause stomach bleeding. Much of this, it must be admitted, was the result of advertising, and canvassing by drug company representatives. One NSAID rapidly bit the dust. Phenylbutazone ('Butazolidin') though very effective as an

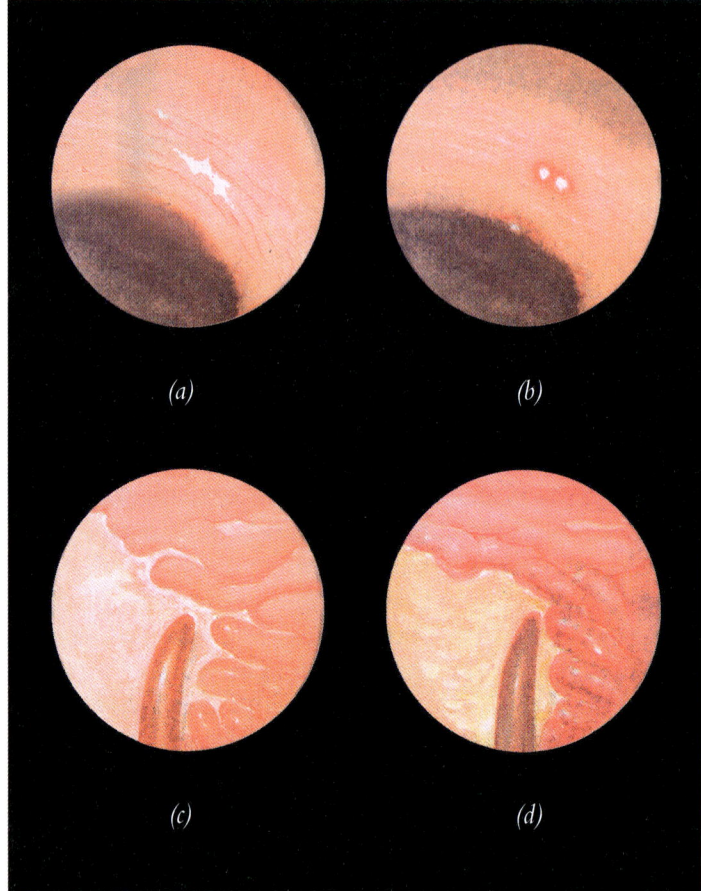

Figure 6.1. View through rigid endoscope (a) adherent barium, (b) Hyperaemia around aspirin tablets, (c) Gastric tube and pool of mucus, (d) Hyperaemia due to mustard. (Reprinted from the Lancet, Douthwaite A.H. & Lintott G.A.M, Gastroscopic observation of the effect of aspirin and certain other substances on the stomach. November 26th, 1938, with permission from Elsevier).

analgesic anti-inflammatory drug, was notorious for its propensity to cause gastro-intestinal bleeding, and also for damaging the bone marrow. It was subsequently withdrawn from the therapeutic armamentarium of the general practitioner, and confined to use by hospital consultants, and then only for the condition known as ankylosing spondylitis. Another rival to aspirin was indomethacin, a more potent anti-inflammatory. Unfortunately, it tended to cause headache in many patients, and also fluid retention (oedema), which could lead to heart failure. This is a property of

Chapter Six – The Fall of Aspirin

all NSAIDs. Additionally, some patients with osteoarthritis of the hip, though initially very pleased with its effectiveness at relieving pain and stiffness, were disappointed to discover after several months that their hip joint had become virtually destroyed. The phrase "indomethacin hip" was coined.

As a junior doctor in the 1960s, the author was frequently involved in the care of patients presenting with *haematemesis* (vomiting of blood), and *melaena* (passage of altered blood in the motions, with the appearance of black tar). The most frequent association was with aspirin ingestion during the past week – though aspirin took various forms. Alka-Seltzer – frequently taken for indigestion, contained aspirin! Many patients didn't realise what they were consuming. The junior doctor undoubtedly got a fairly jaundiced view of the risk associated with aspirin, because the number of cases encountered was really very small when compared with the huge number of people taking over the counter remedies containing aspirin. And aspirin was in competition not only with paracetamol, but also other NSAIDs, claiming to be safer yet equally effective. Investigation in those days was by **barium meal**, which not infrequently revealed gastric or duodenal ulcer, see figures. The first, figure 6.2. shows a large gastric ulcer on the lesser curve of the stomach in a patient, a female

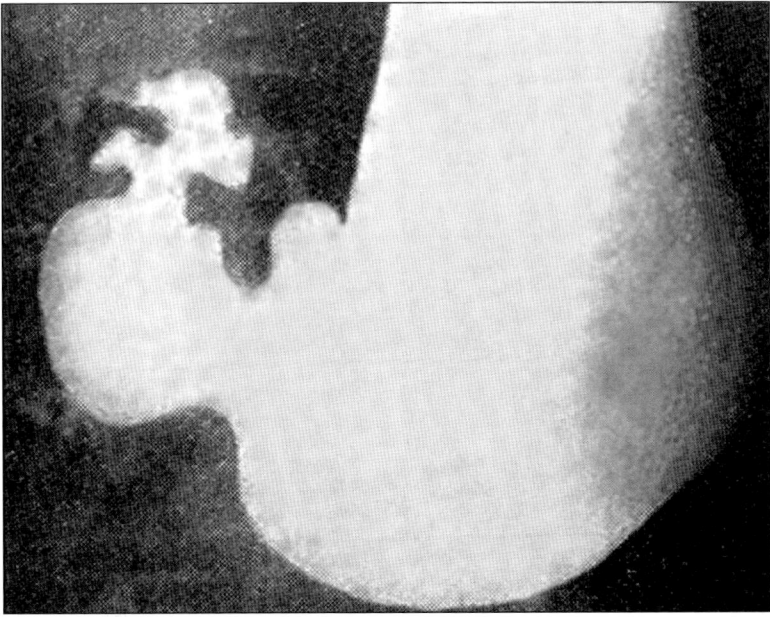

Figure 6.2. Gastric ulcer (depicted by arrow) in a barium meal examination, with clear dramatic evidence of healing. (Reprinted from A Textbook of Medicine, by Cecil R.L. & Loeb R.F, Diseases of the Stomach, page 814, Copyright 1959, with permission from Elsevier).

aged 63 years, with a 35 year history of bouts of epigastric pain i.e. pain felt just below the lower end of the breast bone. Treatment in those days consisted of bed rest, sedation with barbiturates or tranquillizers, admission to hospital and neutralisation of stomach acid. This was achieved by the use of alkalis incorporating substances such as calcium and magnesium carbonate, or aluminium hydroxide. Diet was also important, and consisted of hourly milky drinks (which might include added cream!), followed by soft foods. In some cases, the author recalls patients with persistent pain receiving an intragastric milk drip, via a nasal catheter. The appearance of a duodenal ulcer is shown in the next figure, see figure 6.3.

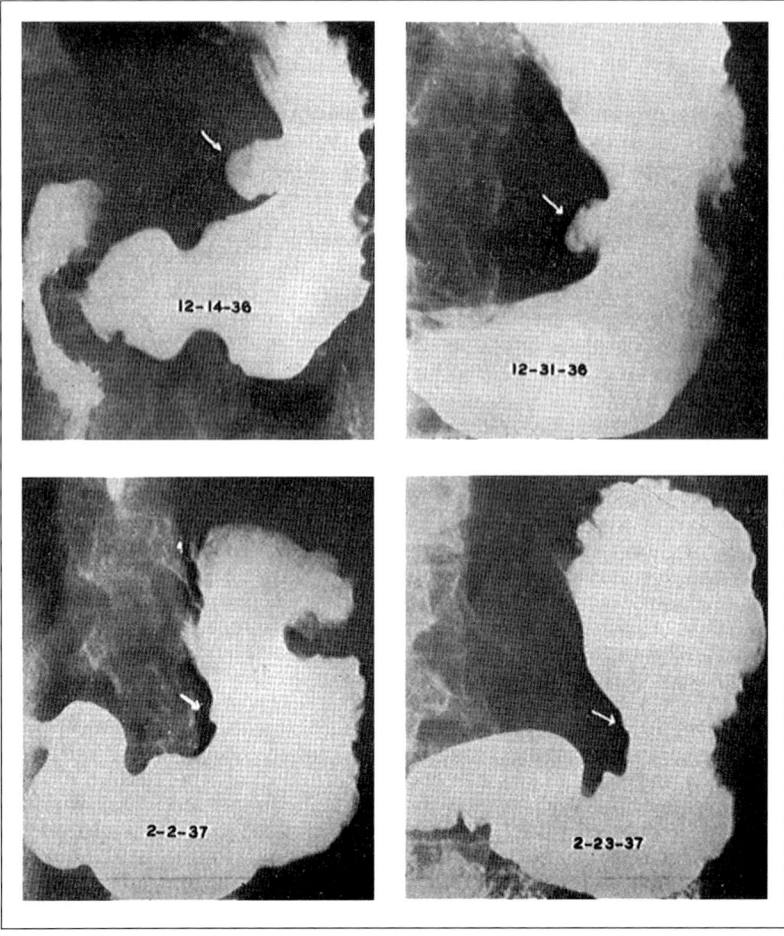

Figure 6.3. Duodenal ulcer, showing the typical trefoil or shamrock deformity. (Reproduced from Bailey & Love's 'A short practice of surgery', 12th edition, 1962, page 734).

Ulcer healing medicines were not yet available, many patients had undergone previous surgery for peptic ulcer, and bore the tell-tale scar on their abdominal wall. Another clue was the presence of arthritic fingers, due to the presence of osteo-or rheumatoid arthritis, diseases for which aspirin was widely used. Further evidence as to the position of aspirin in competition with other drugs may be seen when comparing the occurrence of adverse effects. Using the UK General Practice Research Database, Garcia-Rodriguez and Hernandez-Diaz in 2000–2001, showed that NSAID users had a 4 times greater risk of an upper gastro-intestinal bleed than non-users. But how guilty was aspirin compared to the other NSAIDs? Remember, the other NSAIDs were developed mainly because of the side effects of aspirin, particularly bleeding from the bowel. Evidence from German-speaking countries in Europe gave some very interesting results when looking at *all* adverse effects. In rank order of incidence, the *least* percentage of adverse events being first, the results are tabulated below, see table 6.1 (adapted from Brune et al 1992).

Another way of expressing the relative likelihood of *gastro-intestinal*, as apart from *all* side effects of aspirin and NSAIDs is by a so-called GI Toxicity Index, based on data from the Arthritis, Rheumatism and Ageing Medical Information System (ARAMIS) prospective registry database, see table 6.2 over the page.

However, when modern endoscopic methods are used to look inside the gastro-intestinal tract, a different picture emerges. Using a variety of doses and preparations of aspirin, 22–100% of patients or volunteers had gastric erosions or ulcers. For diflunisal, the figure was 10%, for indomethacin 30%, paracetamol 0% (Lanza et al 1975).

Manufacturers were always on the lookout for drugs which would be more attractive to the public by effectiveness coupled with safety. Two drugs were already on their books, phenacetin (acetanilide in the USA), and paracetamol (acetaminophen in the USA). Aspirin competed by being marketed in various buffered, controlled or sustained release forms, or by 'enteric coating', (designed to delay absorption until after the drug had finished passing through the stomach). Early enteric coatings resulted in very little of the aspirin being absorbed, which rather defeated the object, but this was later circumvented by improved techniques of coating.

With aspirin fast getting a reputation as a potentially dangerous drug, a fact not helped by Reckitt & Colman's advertising of Disprin (a soluble form of aspirin, claimed to be safer than plain aspirin), the market was awaiting a straightforward safe analgesic, cheap yet effective. The path towards this goal started in 1947 at Yale University. Acetanilide, a by-product of the aniline dye industry, had been found to have an anti-pyretic effect, and was marketed as Antifebrine by Kalle & Company. Bayer tried another by-product called acetophenetidin, brand name Phenacetin, claiming it to have a more potent analgesic effect than Antifebrine. Now whilst these drugs did not appear to irritate the stomach, they unfortunately produced another, rather alarming, effect. Many people, taking these drugs on a regular basis, started

The Fall and Rise of Aspirin

Drug	No. adverse events	No. prescriptions	Rank order of unlikelihood
Aspirin	250	1211	1
Naproxen	282	1067	2
Ibuprofen	1110	4037	3
Piroxicam	488	1645	4
Tenoxicam	359	1075	5
Diclofenac	4891	14477	6
Ketoprofen	448	1183	7
Acemetacin	1553	3633	8

Table 6.1. NSAIDs most unlikely to be followed by **any** adverse event.

Drug	No. Patients	Rank order of unlikelihood for GI side effects
Salsalate	187	1
Ibuprofen	577	2
Aspirin	1521	3
Sulindac	562	4
Diclofenac	415	5
Naproxen	1062	6
Tolmetin	243	7
Piroxicam	814	8
Fenoprofen	158	9
Indomethacin	418	10
Ketoprofen	259	11
Meclofenamate	165	12

Table 6.2. Unlikelihood for gastro-intestinal adverse events due to NSAIDs.

turning blue! And furthermore, some developed kidney disease. Doctors called this 'analgesic nephropathy.' What was happening was that these drugs were entering the red blood cells, and changing the haemoglobin (an iron containing protein). The iron within should be in the reduced (ferrous) form, but these drugs oxidised it to the ferric form. The trouble was that haemoglobin with ferric, not ferrous iron, could not carry out its most fundamental task, namely uptake of oxygen from its passage through the lungs. Consequently, as the body's tissues extracted oxygen from undamaged red cells, so the body's arterial system, instead of being replete with oxidised haemoglobin (oxyhaemoglobin), was contaminated with increasing amounts of reduced tainted haemoglobin, called *methaemoglobin*. However, there was soon to emerge another tremendously successful rival, which would potentially finish off aspirin altogether.

Bayer possessed large quantities of another aniline by-product called N-acetyl p-aminophenol. Preliminary studies had appeared to indicate that it caused side effects in people, so it was put on the back burner. Until, in 1946, at Yale University, Lester & Greenberg carried out some experiments prompted by earlier findings that in dogs, the administration of acetanilide led to the appearance of N-acetyl p-aminophenol in blood. So, putting together the knowledge that dogs given a drug which was known to relieve pain and temperature in humans but could turn them blue, was converted in dogs into N-acetyl p-aminophenol, led them to re-examine whether this latter drug might be metabolised the same way in humans, be effective at pain relief, but free from side effects.

So they took two male volunteers, and each swallowed 0.935 grams of acetanilide. Blood samples were drawn at various time intervals, and urine samples were also collected. They found that the main substance detected in the blood and plasma was N-acetyl p-aminophenol, with very little unchanged acetanilide remaining. Similar findings were obtained for acetophenetidin by Brodie and Axelrod in 1949.

The next step came in 1948, when Flinn and Brodie at Columbia University in New York asked the question – if acetanilide is converted to N-acetyl p-aminophenol, and administration of acetanilide leads to relief of pain and temperature, is it the unchanged administered drug which is producing this effect, or is it the metabolite, N-acetyl p-aminophenol? They used twelve normal human females each of whom swallowed 0.325 grams of N-acetyl p-aminophenol. They employed a technique whereby heat was radiated towards the skin, and the volunteer had to state at which time the effect was painful. Some volunteers received placebo (dummy). The results showed a 30% reduction in the pain threshold i.e. the time taken to register that the experience was becoming painful, and for the placebo receivers, 4%. (This might seem a bit puzzling as to why a dummy substance could also lead to pain reduction, but this is well recognised in medicine, that all drugs have a so-called 'placebo-effect', and this needs to be taken into account whenever a drug is being evaluated). How many patent remedies, sold in Health shops, have been subjected to a similar test?

So the conclusion from this was that the pain relief was due to N-acetyl p-aminophenol, and not acetanilide because most of the latter was converted in the body to the former. And, even more importantly, no-one taking the former turned blue! In fact side effects were few and far between. In 1956, the drug was marketed in Britain, by Bayer, under the brand **Panadol**. Initially it was only obtainable with a prescription. Later, it received the generic name **paracetamol**, which was manufactured at a far lower price by generic manufacturers, once the patent had expired. In the USA, it was known as acetaminophen.

The Fall and Rise of Aspirin

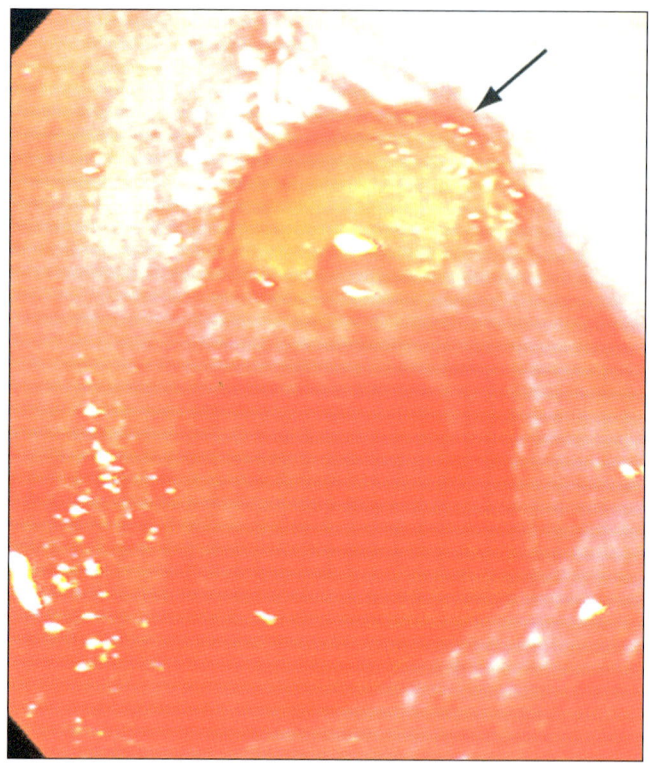

Figure 6.4. A gastric ulcer viewed through a modern endoscope, equipped with a TV camera. (Reproduced from Kumar P. & Clark M, Clinical Medicine, Fifth edition, 2002, page 274, with permission of Elsevier).

Here was a true contender for the aspirin crown. The days of aspirin appeared numbered. By 1970, sales of aspirin and those of paracetamol were very similar. Starting about 50 years later, paracetamol had caught up with aspirin. And the competition from other NSAIDs was hotting up too. Early competitors included phenylbutazone (Butazolidine), which though very effective as a pain killer and anti-inflammatory, was associated with gastro-intestinal haemorrhage, ulcers, and rarely but catastrophically, aplastic anaemia (severe bone marrow depression). Indomethacin (Indocid) was also very effective, particularly for gout, and osteoarthritis of the hip. Unfortunately, it tended to cause headaches in many patients, as well as fluid retention, and acceleration of hip damage, although the pain was blunted. The two big guns were Ibuprofen (Brufen) made by Boots of Nottingham, and Naproxen (Naprosyn), made by Syntex. These drugs combined efficacy with relatively less gastro-intestinal problems. A list of NSAIDs is given opposite, from which it can be

Chapter Six – The Fall of Aspirin

seen that aspirin faced, and continues to face, formidable competition as a pain killer. Salicylate derivatives have not been included.

Benzene acetic acid derivatives
Aceclofenac (*Preservex*)
Bromfenac (*Duract*-USA), withdrawn
Diclofenac (*Voltarol*)
Ibuprofen (*Brufen*)

Oxicams
Ketoprofen (*Orudis*) (*Oruvail*)
Naproxen (*Naprosyn*)
Ampiroxicam (*Flucam*, Japan)
Droxicam (*Drogelon*, Spain)
Lornoxicam (*Xefo*)
Meloxicam (*Mobic*)
Tenoxicam (*Mobiflex*)

Indole/indene derivatives
Acemetacin (*Emflex*)
Indomethacin (*Indocid*)
Sulindac (*Clinoril*)

Fenamates
Meclofenamate sodium
Mefenamic acid (*Ponstan*)

Propionic acid derivatives
Carprofen (taken off the market)
Fenbufen (*Lederfen*)
Flurbiprofen (*Froben*)
Oxaprozin (*Daypro*-USA)
Pirprofen (withdrawn)
Tiaprofenic acid (*Surgam*)
Zaltoprofen (no products listed)

Pyrazolones
Azapropazone (*Rheumox*)
Oxyphenbutazone (*Tanderil*)
Phenylbutazone (*Butazolidine*)

Others
Etodolac (*Lodine*)
Nabumetone (*Relifex*)
Tolmetin (*Tolectin*)

Table 6.3. Major NSAIDs prior to designer Cox-2 selective inhibitors.

In the early 1970s, a form of aspirin called 'Benoral' was marketed by Winthrop pharmaceuticals. It consisted of a compound which, upon entry into the stomach, was split into paracetamol, aspirin, and salicylate. It was marketed as a 'pro-drug' and claimed fewer side effects than normal aspirin. But this was illusory, because larger amounts of the drug were needed to rival the benefit conferred by aspirin, and when this was taken into account, it proved no safer from the point of view of stomach bleeding.

Other salicylates include choline magnesium silicate, diflunisal, and salasalate. Choline magnesium silicate was designed to buffer the acidity of the salicylate. Studies of blood loss after taking these drugs have shown substantially less with them than with aspirin, and virtually nil after paracetamol. There appeared no doubt that, from the point of view of pain relief, aspirin was up to some pretty stiff competition, and it wasn't winning. More was to come.

It was noticed in Sydney, Australia, between 1951 and 1962, that 21 children were admitted to the Royal Alexandra Hospital for Children, suffering from disturbed consciousness, fever, convulsions, vomiting, and various other features. The illness usually started with cough, runny nose, sore throat or earache. Blood tests showed low levels of glucose in both blood and spinal fluid, and changes in various blood chemicals indicative of liver disturbance. 17 children died, and at autopsy, there were unexpected findings. They all had swelling of the brain, slight enlargement of the liver which was bright yellow in colour, with a pale appearance and widening in the outer border (the cortex) of the kidneys. 14 of the 21 were aged below 2 years. The condition started with common respiratory infection features, but the alarm bells rang when the children started vomiting persistently and severely, with onset of altered conscious level. Half became wildly delirious, screamed and were extremely irritable. 17 cases had fits. Irregularities of breathing were noted, and included

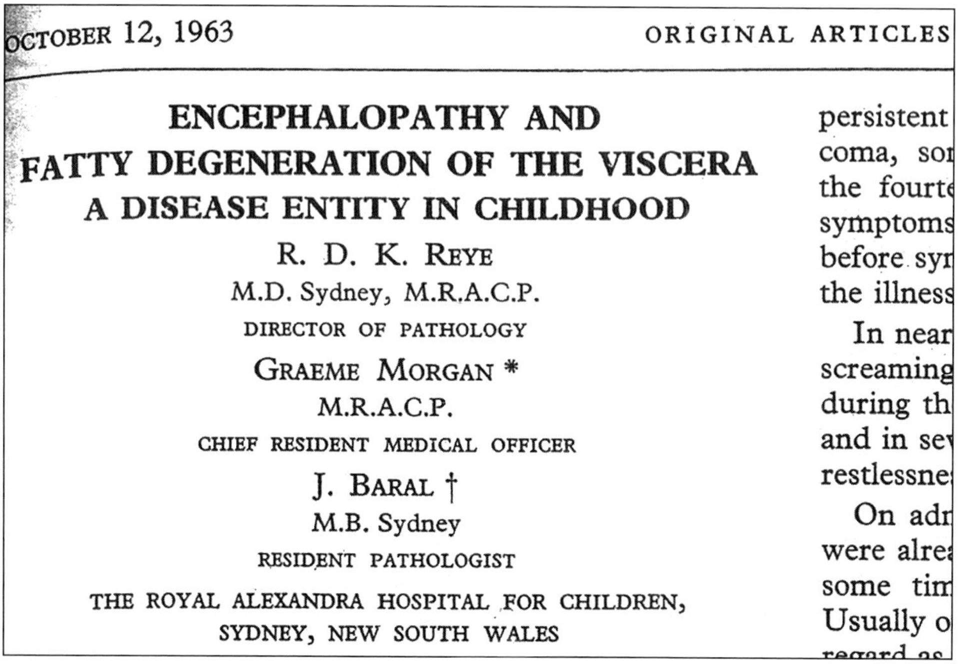

OCTOBER 12, 1963 ORIGINAL ARTICLES

ENCEPHALOPATHY AND FATTY DEGENERATION OF THE VISCERA

A DISEASE ENTITY IN CHILDHOOD

R. D. K. REYE
M.D. Sydney, M.R.A.C.P.
DIRECTOR OF PATHOLOGY

GRAEME MORGAN *
M.R.A.C.P.
CHIEF RESIDENT MEDICAL OFFICER

J. BARAL †
M.B. Sydney
RESIDENT PATHOLOGIST

THE ROYAL ALEXANDRA HOSPITAL FOR CHILDREN, SYDNEY, NEW SOUTH WALES

persistent coma, so the fourt symptoms before syr the illness

In near screaming during th and in se restlessne

On adr were alre some tin Usually o

Figure 6.5. Reye's original paper, from the Lancet, 12th October 1963. (Reproduced from Lancet 2, 1963, Encephalopathy and fatty degeneration of the viscera. A disease entity in childhood. Reye R, Morgan G. & Baral J. 749–752. With permission of Elsevier).

Chapter Six – The Fall of Aspirin

excessive rapidity, or irregularity. One patient stopped breathing altogether, and eventually died despite being put on a ventilator. 12 children had an enlarged liver, detected by palpating the abdomen. In 7 cases, a characteristic posture was noted, namely lying with the elbows bent, the legs held out straight and the hands clenched. Although vomiting stopped after admission to hospital, this could not be regarded as a good sign, because this also was a feature in all those who died. Those who died invariably did so within 2½ days.

The autopsies showed fatty degeneration especially in the liver. Every cell was packed with fatty droplets. When it came to treatment, the outlook initially was one of hopelessness, with intravenous glucose failing to bring the low blood level up to normal. However, when combined with steroids, and in some cases insulin as well, there was more success. These cases were described by Dr. R.D.K. Reye, Director of Pathology, together with Drs. Morgan and Baral, in the Lancet, dated October 12th 1963, see figure 6.5. The gradual accumulation of these cases with their peculiar

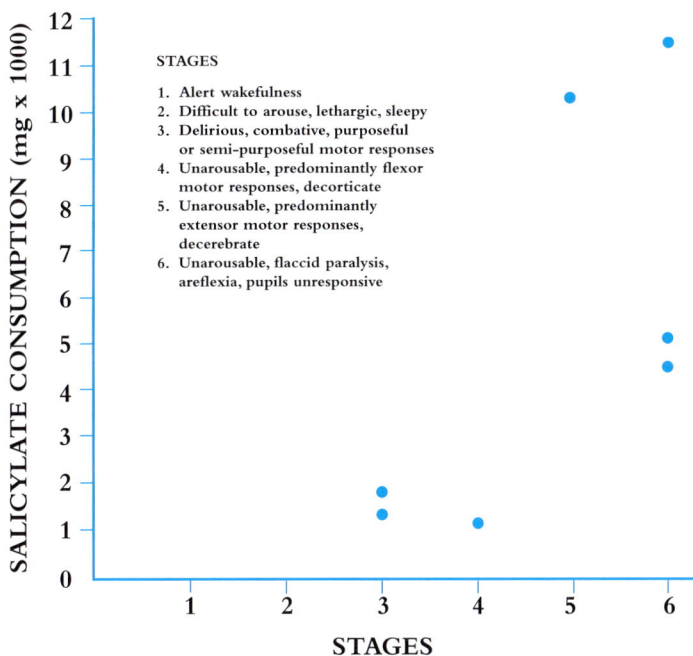

Figure 6.6. Pre-hospitalisation salicylate consumption by children with Reye's syndrome, related to stage of Reye's syndrome at most severe point. Increasing dose of salicylate and severity of Reye's syndrome are directly related. (Reproduced with permission from Pediatrics Vol. 66, Pages 859–864, Copyright 1980, by the American Academy of Pediatrics).

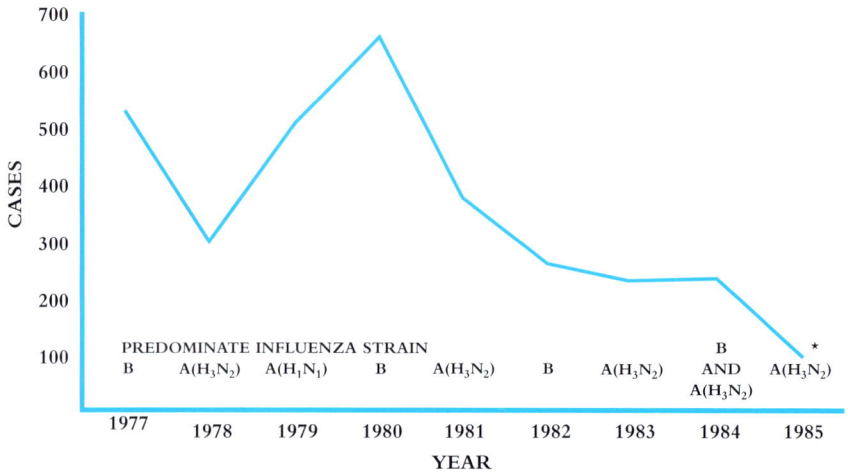

Figure 6.7. Cases of Reye's syndrome reported 1977–1985.

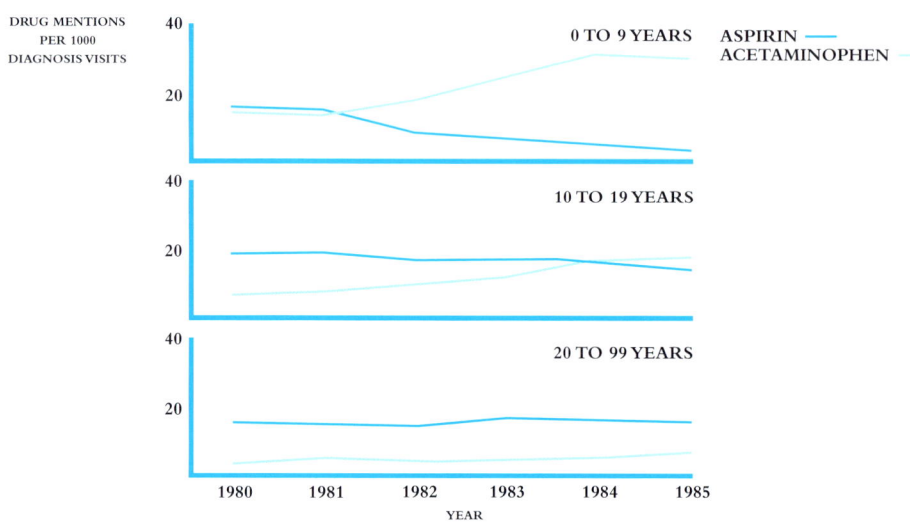

Figure 6.8. Rates of mention of aspirin or acetaminophen (paracetamol) by age groups by year.

Chapter Six – The Fall of Aspirin

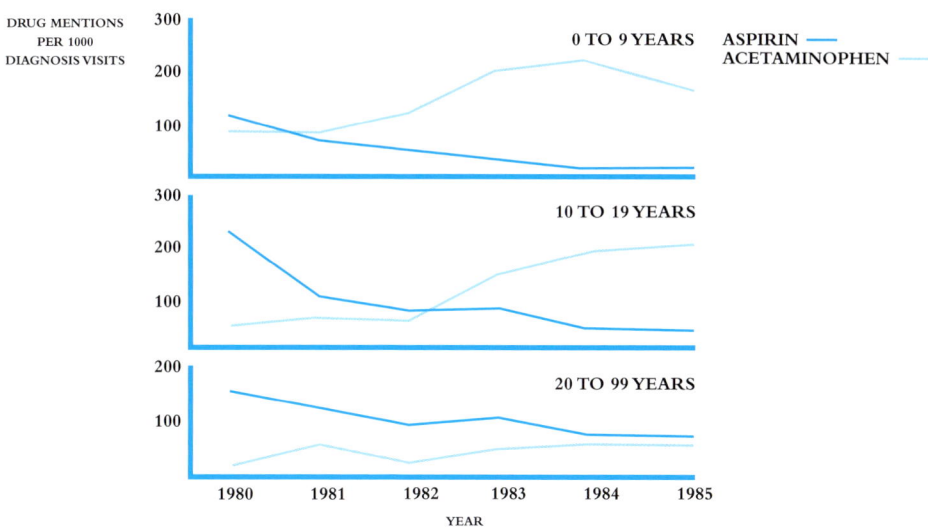

Figure 6.9. Rates of physician mentions of aspirin and acetominophen (paracetamol) for flu and chickenpox, by age group by year.

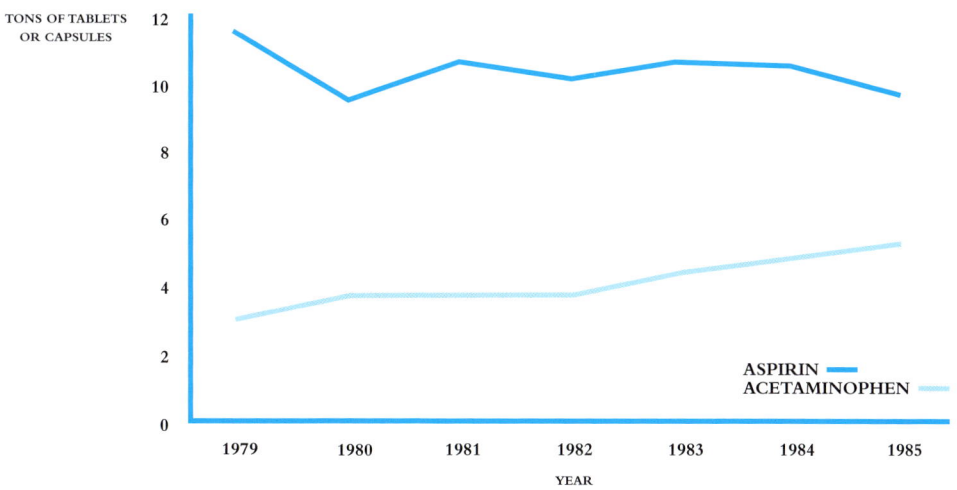

Figure 6.10. Purchases of adult aspirin and acetominophen (paracetamol) by drugstores.

features, led the team to believe they were dealing with a more or less distinct clinical entity, not previously described. After 7 cases had been seen, the cooperation of the Institute of Child Care in Sydney was enlisted. Careful histories were obtained from the homes of the affected children, with particular reference to access to drugs and poisons.

Subsequently a more searching enquiry was carried out by the department of public health in New South Wales. Special attention was focused on possible ingestion of carbon tetrachloride or trichloroethylene (known to be toxic to liver), and to pesticides, which were known to cause high fever (hyperpyrexia). No relationship to any suspected substances was found. The authors stated:

"We have recorded the details of this series because we are convinced that they form a group different from those children in whom fatty changes, especially in the liver, are a secondary manifestation of a variety of diseases. We hope that the experience of others may help us to suggest an answer to the problems of aetiology, prevention, and treatment."

The disorder was subsequently named **Reye's syndrome**. To Dr. Reye, as well as to the rest of the world, its cause remained a mystery.

The next clue came from an outbreak of influenza, investigated in Arizona, because 7 cases developed Reye's syndrome, see figure 6.6. As a control population, 16 ill classmates were chosen (ill with influenza, but not complicated by Reye's syndrome). The whole symptom complex at onset was compared, and found to be similar. All seven cases of Reyes had consumed salicylates, whereas only half of the control group had. Also, the average dose of salicylate taken by them was greater than the control group. Salicylate consumption correlated with severity of Reye's syndrome. The authors stated:

"It is postulated that salicylate, operating in a dose-dependant manner, possibly potentiated by fever, represents a primary causative agent of Reye's syndrome." (Starko et al 1980).

Since 1980, several controlled studies have demonstrated an association between aspirin exposure during a preceding illness and subsequent development of Reyes syndrome. The preceding illnesses included influenza B, influenza A (H_1N_1) or varicella (chicken pox), which were reported to the Center for Disease Control in Atlanta, and showed a marked decline between 1980 and 1985. In 1987, Dr. Arrowsmith and colleagues at the Office of Epidemiology and Biostatistics, in Maryland, reported on "National Patterns of Aspirin Use and Reye Syndrome Reporting, United States, 1980 to 1985." They reviewed reporting trends of aspirin recommendations by physicians, and trends in aspirin purchase at drugstores. They also collected data on acetaminophen (paracetamol). These figures were scrutinised against a backdrop of numbers of reports of Reye's syndrome in the USA between 1977 and 1985 (see figures 6.6.–6.11, reproduced from their paper).

Chapter Six – The Fall of Aspirin

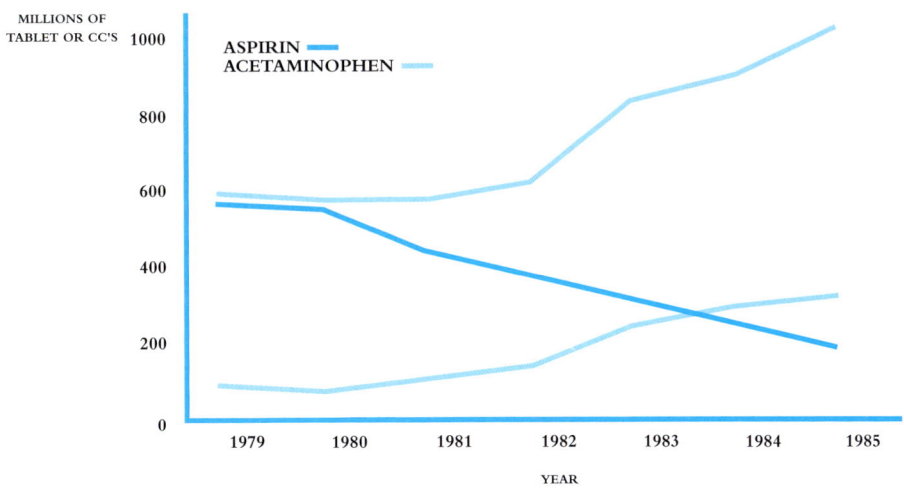

Figure 6.11. Purchases of children's aspirin and acetominophen (paracetamol) by drugstores. (Figures 6.7. – 6.11. inclusive are reproduced with permission from Pediatrics, Volume 79, Pages 858–863, Copyright 1987 by the American Academy of Pediatrics).

It can clearly be seen that cases of Reye's syndrome peaked in 1980, and declined steadily thereafter, see figure 6.7. When rates of physician mention of these drugs for all diagnoses is viewed, it can be seen that in the 0–9 years age group, aspirin prescribing fell gradually after 1981, at the same time as acetaminophen (paracetamol) was on the rise, see figure 6.8. In the 10–19 year group, paracetamol had overtaken aspirin by 1985. By contrast, in the 20–99 years age group, the larger number of aspirin prescriptions was maintained. Similar comparisons for treatment specifically of influenza and chickenpox, see figure 6.9. showed the same direction for the 0–9 years age group. But for the 10–19 years age group, the switch to paracetamol was more dramatic and occurred by 1982, i.e. 3 years earlier than prescriptions for all conditions. In the 20–99 years age group, the numeric superiority of aspirin was, like for all condition prescribing, maintained, but only just.

The data for purchases by drugstores in the USA for adult, see figure 6.10, and for children's aspirin, see figure 6.11. makes interesting reading. But not if one has shares in aspirin manufacture, certainly not for products aimed at children. Whereas adult aspirin sales held up well, those for children plummeted.

The British National Formulary says:

"Owing to an association with Reye's syndrome aspirin-containing preparations should not be given to children under 12 years, unless specifically indicated, e.g. for juvenile arthritis (Still's disease). Reye's syndrome has also been reported very rarely in children over 12 years and aspirin should preferably be avoided during fever or viral infections in children and adolescents over 12 years".

It also says:

"Aspirin should also preferably be avoided during fever or viral infection in children and adolescents over 12 years. Families should be advised that aspirin should not be given to children under 12 years except when prescribed by a doctor and it is best avoided in adolescents with feverish conditions."

Aspirin, it can be seen, was now coming under serious fire not only from NSAIDs, but also from paracetamol. The future was looking decidedly bleak.

Chapter Seven

INFLAMMATION

Inflammation is one of the most important protective processes of the body, and is designed primarily for fending off infections. These can have many causes, including viruses, bacteria, fungae, or parasitic worms. We are all familiar with the main signs of inflammation e.g. when we have a sore throat we are aware of pain, and we can, when looking into the mouth, see swelling of the area including the tonsils. Occasionally it may be accompanied by a fever. The swelling itself may appear red. And the function of the throat i.e. the act of swallowing, may only be accomplished with difficulty.

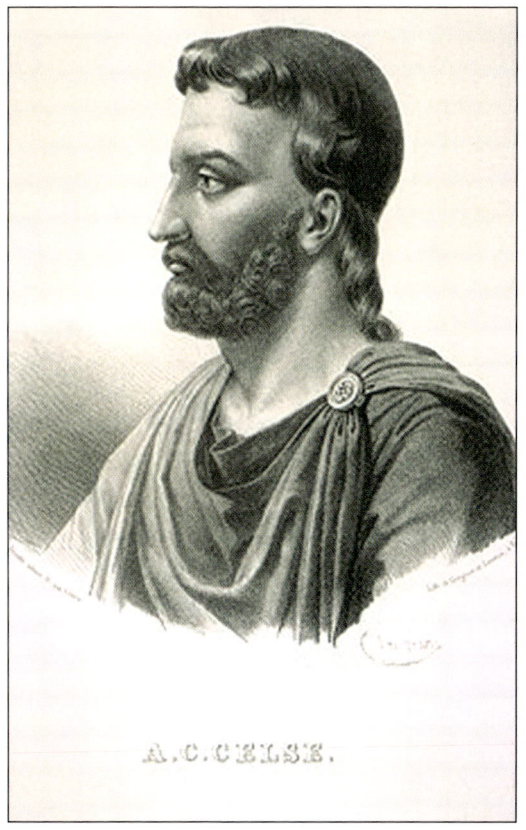

Figure 7.1. Celsus (25BC–50AD).

1. Celsus on inflammation

All these signs of inflammation were originally described by **Aulus Cornelius Celsus**, see figure 7.1, in his work **"De Medicina"** (on Medicine). He was born around 25 BC during the reign of the Emperor Tiberius. There is some dispute as to whether he was actually a physician, or merely the author of an Encyclopedia in six parts, as follows:

Part 1   Agriculture
Part 2   Medicine
Part 3   Military arts
Part 4   Rhetoric
Part 5   Philosophy
Part 6   Jurisprudence

The following extracts are taken from the translation by W.G. Spencer in 1938, and now forming part of the **Loeb Classical Library**, of Harvard University.

The Prooemium, (preamble) states:

"Just as agriculture promises nourishment to the healthy bodies, so does the art of Medicine promise health to the sick. Nowhere is this Art wanting, for the most uncivilised nations have had knowledge of herbs, and other things to hand for the aiding of wounds and diseases. This Art, however, has been cultivated among the

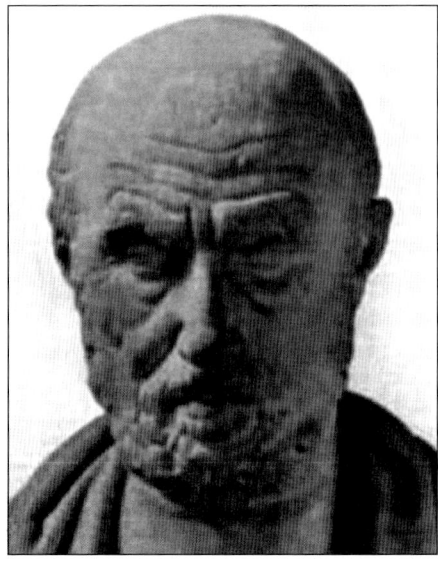

Figure 7.2. Hippocrates of Cos, (470BC–410BC)

Greeks much more than in other nations – not, however, even among them from their first beginnings, but only for a few generations before ours. Hence Aesculapius is celebrated as the most ancient authority, and because he cultivated this science, as yet rude and vulgar, with a little more than common refinement, he was numbered among the gods –

Therefore, even after these I have mentioned, no distinguished men practised the Art of Medicine until literary studies began to be pursued with more attention, which more than anything else are a necessity for the spirit, but at the same time are bad for the body. At first the science of healing was held to be a part of philosophy, so that treatment of disease and the contemplation of the nature of things began through the same authorities; clearly because healing was needed especially by those whose bodily strength had been weakened by restless thinking and night-watching. Hence we find that many who professed philosophy became expert in medicine, the most celebrated being Pythagoras, Empedocles and Democritus. But it was, as some believe, a pupil of the last, Hippocrates of Cos," see figure 7.2,

"a man first and foremost worthy to be remembered, notable both for professional skill and for eloquence, who separated this branch of learning from the study of philosophy –

During the same times the art of Medicine was divided into three parts: one being that which cures through diet, another through medicaments, and the third by hand. The Greeks termed the first *Diathtikh*, the second *Farmakeutikh*, the third *Xeirourgia*."

Following on from this, Celsus implies that the most famous authorities used diet to treat diseases, based upon a "knowledge of nature", without which the Art of Medicine would be "stunted and weak." Others did not see it this way, basing their therapy on practice and experience. They called themselves Empirici or Experimentalists. These opposing points of view are mirrored today in those who assume "knowledge of nature" with the sort of terminology used by those practising or writing about alternative medicine, and present day doctors whose best practise is evidence-based. Such best practise is reviewed by the National Institute of Health and Clinical Excellence (NICE), but whose views are, perhaps of necessity, tempered by economic considerations.

Things now become a little gruesome, as Celsus deduces that in order to cure pain, which originates in "the more internal parts," one needs to know more about the parts themselves. Therefore he approves of the dissection of the dead, but then goes on to applaud the method adopted by Herophilus, which was to take criminals and open them up in order to observe their innards! " – and while these were still breathing, observed parts which beforehand nature had concealed, their position, colour, shape, size, arrangement, hardness, softness, smoothness, relation, processes and depressions of each, and whether any part is inserted into or is received into another." He goes on to question the value of the appearance of inner organs when the revelation will have been preceded by suffering. He reveals that on occasion it is well nigh impossible to observe what goes on whilst the subject is still alive if he dies during the intended procedure:

"Nor is anything more foolish, they say, than to suppose that whatever the condition of the part of a man's body in life, it will also be the same when he is dying, nay when he is already dead; for the belly indeed, which is of less importance, can be laid open with the man still breathing; but as soon as the knife really penetrates to the chest, by cutting through the transverse septum which divides the upper from the lower parts (the Greeks call it *dia/fragma*), the man loses his life at once: so it is only when the man is dead that the chest and any of the viscera come into the view of the medical murderer, and they are necessarily those of a dead, not of a living man. – " (It is only with the aid of general anaesthesia that these objections can nowadays be overcome).

In book 1 (of 8), we read:

"A man in health, who is both vigorous and his own master, should be under no obligatory rules, and have no need, either for a medical attendant, or for a rubber and anointer. – His kind of life should afford him variety; he should be now in the country, now in town, and more often about the farm; he should sail, hunt, rest sometimes, but more often take exercise; for whilst inaction weakens the body, work strengthens it; the former brings on premature old age, the latter prolongs youth.

It is well also at times to go to the bath, at times to make use of cold waters; to undergo sometimes inunction, sometimes to neglect that same; to avoid no kind of food in common use; to attend at times a banquet, at times to hold aloof; to eat more than sufficient at one time, at another no more; to take food twice rather than once a day, and always as much as one wants provided one digests it. But whilst exercise and food of this sort are necessities, those of the athletes are redundant; for in the one class any break in the routine of exercise, owing to necessities of civil life, affects the body injuriously, and in the other, bodies thus fed up in their fashion age very quickly and become infirm. Concubitus" i.e. sex, "indeed is neither to be desired overmuch, nor overmuch to be feared; seldom used it braces the body, used frequently it relaxes. Since, however, nature and not number should be the standard of frequency, regard being had to age and constitution, concubitus can be recognised as harmless when followed neither by languor nor by pain. The use is worse in the day-time, and safer by night; but care should be taken that by day it be not immediately followed by a meal, and at night not immediately followed by work and watching. Such are the precautions to be observed by the strong, and they should take care that whilst in health, their defences against ill-health are not used up. The weak, however, among whom are a large proportion of townspeople, and almost all those fond of letters, need greater precaution, so that care may re-establish what the character of their constitution or of their residence or of their study detracts.

Anyone therefore of these who has digested well may with safety rise early; if too little he must stay in bed, or if he has been obliged to get up early, must go to sleep again; he who has not digested, should lie up altogether, and neither work nor take exercise nor attend to business. He who without heartburn eructates indigested food should drink cold water at intervals and none the less exercise self-control. He should also reside in a house that is light, airy in summer, sunny in winter; avoid the midday sun, the morning and evening chill, also exhalations from rivers and marshes; and he should not often expose himself when the sky is cloudy to a sun that breaks through – lest he should be affected alternately by cold and heat – a thing which excites particularly choked nostrils and running colds. Much more indeed are these things to be watched in unhealthy localities, where they even produce pestilence.

He can tell that his body is sound, if his morning urine is whitish, later reddish; the former indicates that digestion is going on, the latter that digestion is complete. On waking one should lie still for a while, then, except in winter time, bathe the face freely with cold water; when the days are long the siesta should be taken before the midday meal, when short, after it. In winter, it is best to rest in bed the whole night long; if there must be study by lamp-light, it should not be immediately after taking food, but after digestion. He who has been engaged in the day, whether in domestic or on public affairs, ought to keep some portion of the day for the care of the body. The primary care in this case is exercise, which should always precede the taking of food; the exercise should be ampler in the case of one who has laboured less and digested less well. Useful exercises are: reading aloud, drill, handball, running, walking; but this is by no means most useful on the level, since walking up and down hill varies the movement of the body, unless indeed the body is thoroughly weak; but it is better to walk in the open air than under cover; better when the head allows of it, in the sun than in the shade; better under the shade of a wall or of trees than under a roof; better a straight than a winding walk. But the exercise ought to come to an end with sweating, or at any rate lassitude, which should be well this side of fatigue; and sometimes less, sometimes more, is to be done. But in these matters, as before, the example of athletes should not be followed, with their fixed rules and immoderate labour. The proper sequel to exercise is: at times an anointing, whether in the sun or before a brazier; at times a bath, which should be in a chamber as lofty, well lighted and spacious as possible. However, neither should be made use of invariably, but one of the two the oftener, in accordance with the constitution. There is need of a short rest afterwards. Coming to food, a surfeit is never of service, excessive abstinence is often unserviceable; if any intemperance is committed, it is safer in drinking than in eating. It is better to begin a meal with savouries, salads and such-like; and after that meat is to be eaten, best either when roasted or boiled. All preserved fruits are unserviceable for two reasons, because more is taken owing to their sweetness, and even when that is moderate is still digested with some difficulty. Dessert does no those which soothe as well as repress. If pain is greater, rind of poppy-heads is to be boiled in wine, and mixed with wax-salve made up with rose oil; or wax and lard, equal parts, are melted together, and then the wine mixed with these; and as soon as this application becomes hot, it is to be removed and another immediately put on. But if the swellings have grown hard and are painful, the application of a sponge frequently squeezed out of oil and vinegar, or out of cold water, or the application of pitch, wax and alum, equal parts mixed, gives relief. There are also several emollients suitable alike for the hands and feet. But if the pain does not allow of anything being put on, when there is no swelling, the joint should be fomented with a sponge which has been dipped in a warm decoction of poppy-head rind, or of wild cucumber root, next the joints are smeared with saffron, poppy-juice and ewe's milk. But if there is a swelling, this ought to be bathed with a tepid decoction of mastic or some other repressant vervain, and then covered with a medicament composed of bitter almonds pounded up in vinegar, or of white lead, to which has been added the juice of pounded pellitory. The stone, too, which corrodes flesh, which the Greeks call *sarcophagos*, is carved out so as to admit the feet; when these are painful, they are inserted and held there, and are usually relieved. In Asia Minor Assian limestone is held in esteem for this purpose. When pain and inflammation have subsided, which should happen within forty days, unless the patient is in fault, gentle exercise, spare diet, soothing anointings, are to be employed, provided that also then the joints may be rubbed with an anodyne salve or with a liquid wax-salve of cyprus oil. But riding on horseback is harmful for those with podagra. Those, too, in whom joint-pains tend to recur at certain seasons ought both to take precautions beforehand as to their

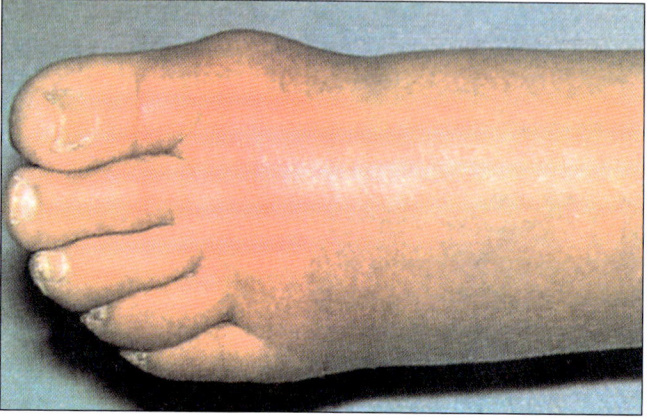

Figure 7.3. Acute gout involving mainly the big toe. Also termed 'podagra.'
(From 'Clinical Medicine' by Forbes and Jackson, 2nd Edition 1997, Mosby-Wolfe.
(Reproduced with permission from Elsevier).

diet, lest there should be a surfeit of harmful material in the body, and to use an emetic the most frequently; and those in any anxiety as to their body should make use of clystering, or of purgation by milk. This treatment for those with podagra was rejected by Erasistratus, lest a flux directed downwards might fill up the feet, though it is evident that any purgation extracts, not only from the upper parts, but also from the lower as well."

In figure 7.3. we see clearly depicted, the signs of inflammation in a patient affected by the gout (podagra). Curiously, aspirin is ineffective against the gout itself, due to an excessive concentration of uric acid in the blood. At low doses, aspirin reduces the rate at which the kidneys excrete uric acid, but at very high doses, it promotes excretion.

There now follows an academic description of inflammation, written in medical terms. It has been downloaded from the web-site of the Pathology Department of the University of Birmingham (the author's alma mater), and acknowledged. Some additional comments have been made when considered appropriate.

Introduction (from medweb. Bham.ac.uk – with thanks)

Inflammation is the response of living tissue to damage. The acute inflammatory response has 3 main functions:

1. The affected area is occupied by a transient material called the acute inflammatory exudate. The exudate carries proteins, fluid and cells from local blood vessels into the damaged area to mediate local defenses.
2. If an infective causitive agent (e.g. bacteria) is present in the damaged area, it can be destroyed and eliminated by components of the exudate.
3. The damaged tissue can be broken down and partially liquefied, and the debris removed from the site of damage.

Acute inflammation may be due to physical damage, chemical substances, micro-organisms or other agents. The inflammatory response consists of changes in blood flow, increased permeability of blood vessels and escape of cells from the blood into the tissues. The changes are essentially the same whatever the cause and wherever the site.

Acute inflammation is short-lasting, lasting only a few days. If it is longer lasting however, then it is referred to as chronic inflammation. Various examples of acute inflammation that you may be aware of are sore throat, reactions in the skin to a scratch or a burn or insect bite, and acute hepatitis and so on. However, there are occasional historical exceptions such as pneumonia, inflammation of the lung rather than present day terms like pneumonitis and pleurisy, and inflammation of the pleura, rather than pleuritis.

The Fall and Rise of Aspirin

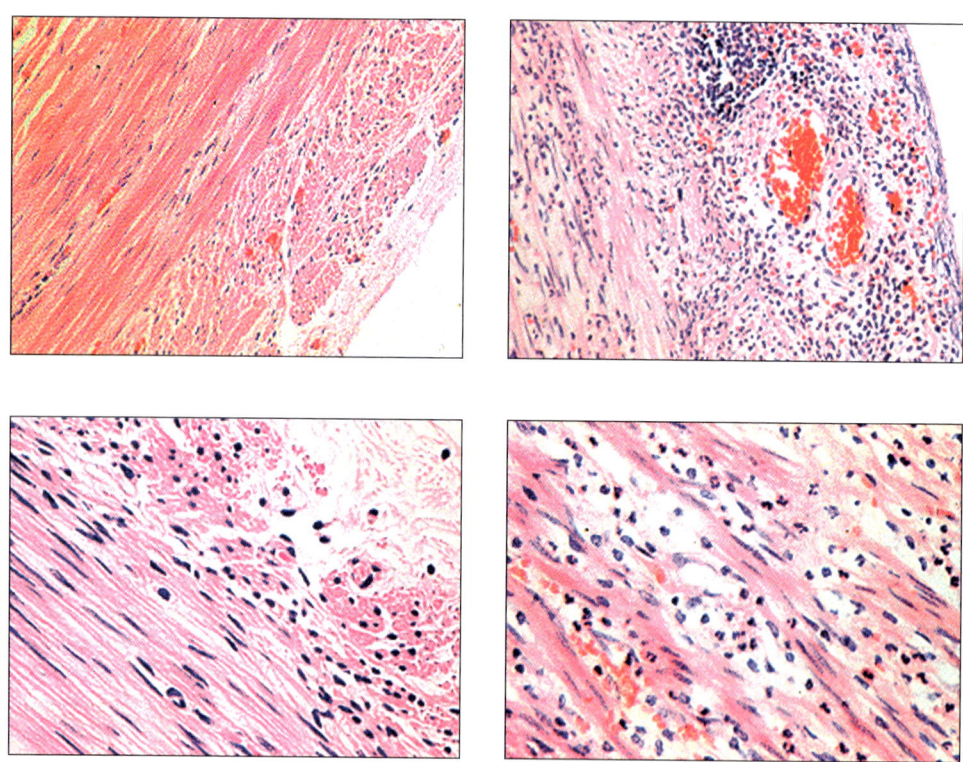

Top Left: Figure 7.4. This slide shows the muscle coats and peritoneum of a normal appendix. The peritoneal surface runs diagonally across the upper right hand corner. It is covered by a layer of mesothelial cells (not apparent in this picture) underlying which is a layer of pale staining fibrous tissue in which are a few small blood vessels. The outer longitudinal and inner circular muscle coats consist of smooth muscle with a few small blood vessels.

Top Right: Figure 7.5. This slide shows the same area in an acutely inflamed appendix. The changes are striking. The peritoneum is widened by an increase in tissue fluid (oedema) and by many inflammatory cells. In addition, the blood vessels are dilated. The muscle coat also shows oedema which has caused separation of the muscle fibres. There are numerous inflammatory cells between the muscle fibres.

Bottom Left: Figure 7.6. This slide shows a higher magnification view of the muscle coats of the normal appendix.

Bottom Right: Figure 7.7. This slide shows a high magnification view of the same area in an acutely inflamed appendix. The muscle fibres have been separated by oedema and numerous inflammatory cells. At this magnification it can be seen that most of the inflammatory cells are neutrophil polymorphs having the characteristic lobed nucleus.

Causes of Acute Inflammation
Microbial infections
One of the commonest causes of inflammation is microbial infection. Viruses lead to death of individual cells by intracellular multiplication. Bacteria release specific exotoxins – chemicals synthesised by them which specifically initiate inflammation or endotoxins, which are associated with their cell walls and only released when the bacteria die. Additionally, some organisms cause immunologically-mediated inflammation through hypersensitivity reactions. Parasitic infections and tuberculous inflammation are instances where hypersensitivity is important.

Hypersensitivity reactions
A hypersensitivity reaction occurs when an altered state of immunological responsiveness causes an inappropriate or excessive immune reaction which, though intended to eliminate harmful agents such as germs, damages the host's tissues. The types of reaction are classified here, but all have cellular or chemical mediators similar to those involved in inflammation.

Physical agents
Tissue damage leading to inflammation may occur through physical trauma, ultraviolet or other ionising radiation, burns or excessive cooling ('frostbite').

Irritant and corrosive chemicals
Corrosive chemicals (acids, alkalis, oxidising agents) provoke inflammation through gross tissue damage. However, infecting agents may release specific chemical irritants which lead directly to inflammation.

Tissue necrosis
Death of tissues from lack of oxygen or nutrients resulting from inadequate blood flow (infarction) is a potent inflammatory stimulus. The edge of a recent infarct often shows an acute inflammatory response.

Clinical Aspects of Acute Inflammation
The four principal effects of acute inflammation were described nearly 2,000 years ago by **Celsus**:

Redness (rubor)
An acutely inflamed tissue appears red, for example skin affected by sunburn, cellulitis due to bacterial infection or acute conjunctivitis. This is due to dilatation of small blood vessels within the damaged area.

Heat (calor)
Increase in temperature is seen only in peripheral parts of the body, such as the skin. It is due to increased blood flow (hyperaemia) through the region, resulting in vascular dilatation and the delivery of warm blood to the area. Systemic fever, which results from some of the chemical mediators of inflammation, also contributes to the local temperature.

Swelling (tumor)
Swelling results from oedema, the accumulation of fluid in the extra vascular space as part of the fluid exudate, and to a much lesser extent, from the physical mass of the inflammatory cells migrating into the area.

Pain (dolor)
For the patient, pain is one of the best known features of acute inflammation. It results partly from the stretching and distortion of tissues due to inflammatory oedema and, in particular, from pus under pressure in an abscess cavity. Some of the chemical mediators of acute inflammation, including bradykinin, the prostaglandins and serotonin, are known to induce pain.

Loss of function
Loss of function, a well-known consequence of inflammation, was added by Virchow (1821–1902) to the list of features drawn up by Celsus. Movement of an inflamed area is consciously and reflexly inhibited by pain, while severe swelling may physically immobilise the tissues.

Clinical indications of acute inflammation
Clinical indications of an acute inflammatory process include:

- General malaise.
- Fever.
- Pain, often localised to the inflamed area, e.g. the right iliac fossa in acute appendicitis.
- Rapid pulse rate.

Laboratory investigations usually reveal:

- A raised neutrophil count in the peripheral blood.
- An increased erythrocyte sedimentation rate (ESR).

An increase in the concentration of acute-phase proteins in the blood. These are normally present in small concentrations, but this increases dramatically in response to acute inflammation. Produced by the liver, they are induced by circulating IL–1. Specific examples, the most common being C-reactive protein, may be measured in blood to monitor inflammatory processes.

Progression to Chronic Inflammation
If the agent causing acute inflammation is not removed, the acute inflammation may progress to the chronic stage. In addition to organisation of the tissue just described, the character of the cellular exudate changes, with lymphocytes, plasma cells and macrophages (sometimes including multi nucleate giant cells) replacing the neutrophil polymorphs. Often, however, chronic inflammation occurs as a primary event, there being no proceeding period of acute inflammation.

Systemic effects of acute inflammation
Apart from the local features of acute and chronic inflammation described above, an inflammatory focus produces systemic effects.

Pyrexia
Polymorphs and macrophages produce compounds known as endogenous pyrogens which act on the hypothalamus to set the thermoregulatory mechanisms at a higher temperature. Release of endogenous pyrogen is stimulated by phagocytosis, endotoxins and immune complexes.

Constitutional symptoms
Constitutional symptoms include malaise, anorexia and nausea. Weight loss is common when there is extensive chronic inflammation. For this reason, tuberculosis used to be called 'consumption'.

Reactive hyperplasia of the reticulo-endothelial system
Local or systemic lymph node enlargement commonly accompanies inflammation, while splenomegaly is found in certain specific infections (e.g. malaria, infectious mononucleosis).

Haematological changes
Increased erythrocyte sedimentation rate. An increased erythrocyte sedimentation rate is a non-specific finding in many types of inflammation.

Leukocytosis. Neutrophilia occurs in pyogenic infections and tissue destruction; eosinophilia in allergic disorders and parasitic infection; lymphocytosis in chronic infection (e.g. tuberculosis), many viral infections and in whooping cough; and monocytosis occurs in infectious mononucleosis and certain bacterial infections (e.g. tuberculosis, typhoid). *Anaemia.* This may result from blood-loss in the inflammatory

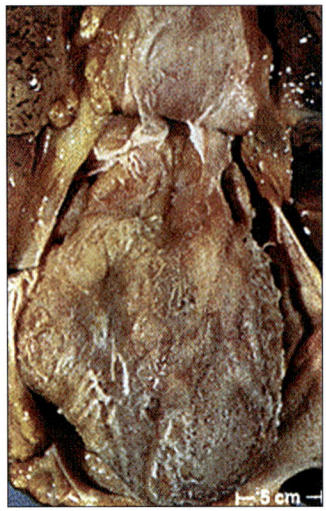 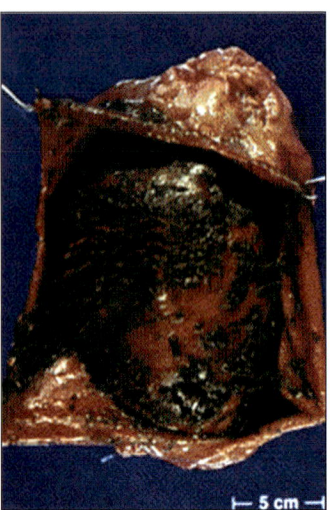

Left: Figure 7.8. Fibrinous inflammation. Right: Figure 7.9. Haemorrhagic inflammation.

exudate (e.g. in ulcerative colitis), haemolysis (due to bacterial toxins), and 'the anaemia of chronic disorders' due to toxic depression of the bone marrow, or lack of stimulation by a substance produced in the kidney called erythropoietin.

Amyloidosis
Longstanding chronic inflammation (for example, in rheumatoid arthritis, tuberculosis and bronchiectasis), by elevating serum amyloid A protein (SAA), may cause amyloid to be deposited in various tissues resulting in secondary (reactive) amyloidosis.

Macroscopic appearance of acute inflammation
The cardinal signs of acute inflammation are modified according to the tissue involved and the type of agent provoking the inflammation. Several descriptive terms are used for the appearances.

Serous inflammation
In serous inflammation, there is abundant protein-rich fluid exudate with a relatively low cellular content. Examples include inflammation of the serous cavities, such as peritonitis, and inflammation of a synovial joint, acute synovitis. Vascular dilatation may be apparent to the naked eye, the serous surfaces appearing injected, i.e. having dilated, blood-laden vessels on the surface, (like the appearance of the conjunctiva in 'blood-shot' eyes).

Chapter Seven – Inflammation

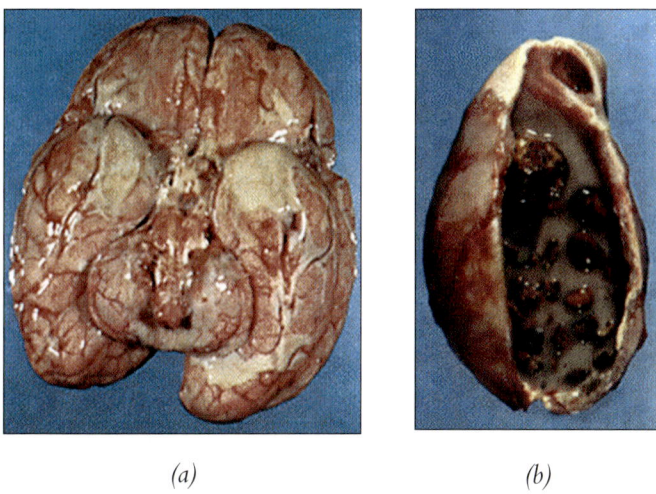

(a) (b)

Figure 7.10. Suppurative inflammation.

Catarrhal inflammation
When mucus hypersecretion accompanies acute inflammation of a mucous membrane, the appearance is described as catarrhal. The common cold is a good example.

Fibrinous inflammation (Figure 7.8.)
When the inflammatory exudate contains plentiful fibrinogen, this polymerises into a thick fibrin coating. This is often seen in acute pericarditis (inflammation of the membranes surrounding the heart), and gives them a 'bread and butter' appearance.

Haemorrhagic inflammation (Figure 7.9.)
Haemorrhagic inflammation indicates severe vascular injury or depletion of coagulation factors. This occurs in acute pancreatitis due to proteolytic destruction of vascular walls, and in meningococcal septicaemia due to disseminated intravascular coagulation.

Suppurative (purulent) inflammation (Figure 7.10.)
The terms 'suppurative' and 'purulent' denote the production of pus, which consists of dying and degenerate neutrophils, infecting organisms and liquefied tissues. Figure 7.10. (a) shows the brain surrounded by pus in the meninges (meningitis) or pleura (the lung lining). The pus may become walled-off by granulation tissue or fibrous tissue to produce an abscess (a localised collection of pus in a tissue). If a hollow viscus fills with pus, this is called an empyema, for example, empyema of the gall bladder figure 7.10. (b) or of the appendix.

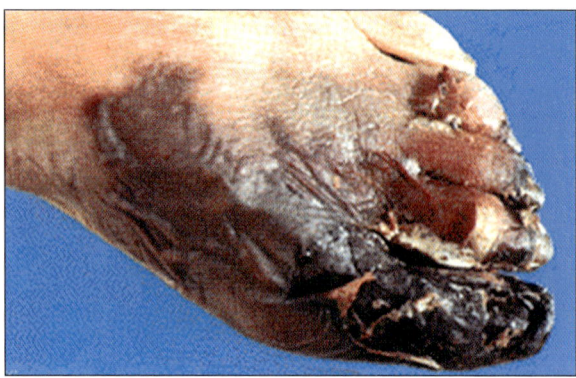

Figure 7.11. Necrotising (gangrenous) inflammation.

Membranous inflammation
In acute membranous inflammation, an epithelium becomes coated by fibrin, desquamated epithelial cells and inflammatory cells. An example is the grey membrane seen in pharyngitis or laryngitis in diptheria, itself due to a bacterium called *Corynebaceterium diphtheriae*.

Pseudomembranous inflammation
The term 'pseudomembranous' describes superficial mucosal ulceration with an overlying slough of disrupted mucosa, fibrin, mucus and inflammatory cells. This is seen in pseudomembranous colitis due to *Clostridium difficile* colonisation of the bowel, usually following broad-spectrum antibiotic treatment.

Necrotising (gangrenous) inflammation (Figure 7.11.)
High tissue pressure due to oedema may lead to vascular occlusion and thrombosis, which may result in widespread septic necrosis of the organ. The combination of necrosis and bacterial putrefaction is gangrene. Gangrenous appendicitis is a good example.

Effects of Acute Inflammation
The systemic effects of acute inflammation have been discussed. The local effects are usually clearly beneficial, for example the destruction of invading micro-organisms; but at other times they appear to serve no obvious function, or may even be positively harmful.

Beneficial effects
Both the fluid and cellular exudates may have useful effects. Beneficial effects of the fluid exudate are as follows:

Dilution of toxins. Dilution of toxins, such as those produced by bacteria, allows them to be carried away in lymphatics.

Entry of antibodies. Increased vascular permeability allows antibodies to enter the extravascular space, where they may lead either to lysis of micro-organisms, through the participation of complement, or to their phagocytosis by opsonisation. Antibodies are also important in neutralisation of toxins.

Drug transport. The fluid carries with it therapeutic drugs such as antibiotics to the site where bacteria are multiplying.

Fibrin formation. Fibrin formation from exuded fibrinogen may impede the movement of micro-organisms, trapping them and so facilitating phagocytosis.

Delivery of nutrients and oxygen. Delivery of nutrients and oxygen, essential for cells such as neutrophils which have high metabolic activity, is aided by increased fluid flow through the area.

Stimulation of immune response. The drainage of this fluid exudate into the lymphatics allows particulate and soluble antigens to reach the local lymph nodes where they may stimulate the immune response.

The role of neutrophils in the cellular exudate will now be described. They have a life-span of only 13 days and must be constantly replaced. Most die locally, but some leave the site via the lymphatics. Blood monocytes also arrive at the site and, on leaving the blood vessels, transform into macrophages, becoming more metabolically active, motile and phagocytic. Swallowing and killing ('phagocytosis') of micro-organisms is enhanced by coating ('opsonisation') by antibodies or by a cascading system of proteins ('complement') leading to death of bacteria by puncturing their membrane as a consequence of the last components of the sequence, termed the 'membrane attack complex'. In most acute inflammatory reactions, macrophages play a lesser role in phagocytosis compared with that of neutrophil polymorphs. They appear late in the response and are usually responsible for clearing away tissue debris and damaged cells.

Both neutrophils and macrophages may discharge their lysosomal enzymes into the extracellular fluid by exocytosis, or the entire cell contents may be released when the cells die. Release of these enzymes assists in the digestion of the inflammatory exudate.

Harmful effects

The release of lysosomal enzymes by inflammatory cells may also have harmful effects:

Digestion of normal tissues. Enzymes such as collagenases and proteases may digest normal tissues, resulting in their destruction. This may result particularly in vascular damage, for example in type III hypersensitivity reactions in which antibodies latch on to the antigens which stimulated their production and circulate together, ending up on a basement membrane of cells e.g. those lining the filters in the kidneys, starting the complement cascade sequence and causing tissue damage, in this case termed 'glomerulonephritis'.

Swelling. The swelling of acutely inflamed tissues may be harmful: for example, the swelling of the epiglottis in acute epiglottitis in children due to Haemophilus influenzae infection may obstruct the airway, resulting in death. Inflammatory swelling is especially serious when it occurs in an enclosed space such as the cranial cavity. Thus, acute meningitis or a cerebral abscess may raise intracranial pressure to the point where blood flow into the brain is impaired, resulting is ischaemic damage, or may force the cerebral hemispheres against the tentorial orifice and the cerebellum into the foramen magnum (pressure coning).

Inappropriate inflammatory response. Sometimes, acute inflammatory responses appear inappropriate, such as those which occur in type I hypersensitivity reactions (e.g. hay fever) where the provoking environmental antigen (e.g. pollen) otherwise poses no threat to the individual. Such allergic inflammatory responses may be life-threatening, for example extrinsic asthma.

Early Stages of Acute Inflammation
In the early stages, oedema fluid, fibrin and neutrophil polymorphs accumulate in the extracellular spaces of the damaged tissue. The presence of the cellular component, the neutrophil polymorph, is essential for a histological diagnosis of acute inflammation. The acute inflammatory response involves three processes:

- changes in vessel calibre and, consequently, flow.
- increased vascular permeability and formation of the fluid exudate.
- formation of the cellular exudate by emigration of the neutrophil polymorphs into the extravascular space.

Briefly, the steps involved in the acute inflammatory response are:

1. Small blood vessels adjacent to the area of tissue damage initially become dilated with increased blood flow, then flow along them slows down.
2. Endothelial cells swell and partially retract so that they no longer form a completely intact internal lining.
3. The vessels become leaky, permitting the passage of water, salts, and some small proteins from the plasma into the damaged area (exudation). One of the main proteins to leak out is the small soluble molecule, fibrinogen.
4. Circulating neutrophil polymorphs initially adhere to the swollen endothelial cells (margination), then actively migrate through the vessel basement membrane (emigration), passing into the area of tissue damage.
5. Later, small numbers of blood monocytes (macrophages) migrate in a similar way, as do lymphocytes.

Changes in Vessel Calibre
The microcirculation consists of the network of small capillaries lying between arterioles, which have a thick muscular wall, and thin-walled venules. Capillaries have no smooth muscle in their walls to control their calibre, and are so narrow that red blood cells must pass through them in single file. The smooth muscle of arteriolar walls forms pre-capillary sphincters which regulate blood flow through the capillary bed. Flow through the capillaries is intermittent, and some form preferential channels for flow while others are usually shut down.

In blood vessels larger than capillaries, blood cells flow mainly in the centre of the lumen (axial flow), while the area near the vessel wall carries only plasma (plasmatic zone). This feature of normal blood flow keeps blood cells away from the vessel wall. Changes in the microcirculation occur as a physiological response; for example, there is hyperaemia in exercising muscle and active endocrine glands. The changes following injury which make up the vascular component of the acute inflammatory reaction were described by Lewis in 1927 as 'the triple response to injury': a flush, a flare and a wheal. If a blunt instrument is drawn firmly across the skin, the following sequential changes take place:

- A momentary white line follows the stroke. This is due to arteriolar vasoconstriction, the smooth muscle of arterioles contracting as a direct response to injury.
- The flush: a dull red line follows due to capillary dilatation.
- The flare: a red, irregular, surrounding zone then develops, due to arteriolar dilatation. Both nervous and chemical factors are involved in these vascular changes.
- The wheal: a zone of oedema develops due to fluid exudation into the extravascular space.

The initial phase of arteriolar constriction is transient, and probably of little importance in acute inflammation. The subsequent phase of vasodilatation (active hyperaemia) may last from 15 minutes to several hours, depending upon the severity of the injury. There is experimental evidence that blood flow to the injured area may increase up to ten-fold. As blood flow begins to slow again, blood cells begin to flow nearer to the vessel wall, in the plasmatic zone rather than the axial stream. This allows 'pavementing' of leukocytes (their adhesion to the vascular epithelium) to occur, which is the first step in leukocyte emigration into the extravascular space. The slowing of blood flow which follows the phase of hyperaemia is due to increased vascular permeability, allowing plasma to escape into the tissues while blood cells are retained within the vessels.

Increased vascular permeability

Small blood vessels are lined by a single layer of endothelial cells. In some tissues, these form a complete layer of uniform thickness around the vessel wall, while in other tissues there are areas of endothelial cell thinning, known as fenestrations. The walls of small blood vessels act as a microfilter, allowing the passage of water and solutes but blocking that of large molecules and cells. Oxygen, carbon dioxide and some nutrients transfer across the wall by diffusion, but the main transfer of fluid and solutes is by ultrafiltration, as described by Starling. The high colloid osmotic pressure inside the vessel, due to plasma proteins, favours fluid return to the vascular compartment. Under normal circumstances, high hydrostatic pressure at the arteriolar end of capillaries forces fluid out into the extravascular space, but this fluid returns into the capillaries at their venous end, where hydrostatic pressure is low. In acute inflammation, however, not only is capillary hydrostatic pressure increased, but there is also escape of plasma proteins into the extravascular space, increasing the colloid osmotic pressure there. Consequently, much more fluid leaves the vessels than is returned to them. The net escape of protein-rich fluid is called exudation; hence, the fluid is called the fluid exudate.

Factors involved in vascular permeability in acute inflammation

There are two mechanisms for increased permeability of small vessels following tissue damage.

- Toxins and physical agents may cause necrosis of vascular endothelium, leading to abnormal leakage (non-mediated vascular leakage).
- Chemical mediators of acute inflammation may cause retraction of endothelial cells, leaving intercellular gaps (mediated vascular leakage).

Experimental work has isolated three patterns of increased leakage of fluid from vessels, which occur at different times following injury.

1. An immediate response that is transient, lasts for 30–60 minutes, and is mediated by histamine acting on endothelium.
2. A delayed response that starts 2–3 hours after injury and lasts for up to 8 hours. This is mediated by factors synthesized by local cells, e.g. bradykinin; factors derived from complement; and factors released from dead neutrophils in the exudate.
3. An immediate response that is prolonged for over 24 hours and is seen if there has been direct necrosis of endothelium, e.g. in a burn or by a chemical toxin.

In disease it is likely that all three responses are activated, with an immediate prolonged response close to the centre of damage, and mediated responses at the interface between the damaged and healthy tissues.

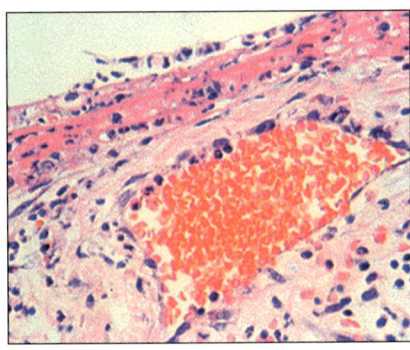 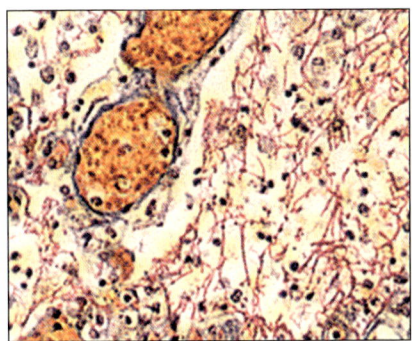

Left: Figure 7.12. This slide shows the peritoneal surface of an acutely inflamed appendix. The pink layer on the peritoneal surface consists of fibrin in which cells are enmeshed. Right: Figure 7.13. This slide shows pink staining threads of fibrin with leucocytes in alveoli of the lung, in a case of pneumonia (pneumonitis in current terminology).

Features of the Fluid Exudate

The increased vascular permeability means that large molecules, such as proteins, can escape from vessels. Hence, the exudate fluid has a high protein content of up to 50 g/l. The proteins present include immunoglobulins, which may be important in the destruction of invading micro-organisms, and coagulation factors, including fibrinogen, which result in fibrin deposition on contact with the extravascular tissues. Hence, acutely inflamed organ surfaces are commonly covered by fibrin: the fibrinous exudate. There is a considerable turnover of the inflammatory exudate it is constantly drained away by local lymphatic channels to be replaced by new exudate.

Ultrastructural basis of increased vascular permeability

The ultrastructural basis of increased vascular permeability was originally determined using an experimental model in which histamine, one of the chemical mediators of increased vascular permeability, was injected under the skin. This caused transient leakage of plasma proteins into the extravascular space. Electron microscopic examination of venules and small veins during this period showed that gaps of 0.1–0.4µm in diameter had appeared between endothelial cells. These gaps allowed the leakage of injected particles, such as carbon, into the tissues. The endothelial cells are not damaged during this process. They contain contractile proteins such as actin, which, when stimulated by the chemical mediators of acute inflammation, cause contraction of the endothelial cells, pulling open the transient pores. The leakage induced by chemical mediators, such as histamine, is confined to venules and small veins. Although fluid is lost by ultrafiltration from capillaries, there is no evidence that they too become more permeable in acute inflammation.

In addition to the transient vascular leakage caused by some inflammatory stimuli, certain other stimuli, e.g. heat, cold, ultraviolet light and X-rays, bacterial toxins and corrosive chemicals, cause delayed prolonged leakage. In these circumstances, there is direct injury to endothelial cells in several types of vessels within the damaged area.

The relative importance of chemical mediators and of direct vascular injury in causing increased vascular permeability varies according to the type of tissue. For example, vessels in the central nervous system are relatively insensitive to the chemical mediators, while those in the skin, conjunctiva and bronchial mucosa are exquisitely sensitive to agents such as histamine.

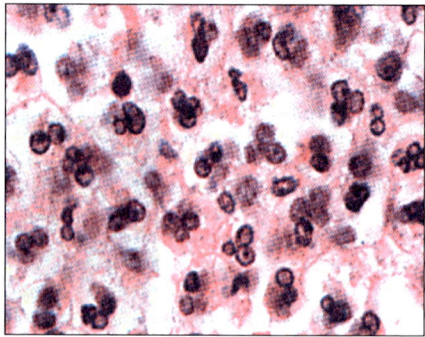

Figure 7.14. High-magnification of pus in the lumen of the appendix. Pus consists of living and degenerate neutrophil polymorphs together with liquefied tissue debris.

Formation of the Cellular Exudate

The accumulation of neutrophil polymorphs within the extracellular space is the diagnostic histological feature of acute inflammation.

The neutrophil is the main cell to mediate the effects of acute inflammation. If tissue damage is slight, an adequate supply is derived from normal numbers circulating in blood. If tissue damage is extensive, stores of neutrophils, including some immature forms, are released from bone marrow to increase the absolute count of neutrophils in the blood. To maintain the supply of neutrophils, growth factors derived from the inflammatory process stimulate division of myeloid precursors in the bone marrow, thereby increasing the number of developing neutrophils.

- The main cellular events in acute inflammation, all of which are caused by chemical mediators, are as follows:
- The normally inactive endothelium has to be activated to allow adhesion of neutrophils.
- Normally inactive neutrophils have to be activated to enhance their capacity for phagocytosis, bacterial killing, and generation of inflammatory mediators.
- Neutrophils have to develop the ability to move actively, in a directional fashion, from vessels towards the area of tissue damage. Normally inactive neutrophils have to be activated to enhance their capacity for phagocytosis, bacterial killing, and generation of inflammatory mediators. Neutrophils have to develop the ability to move actively, in a directional fashion, from vessels towards the area of tissue damage.

Chapter Seven – Inflammation

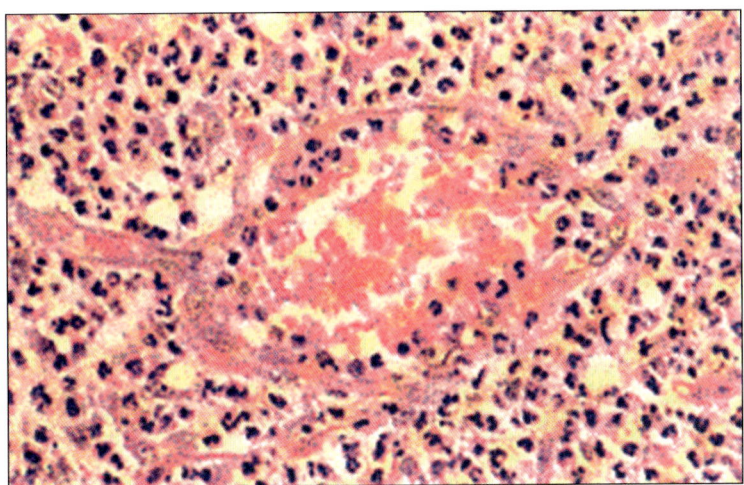

Figure 7.15. A capillary surrounded by polymorphonuclear leucocytes in an area of inflammation in the lung. Leucocytes are adherent to the vascular endothelium (margination), from here they will migrate into the surrounding tissue.

Margination of neutrophils (Figure 7.15.)
In the normal circulation, cells are confined to the central (axial) stream in blood vessels, and do not flow in the peripheral (plasmatic) zone near to the endothelium. However, loss of intravascular fluid and increase in plasma viscosity with slowing of flow at the site of acute inflammation allow neutrophils to flow in this plasmatic zone. The adhesion of neutrophils to endothelium causes them to aggregate along the vessel walls in a process termed **margination**.

Pavementing of neutrophils (Figure 7.16.)
The adhesion of neutrophils to the vascular endothelium which occurs at sites of acute inflammation is termed '**pavementing**' of neutrophils. Neutrophils randomly contact the endothelium in normal tissues, but do not adhere to it. However, at sites of injury, pavementing occurs early in the acute inflammatory response and appears to be a specific process occurring independently of the eventual slowing of blood flow. The phenomenon is seen only in venules. Its mechanism remains a mystery, since no ultrastructural changes have been detected in the endothelial cells to which the leukocytes adhere.

Neutrophil emigration (Figure 7.17.)
Leukocytes migrate by active amoeboid movement through the walls of venules and small veins, but do not commonly exit from capillaries. Electron microscopy shows

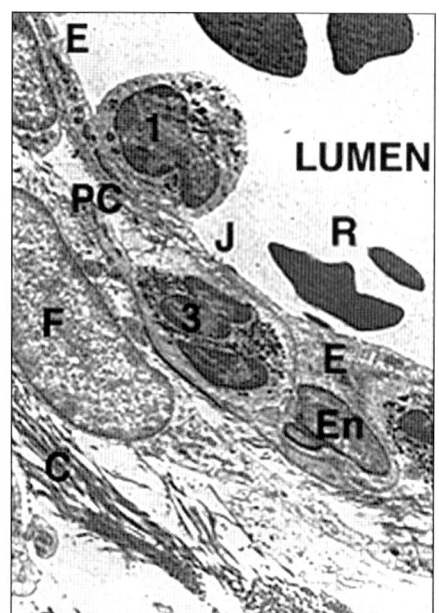 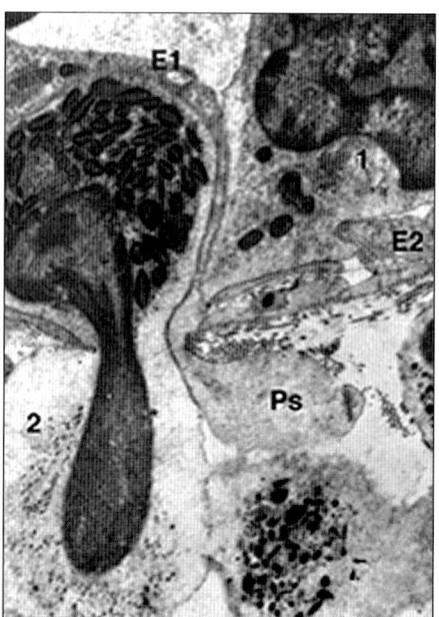

Left: Figure 7.16. Pavementing of neutrophilis.
Right: Figure 7.17. Neutrophil emigration.

that neutrophil and eosinophil polymorphs and macrophages can insert foot like processes ('pseudopodia') between endothelial cells, migrate through the gap so created between the endothelial cells, and then on through the basal lamina into the vessel wall. The defect appears to be self-sealing, and the endothelial cells are not damaged by this process.

Diapedesis

Red cells may also escape from vessels, but in this case the process is passive and depends on hydrostatic pressure forcing the red cells out. This process is called diapedesis, and the presence of large numbers of red cells in the extravascular space implies severe vascular injury, such as a tear in the vessel wall.

Later Stages of Acute Inflammation Chemotaxis of neutrophils

The movement of neutrophils from the vessel lumen into into a damaged area is induced by substances known as **chemotactic factors**, which diffuse from the area of tissue damage. Time-lapse cinephotography in experiments shows apparently purposeful migration of neutrophils along a concentration gradient. The main neutrophil chemotactic factors are:

- C5a (the 'a' fragment of the 5th component of the complement system produced by activation of C5 by the preceding complement component (itself the product of interaction of C1, C4, and C2)
- LTB4 (=leukotriene B4)
- Bacterial components

These factors bind to receptors on the surface of neutrophils and activate secondary messenger systems, stimulating increased cytosolic calcium, with resulting assembly of cytoskeletal specializations involved in motility.

It is not known whether chemotaxis is important in vivo. Neutrophils may possibly arrive at sites of injury by random movement, and then be trapped there by immobilising factors (a process analogous to the trapping of macrophages at sites of delayed-type hypersensitivity by migration inhibitory factor).

Role of the Neutrophil Polymorph

The neutrophil polymorph is the characteristic cell of the acute inflammatory infiltrate. The actions of this cell will now be considered.

Movement

Contraction of cytoplasmic microtubules and gel/sol changes in cytoplasmic fluidity bring about amoeboid movement. These active mechanisms are dependent upon calcium ions and are controlled by intracellular concentrations of cyclic nucleotides. The movement shows a directional response (chemotaxis) to various chemicals.

Adhesion to micro-organisms

Micro-organisms are opsonised (from the Greek word meaning 'to prepare for the table'), or rendered more amenable to phagocytosis, either by immunoglobulins or by complement components. Bacterial lipopolysaccharides activate complement via the alternative pathway, generating component C3b which has opsonising properties. In addition, if antibody binds to bacterial antigens, this can activate complement via the classical pathway, also generating C3b. In the immune individual, the binding of immunoglobulins to micro-organisms by their Fab components leaves the Fc component exposed. Neutrophils have surface receptors for the Fc fragment of immunoglobulins, and consequently bind to the micro-organisms prior to ingestion.

Phagocytosis

The process whereby cells (such as neutrophil polymorphs and macrophages) ingest solid particles is termed phagocytosis. The first step in phagocytosis is adhesion of the particle to be phagocytosed to the cell surface. This is facilitated by opsonisation. Opsonisation can be aided by complement or antibody. Antibodies latch on to antigens (the bit of the germ which they happen to fit), and then using the other end of the antibody molecule, attach to the phagocytic cell's anchoring point for antibodies. Thus is the germ pulled screaming and writhing into the cell designed to devour it. Just as we need enzymes to digest food, so do the phagocytic cells. These enzymes are present inside little sachets called 'lysosomes'. The phagocyte then ingests the attached particle by sending out pseudopodia around it. These meet and fuse so that the particle lies in a phagocytic vacuole (also called a phagosome) bounded by cell membrane. Lysosomes, membrane-bound packets containing the toxic compounds described below, then fuse with phagosomes to form phagolysosomes. It is within these that intracellular killing of micro-organisms occurs.

Intracellular killing of micro-organisms

Neutrophil polymorphs are highly specialised cells, containing noxious microbial agents, some of which are similar to household bleach. The microbial agents may be classified as:

- those which are oxygen-dependent.
- those which are oxygen-independent.

Oxygen-dependent mechanisms. The neutrophils produce hydrogen peroxide which reacts with myeloperoxidase in the cytoplasmic granules in the presence of halide, such as chlorine ('Cl'), to produce a potent microbial agent. Other products of oxygen reduction also contribute to the killing, such as peroxide anions, hydroxyl radicals, and singlet oxygen.

Oxygen-independent mechanisms. These include lysozyme (muramidase), lactoferrin which chelates iron required for bacterial growth, cationic proteins, and the low pH inside phagocytic vacuoles.

Release of lysosomal products

Release of lysosomal products from the cell damages local tissues by proteolysis by enzymes such as elastase and collagenase, activates coagulation factor XII, and attracts other leukocytes into the area. Some of the compounds released increase vascular permeability, while others are pyrogens, producing systemic fever (the 'agues' of former times, see chapter 2), by acting on the hypothalamus.

Chemical Mediators of Acute Inflammation

The spread of the acute inflammatory response following injury to a small area of tissue suggests that chemical substances are released from injured tissues, spreading outwards into uninjured areas. These chemicals, called endogenous chemical mediators, cause vasodilatation, emigration of neutrophils, chemotaxis and increased vascular permeability.

Chemical mediators released from cells

Histamine. This is the best-known chemical mediator in acute inflammation. It causes vascular dilatation and the immediate transient phase of increased vascular permeability. It is stored in mast cells, basophil and eosinophil leukocytes, and platelets. Histamine release from those sites (for example, mast cell degranulation) is stimulated by complement components C3a and C5a, and by lysosomal proteins released from neutrophils.

Lysosomal compounds. These are released from neutrophils and include cationic proteins, which may increase vascular permeability, and neutral proteases, which may activate complement.

***Prostaglandins.* These are a group of long-chain fatty acids derived from arachidonic acid and synthesised by many cell types. Some prostaglandins potentiate the increase in vascular permeability caused by other compounds. Others include platelet aggregation (prostaglandin 1. is inhibitory while prostaglandin A2 is stimulatory).** *Part of the anti-inflammatory activity of drugs such as aspirin and the non-steroidal anti-inflammatory drugs is attributable to inhibition of one of the enzymes involved in prostaglandin synthesis.*

Leukotrienes. These are also synthesised from arachidonic acid, especially in neutrophils, and appear to have vasoactive properties. SRS-A (slow reacting substance of anaphylaxis), involved in type I hypersensitivity, e.g. allergic asthma, is a mixture of leukotrienes. Drugs active against leukotriene receptors, or against the synthesis of leukotriene itself are used in the treatment of asthma.

5-hydroxytryptamine (serotonin). This is present in high concentration in mast cells and platelets. It is a potent vasoconstrictor (causes rapid narrowing of the diameter of blood vessels, by a contraction of muscle fibres within the blood vessel wall).

Lymphokines. This family of chemical messengers released by lymphocytes. Apart from their major role in type IV hypersensitivity, lymphokines may also have vasoactive or chemotactic properties.

Plasma factors

The plasma contains four enzymatic cascade systems: complement, the kinins, the coagulation factors and the fibrinolytic system (designed to unclot clots, nature's Dyno-Rod!) which are inter-related and produce various inflammatory mediators.

Complement system. The complement system is a cascade system of enzymatic proteins. It can be activated during the acute inflammatory reaction in various ways:

- In tissue necrosis, enzymes capable of activating complement are released from dying cells.
- During infection, the formation of antigen–antibody complexes can activate complement via the classical pathway, while the endotoxins of Gram-negative bacteria activate complement via the alternative pathway.
- Products of the kinin, coagulation and fibrinolytic systems can activate complement.
- A more recently described system, the mannan binding lectin pathway of complement activation, which involves the mannose found in the cell walls of certain bacteria.

The products of complement activation most important in acute inflammation include:

- C5a: chemotactic for neutrophils; increases vascular permeability; releases histamine from mast cells.
- C3a: similar properties to those of C5a, but less active.
- C567: chemotactic for neutrophils (pulls them in by chemical attraction).
- C56789: cytolytic activity (kills bacteria by puncturing their cell wall membrane).
- C4b, 2a, 3b: opsonisation of bacteria (facilitates phagocytosis by macrophages).

Kinin system. The kinins are peptides of 9–11 amino acids; the most important vascular permeability factor is bradykinin. The kinin system is activated by coagulation factor XII. Bradykinin is also a chemical mediator of the pain which is a cardinal feature of acute inflammation.

Coagulation system. The coagulation system is responsible for the conversion of soluble fibrinogen into fibrin, a major component of the acute inflammatory exudate. The blood clotting and the inflammation processes share certain components.

Coagulation factor XII (the Hageman factor), once activated by contact with extracellular materials such as basal lamina, and various proteolytic enzymes of bacterial origin, can activate the coagulation, kinin and fibrinolytic systems.

Fibrinolytic system. Plasmin is responsible for the lysis of fibrin into fibrin degradation products, which may have local effects on vascular permeability.

Chronic inflammation

The function of acute inflammation is to counteract infection. In the course of achieving this there is inevitably some discomfort, or pain, and feeling ill (malaise). But not all infectious agents succumb to acute inflammation. As an example let us consider the agent responsible for tuberculosis – *Mycobacterium tuberculosis.* This disease, which the medical profession tapped itself on the back as having been rendered curable, and one day to be eradicated, is now returning with a vengeance. It is a bacterial disease, so why can it not be eradicated by the acute inflammatory process described above? The answer lies in the fact that it possesses a waxy coat which renders it non-susceptible to the whole array of enzymes released by engulfing neutrophils. In diseases such as this, where the offending agent persists, it is sooner or later detected by the roving policemen, in this case lymphocytes. These cells are designed to react to resistant bacteria, and to viruses, by collaborating with other cells, called macrophages, the result of which is that the lymphocytes signal to the macrophages, up-regulating their enzymes. In this way, these cells, which have engulfed the organisms, may be able to kill them – but not always. If not, then the body resorts to a policy of containment, by which a fibrous wall is built around the cells including the mycobacteria. The mycobacteria actually die by a process called caseous necrosis. Many macrophages fuse with other macrophages giving rise to so-called 'giant cells.' The aforementioned fibrous wall may undergo calcification, which renders it visible under X-ray examination. The process lasts for years, and is known as chronic inflammation. Other diseases, some of which have unknown causes, are typified by chronic inflammation. Examples include rheumatoid arthritis, Crohn's disease (chronic bowel inflammation anywhere in the intestine, but typically the ileum), and ulcerative colitis (which, as its name implies, is an ulcerating inflammation in the colon). Of these, rheumatoid arthritis used to be treated with high doses of aspirin, which relieved pain and, to a certain degree, inflammation in the joints. But plain aspirin is of no value in Crohn's disease, or ulcerative colitis. However, by chemical manipulation, some derivatives of aspirin have been synthesised, and these have a very important part to play in the management of these conditions. These will be described in more detail in the next chapter. And the mode of action of aspirin, to be described in the chapter on enlightenment, will hopefully be more readily understood once the basics of the inflammatory process described above, have been grasped.

Chapter Eight

ASPIRIN DERIVATIVES

In this chapter, we will describe the contributions of aspirin-related drugs in the treatment of tuberculosis, chronic inflammatory bowel disease, rheumatoid arthritis, and certain skin disorders.

Tuberculosis
It is a fact of medical history, that the use to which a remedy is first put is not necessarily its only use. For centuries, remedies found to work (after a fashion), in one condition, are tried in another. And, surprise surprise, they either work, or don't work, or work but produce undesirable side effects, or don't produce any benefit, only side effects. By manipulating the dose and timing, some progress and increased understanding of how best to administer a drug is achieved. This principle was followed by William Withering (1741–1799), in the use of foxglove leaf to treat 'dropsy' (an accumulation of fluid in the tissues of the body, usually due to heart failure). He carefully charted the dose, and the effects both beneficial and otherwise. He then back titrated the dose until he found the minimum dose that would produce the desired but little or none of the adverse effects. This is nowadays carried out in the form of drug trials. Subsequently, more active derivatives were found (the cardiac glysosides), from which the most commonly used (digoxin), was prepared by Sidney Smith, in the laboratories of Wellcome at Dartford, in the 1930s. In the 1950s, cortisone was used in the treatment of rheumatoid arthritis. The results were truly amazing, and its discoverers, Hench and Kendall received Nobel prizes. Unfortunately this initial enthusiasm was soon tempered by the appearance of severe side effects. Not deterred, cortisone was tried in many other conditions, and in its current form, prednisolone, is still an enormously successful and life-saving drug in conditions such as pemphigus (a blistering skin disorder), and systemic lupus erythematosus – also known as 'SLE' an auto-immune disease. Similarly, following on the discovery of salicin in the bark of the willow, and in various plants, the acetylation process applied to it was found to result in a drug that was, and still is, highly acceptable. But it did not stop there. Firstly, therefore let us look at tuberculosis.

The story began in August 1940. The war was raging in Europe. France had been overrun by Germany, and in July, the Royal Navy removed the threat of French ships falling into the hands of the Germans by sinking them in Algeria. In so doing, 1000 Frenchmen died. America had not entered the war. It was experiencing difficulties in selling arms to Britain by neutrality acts previously passed by Congress. President Roosevelt was none too keen to upset Congress, as he was running for his third term the following January. Preserving a neutral stance was (initially), the name of the game.

Meanwhile, at Duke University in North Carolina, a pharmacologist and cell biologist called **Frederick Bernheim** was at work in his laboratory. He had predicted an upsurge in cases of tuberculosis (TB) as a consequence of the war, see figure 8.1.

He was intrigued by the fact that, unlike most other bacteria, the germ (bacterium) responsible for TB, the tubercle bacillus, did not oxidise carbohydrates, amino or hydroxy acids when they were all mixed together. But, when sodium salicylate was added, it more than doubled the oxygen intake. This article appeared in the learned journal Science on August 30th 1940. At the time, TB was incurable, and the cause of millions of deaths (in fact it still does, but that is another story of Man's inhumanity to Man, commercial greed and Capitalism, because there is a cure). Be that as it may, the bacterium is resistant to our immune responses, not least because it possesses a strong waxy coating, thus enabling it to resist phagocytosis (see 'inflammation'). Like fishing for pike, to land one you need to know how it ticks. Likewise for TB. The information that it could be tempted to increase its oxygen utilisation by one means, meant that there was a possibility of exploiting this property, perhaps by tempting it with a drug which promised easy oxygen utilisation, but when it came to the crunch, barred it. In pharmacological parlance, this is known as competitive inhibition. It was the principle employed in the synthesis of the sulphonamide drugs, the predecessors to the antibiotics. Another physician and scientist, **Jurgen Lehmann** (1898–1989), see figure 8.2, was to advance the work using the data and principles demonstrated by Bernheim. In the case of the sulphonamides, it had been shown that placing an amino group in the para position to the carboxyl group of the benzene ring had the effect of depriving bacteria of their folic acid. Why not do the same with the salicylic acid molecule and try it in TB? The result was para-aminosalicylic acid, the amino (NH_2) group in the number 4 position (para to the COOH) on the benzene ring, as shown in the diagram, figure 8.3.

Most physicians when asked about the first effective drug to be used against tuberculosis would reply "streptomycin". And indeed, its discoverer, **Selman Waksman** was awarded the Nobel prize in 1952 for his contribution to the effective treatment of tuberculosis. But it can be shown that the first effective drug to be tried was in fact 4-aminosalicylic acid, also called para-aminosalicylic acid, or PAS. It was used by Lehmann. He was chief of the Sahlgrenska Hospital laboratory in Gothenburg. In March 1943 he wrote to the drug firm called Ferrosan in Malmo, and asked them to assist in producing sufficient quantities to be used in a clinical trial. He first demonstrated the inhibitory effect of the drug on the growth of the tubercle bacillus in the laboratory. It was tried in animal experiments, and no serious side effects were observed. The first human to be treated was a child with a tuberculous fistula in a hospital in Gothenburg. The drug was applied directly ("topically") as a

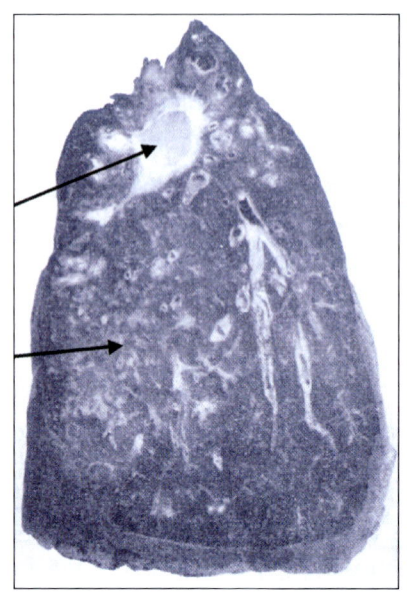

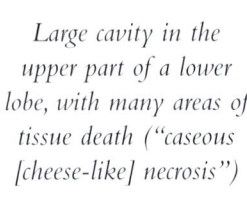
Large cavity in the upper part of a lower lobe, with many areas of tissue death ("caseous [cheese-like] necrosis")

Figure 8.1. Cavitating tuberculosis of the lung.
(Modified, reproduced with thanks from 'A Short Practice of Surgery', Bailey & Love, 12th edition, 1962, H.K. Lewis & Co. Ltd, with permission of Elsevier).

10% solution to the fistulous area. A second child with a similar condition was treated. The results were beneficial in both cases. Later, in March 1944, together with **Dr. Gylfe Vallentine** at the Renstrom Sanatorium, they treated cases of tuberculous empyema, i.e. pus within the pleural cavity, which lines the outer border of the lungs, by direct instillation of PAS solution into the pleural cavities. They noticed a reduction in fever, and concluded that the drug was also being absorbed from the pleural tissue. This suggested that perhaps the drug could be given orally, if absorption was a possibility. The first case thus treated was on October 30th 1944. It was only 8 months later than the first topical application, and 1 month later than the first oral administration of PAS, that streptomycin (an injectable drug) was first administered.

Lehmann knew he was on to something, and in the first week of January 1946, he published a preliminary communication in the journal Lancet. (Incidentally, on January 1st, test flights from London's newest airport started, known as Heath Row (2 words). And on January 3rd, Aneurin Bevan, Health Minister, speaking to 2,000 children, said that illness and death rates were lower than in 1944, but that tuberculosis and venereal disease remained problem areas. He undertook to transform the then existing haphazard system of health care delivery into a single comprehensive National Health Service, which would care for all regardless of their

Chapter Eight – Aspirin Derivatives

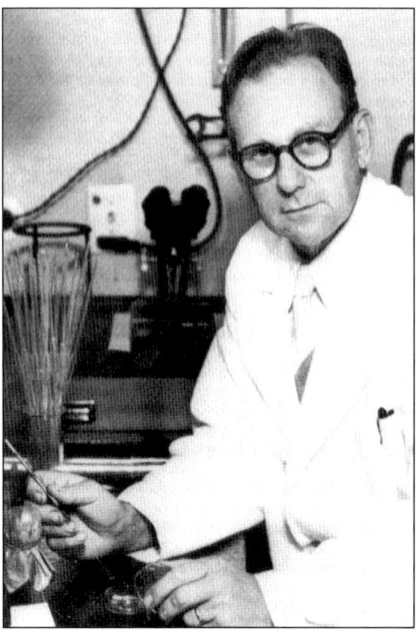

Figure 8.2. Jurgen Lehmann, (1898–1989).
(With permission of the South African Medical Journal).

wealth (or lack of it). Doctors would remain independent, but be expected to cooperate. One wonders, having experienced so-called sex-education in the 1950s quite how venereal disease would have been explained to the children, but that is another matter! Lehmann wrote as follows:

"In 1940, Bernheim showed that salicylic (2-hydroxy-benzoic) acid and benzoic acid increase the oxygen consumption and carbon dioxide production of the tubercle bacillus, whereas the homologues 3- and 4-hydroxybenzoic acid were inactive. It was concluded that salicylic and benzoic acids were oxidised as metabolites and that similar chemical configurations possibly play a part in the metabolism of the bacillus.

On the basis of these experiments I have investigated more than 50 derivatives of benzoic acid with the purpose of finding a substance possessing bacteriostatic properties against the tubercle bacillus. The substances were synthesised by K.G. Rosdahl, of Ferrosan Co., Malmo. –

The most active substance found was 4-aminosalicylic acid (*p*-aminosalicylic acid) – *Animal experiments* showed that 4-aminosalicylic acid was not toxic to rats – *Clinical trial.* – The treatment of tuberculosis in man was started parallel with the animal experiments. Tuberculous abscesses – have been treated – and showed healing after some months even when they had remained unchanged for 3–6 months before treatment. It has been given by mouth to 20 patients since March, 1944, at the Renstroemska Sanatorium in Gothenburg (Superintendent Dr. G. Vallentin). – periods of 8 days treatment were followed by free intervals of 8 days. – In many cases, however, a prompt fall in temperature – temporary or permanent – coincided with the periods of treatment and was accompanied by improvement in the patient's general condition as indicated by a gain in appetite and weight, an increase in the red cells and a decrease in the sedimentation rate."

2 case descriptions followed. The first case was that of a woman aged 24 years with acute pulmonary tuberculosis of about 2 months duration, with a fever ranging between 97.5°F and 101.5°F, see figure 8.4.

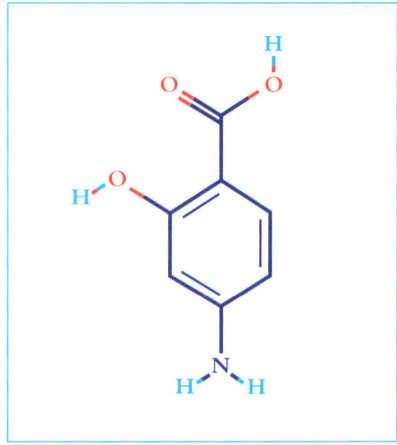

Figure 8.3. 4-aminosalicylic acid (para-amino salicylic acid syn. 'PAS').

It can be seen that her fever had gone by Christmas day, that her weight increased, and that the sedimentation rate of 44 mm per hour on 20th December (upper limit of normal 12 mm) had fallen to 7 mm on January 10th. He went on to remark:

"None of the usual effects of salicylates (sweats, ear symptoms), were observed even with a high dose of p-aminosalicylic acid (15 grams daily). The fall in temperature was therefore thought not to be due to a salicylate effect." (The sedimentation rate is a measurement of inflammation, because inflammatory proteins affect the rate at which red blood cells fall through a vertical column of plasma under the influence of gravity. Thus, after standing a column of blood upright for an hour, one measures, in millimetres, how far down the tube the cells have settled). This last remark was clearly directed at the Swedish critics who, perhaps understandably, ascribed the fever lowering effect to an aspirin like property, based on knowledge of the drug's similarity to aspirin. The 'ear symptoms' alluded to, were tinnitus – a ringing noise in the ears well recognised when patients receive high dose aspirin, as used to be the case in the treatment of acute rheumatic fever, and at one time, rheumatoid arthritis. But molecular similarity by no means guarantees similarity of action. Quite the contrary, such is the way of things. For instance, in the case of the female hormone oestriol, the only difference from testosterone is that the former possesses one more hydroxyl (OH) group at position 16, and one more hydrogen at position 3 on the steroid molecule. Yet these hormones are responsible for development of secondary sexual characteristics, such as breast enlargement, characteristic deposition of body fat giving the typical female figure, and menstruation. Testosterone on the other hand leads to increased muscle strength, beard growth, deepening of the voice, and testicular enlargement.

Chapter Eight – Aspirin Derivatives

Now, as is well known, all drugs can have side effects. And streptomycin was handicapped by the fact that it could damage the hearing and balance mechanism of the inner ear through its effects on the 8th cranial nerve. However, in patients critically ill with tuberculous meningitis, there was little to lose, and it was found that by injecting streptomycin directly into the brain and spinal cord linings ("meninges"), lives were saved. Clearly there was rivalry between the American and Scandinavian camps, so it must have been particularly galling when some of the Swedish physicians attending the Scandinavian Tuberculosis Doctors' meeting in Gothenburg in the summer of 1946, attributed the temperature lowering effect of PAS in cases of TB not to its postulated anti-TB effect, but to the anti-pyretic ("fever lowering") effect well recognised as a property of aspirin. However, further evidence of its effectiveness was not long in coming. In 1948, Carstensen and Sjolin published their results in which they described the dramatic effect of PAS in patients with intestinal tuberculosis. Patients who were very ill, emaciated and feverish, became free of their fever after a few weeks (itself proof that it wasn't working like aspirin, which for people with influenza, or common cold, would relieve fever within hours). But the trial to end this argument was a centralised controlled trial by the Therapeutic Trials Committee of the Swedish National association against Tuberculosis, published in the American Reviews of Tuberculosis in 1950. It was titled "Para-aminosalicylic acid treatment for pulmonary tuberculosis." PAS was shown to have a beneficial effect on the extent of lung involvement as seen on chest X-ray, the disappearance of the tubercle bacilli from sputum of patients, increase in

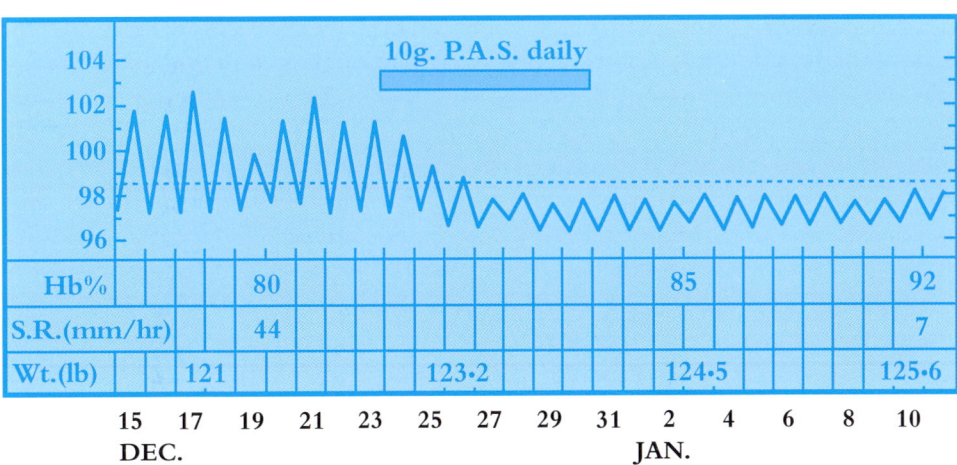

Figure 8.4. Temperature chart in case 1, showing the effect of the third course of para-aminosalicylic acid. (From Lehmann J, (1946) Para-amino salicylic acid in the treatment of tuberculosis. Lancet 1: 15–16). Reproduced with permission of Elsevier.

body weight, reduction of fever, and reduction in the blood sedimentation rate (a non-specific test for inflammation).

In the same year, the Medical Research Council in Britain published their investigation titled "Treatment of pulmonary tuberculosis with streptomycin and para-amino-salicylic acid" in the British Medical Journal on Saturday 11th November. (On November 2nd, George Bernard Shaw had died at his home in Hertfordshire). The study was a controlled trial, and one of its declared objectives was to assess the value of PAS because of the current controversy. The work was carried out at several centres, including the Brompton Hospital in London, Clare Hall County Hospital in Hertfordshire, Colindale Hospital London, Fazakerley Sanatorium, Liverpool, Harefield County Hospital, Middlesex, King George V Sanatorium, Surrey, the London Chest Hospital, London, the London Hospital Annexe, Essex, Sully Hospital, Glamorgan and Yardley Green Hospital, Birmingham. An essential part of the study was the statistical interpretation of the results, and for this purpose, Professor Bradford Hill, the doyen of statistics, was employed. In a controlled trial, the ideal situation is to compare the effect of the trial drug with an identical 'dummy' drug. (In fact, in 1948, the Medical Research Council did in fact carry out a comparison of streptomycin plus bed-rest, versus bed-rest alone, in patients with tuberculosis. They found that after 6 months, four times as many patients treated with bed-rest alone had died compared to those receiving streptomycin, but by 12 months, only twice as many died. Gruesome details, but invaluable, because they demonstrated, sadly, that the tubercle organism was capable of becoming resistant to streptomycin). But tuberculosis is a potentially lethal disease, and it was considered unethical in 1950 to treat patients with a dummy placebo. So they decided, perhaps with tongue in cheek (because some thought PAS was simply aspirin by any other word), to employ PAS as comparator. And with considerable foresight, they included a group who received both streptomycin and PAS. This was because it had earlier been suggested by Westergren, in 1946, that combined therapy might yield better results. Subsequently, Dunner, Brown, and Wallace in 1949, at the seventh streptomycin conference in Denver, Colorado, presented data to support the contention that the problem of drug resistance (to streptomycin), was prevented when it was given in combination with PAS. Additionally, because the criteria for inclusion into the study were identical in 1948 and 1950, they were able to use the 1948 placebo-treated patients (bed-rest only), as controls for all the 1950 participants. The patients included all had acute progressive bilateral (both lungs) tuberculosis. They were aged 15 to 30 years, and considered unsuitable for the then alternative form of treatment, collapse therapy. (Collapse therapy consisted of introducing air into the lining surrounding the lung, causing it to collapse like a squashed sponge. In this way there would be less air to nourish the bacteria, and less likelihood of the bacteria spreading. But it could lead to haemorrhage, or chronic infection by non-tuberculous bacteria – 'empyema' – or an unhealed communication through the skin – 'fistula').

166 patients were available for analysis of the results. 17 had dropped out for various reasons, 12 never entered the study, 5 were later excluded. The allocation of treatment was made on a random basis i.e. certain numbers were allocated to each of the designated treatments, and the patients received a number by lottery. This ensured no bias, but ran the risk of chance leading to uneven distribution of patients to one or other group. In the event, the distribution was, by good fortune, about equal. Interestingly, patients were not told they were taking part in a special investigation. (Nowadays, this would be considered unethical, but Life – and the practice of Medicine – was simpler in those days. In today's world, such a trial would be subject to close scrutiny by a national ethics committee, as well as a local one. Then, informed consent would have to be obtained. Also, all patients allocated to the study would be evaluated at the end of the study, even if they had, for whatever reason, dropped out. This is known as 'intention to treat' analysis, and avoids bias by excluding for instance, patients who deviated from the trial protocol). 59 patients received PAS, 54 streptomycin, and 53 both. At the end of the trial, patients treated with PAS alone, fared much better than their controls treated by bed-rest in the earlier (1948) study. X-ray changes of improvement were found in more patients receiving streptomycin, especially those with fever. Triumphantly, the outstanding effect of PAS was that, given in combination with streptomycin, the emergence of resistant strains fell from 67% (33 of 49) to 10.5% (5 of 48). So, the conclusion was that, PAS itself was less effective than streptomycin, but without the addition of PAS, streptomycin was relatively ineffective on account of the emergence of drug resistance. The doubting (mainly Swedish) doctors, were silenced. Jurgen Lehmann's contribution was shown to be highly significant, the equal of the Nobel prize winning Selman Waksman.

This trial underscored the value of combination therapy, nowadays the cornerstone of treatment of many diseases. By way of military analogy, it involves coming at the enemy from several directions. Dosages of individual drugs can thereby be reduced for equivalent effect, and with it, the likelihood of side effects. Eventually, triple therapy became the norm for treating tuberculosis, the drugs being streptomycin, PAS and isoniazid. However, over time, other drugs have emerged, and PAS no longer figures in modern treatment strategies.

Chronic inflammatory bowel disease and rheumatoid arthritis

Now let us take a look at the involvement of aspirin derivatives in rheumatoid arthritis, and chronic inflammatory bowel disease (Crohn's disease, and ulcerative colitis).

Rheumatoid arthritis is a chronic inflammatory condition involving almost any joints of the body but particularly the hands, feet, and wrists. It can come on at any age, and can start suddenly or extremely gradually. Its final effects can range from spontaneous remission to total loss of independence and being crippled. In certain cases, particularly those where there is inflammation of small arteries ("vasculitis"), the outlook is particularly poor, unless controlled with steroids and immunosuppressive drugs. Originally the approach to treatment was to reduce pain and to some extent inflammation. Aspirin was the most widely used drug for this purpose. But it became clear that more than symptomatic relief was needed. This led to the emergence of so-called 'disease-modifying drugs' or DMARD's. Another offshoot of aspirin was born in the 1930s. **Nanna Svartz**, a professor at the renowned Karolinska Institute in Stockholm, was interested in the treatment of rheumatoid arthritis. The cause of this disease was, and still is, unknown. However, at the time, there was a body of evidence (now disproved) that streptococcal infection was involved. Antibiotics were not yet on the scene, but their predecessors, the sulphonamides, were. Nanna Svartz predicted that a drug regimen consisting of a salicylate plus a sulphonamide, might be a good way of treating this crippling disease. But she then went a step further by chemically combining the two. She worked in collaboration with the pharmaceutical firm Pharmacia. They produced various combinations, of which the most interesting and useful, was a combination of 5-aminosalicylic acid, and sulphapyridine. (By way of comparison, it will be recalled from the foregoing pages, that PAS was 4-aminosalicylic acid). 5-aminosalicylic acid was shown to penetrate well into connective tissue, so might particularly help joints. The drug was known as salicylazosulphapyridine, and was given the proprietary (or trade) name salazopyrin. Its current generic name in the UK is sulphasalazine, see figure below.

Svartz treated more than 400 patients between 1940 and 1946. She reported a favourable outcome in 63%. Another study from America supported these findings (Kuzell & Gardner 1950).

As an intriguing parallel to this scientific story lies an intriguing political question. The world is aware of the Swedish hero, Raoul Wallenberg, who was sent in 1944 by the Swedish Foreign Minister, to Budapest to try to save the Jewish community there. He had several face to face confrontations with Adolf Eichmann, the architect of the Nazi's "Final Solution". It is believed that by his courage, initiative, and daring bravado, he helped save many thousands of Jews from transfer to the death camps. On January 10th 1945, when advised by his colleagues to return swiftly to Stockholm, because by now the Russians had invaded Hungary, he refused saying that he had not yet completed his quest. A week later he was arrested by the Soviets, and taken to Moscow in "protective custody". He was never released. The Russians eventually claimed he had died in his prison cell in 1947. However, Nanna Svartz made a statement to a special Swedish group investigating her credibility in the matter, because she claimed to have been told by Professor Aleksandr Miasnikov, a prominent Soviet medical official in 1961, that Wallenberg was still alive and being kept in a mental hospital. This was subsequently denied by Miasnikov, who interestingly died shortly afterwards. But the whole Wallenberg case and Svartz's involvement caused considerable Soviet ructions. Now to return to salazopyrin!

Worryingly a study carried out in Edinburgh (Sinclair & Duthie 1948), reported that salazopyrin conferred no benefit in patients with rheumatoid arthritis over aspirin, and less than the benefit obtained by the use of gold injections. By inference, they were implying that salazopyrin owed its (mild) beneficial effect in rheumatoid arthritis to its aspirin effect. It is very interesting that this bears a distinct similarity to the scepticism levelled at PAS and the reduction of fever in tuberculosis. 2 years later, and cortisone came on the scene. This was the 'miracle' drug, and no-one remained interested in salazopyrin in rheumatoid arthritis for 30 years. Then in 1978, **Dr. Brian McConkey**, a physician at what was then the Dudley Road Hospital, in Birmingham (and incidentally where the author was employed for his first house-physician's job in 1964), reported a trial of this drug in 68 patients with rheumatoid arthritis treated for more than 1 month, and 31 for more than 1 year. Improvement of the various measures of inflammation, including the erythrocyte sedimentation rate were observed. Subsequent trials (Neumann, Grindulis, Hubbal et al 1983; Carroll, Tinsley, Humphries et al 1983; Pullar, Hunter & Capell 1983; Pinals, Kaplan, Lawson et al 1986), confirmed the effectiveness of this drug. It differed from the effect of aspirin in the following important ways:

1. Aspirin was rapid in onset (within minutes or hours), whereas salazopyrin took 8 weeks or so.
2. Salazopyrin affected inflammatory markers (for instance the erythrocyte sedimentation rate, or 'ESR') more than aspirin.
3. Salazopyrin, if stopped, maintained its beneficial effects for weeks, whereas aspirin's benefits after cessation, lasted only hours.

Following this, salazopyrin for a while moved into the number one place for the so-called 'disease-modifying drugs' used for rheumatoid arthritis. It is still much used, but has been largely supplanted by methotrexate. However, it is still in common use for treating rheumatoid arthritis, unlike PAS in tuberculosis.

The drug is broken down in the intestine by bacteria, which snip away at the azo link, releasing the parent molecules, sulphapyridine and 5-aminosalicylic acid. Svartz had observed that the 5-aminosalicylic acid part would penetrate into the soft tissues of the body by absorption from the intestine. Interestingly, administering 5-aminosalicylic acid orally was shown to be of no value in treating rheumatoid arthritis, though aspirin is. But, even more strange to report, it has been found to be of use in the treatment of chronic inflammatory bowel disease. Returning to rheumatoid arthritis, the observation that 5-amino-salicylic acid was not beneficial led some to pre-suppose that therefore the undoubted benefit of sulphasalazine lay in the sulphapyridine moiety. Indeed, giving patients sulphapyridine did have slight beneficial effects, but not as much as sulphasalazine, and it was far less well tolerated. Several theories have been put forward as to the mode of action of sulphasalazine in rheumatoid arthritis, including that of the author. These are reviewed by Smedegard and Bjork (1995).

Chronic inflammatory bowel disease (IBD), is the term used to cover ulcerative colitis and Crohn's disease. The former is characterised by severe diarrhoea with the passage of blood and mucus. It can lead to severe anaemia and weight loss, and depletion of the body's salts (electrolyte depletion). Treatment used to consist of steroid enemas, sulphasalazine, blood transfusions and intravenous salt solutions. In extreme cases, it may be necessary to remove the diseased section of the intestine, bringing the undiseased portion out through the skin, to empty into a special 'stoma bag'. It was therefore of considerable interest when it emerged that the benefit conferred by sulphasalazine could be mimicked by its salicylate component alone. It can be taken as tablets or enemas. The evidence for the effective moiety within sulphasalazine was due to the work of Azad Khan and colleagues (1977). In a controlled blind clinical trial of patients with ulcerative colitis, and in which there were 3 groups of patients treated with retention enemas of either sulphasalazine, sulphapyridine, or 5-aminosalicylic acid for 14 days, it was found on microscopic examination of the rectal lining that it was the first and last named alone which exerted benefit. Subsequently another trial demonstrated effectiveness of orally administered 5-amino-salicylic acid (Dew et al 1982).

Crohn's disease is characterised by bouts of cramping abdominal pain, diarrhoea with fever and weight loss. Whereas ulcerative colitis, as its name implies, is confined

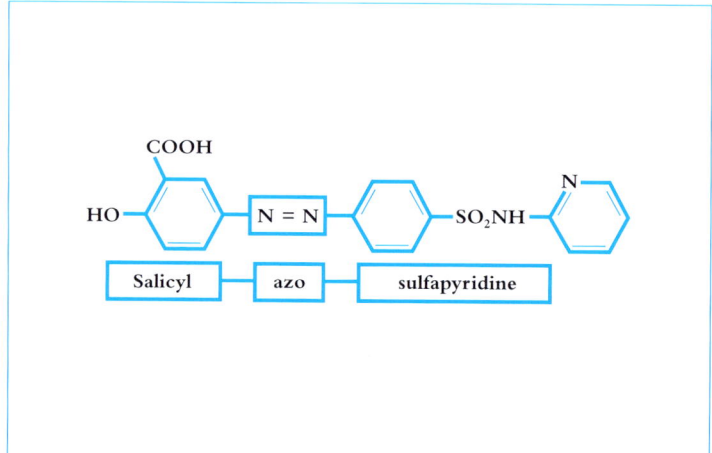

Figure 8.5. 5-aminosalicylic acid linked to a sulphonamide gave salazopyrin (sulphasalazine).

Chapter Eight – Aspirin Derivatives

to the colon, Crohn's can occur anywhere in the gastro-intestinal tract, but most typically in the ileum. When it involves the colon, it too is amenable to treatment with mesalazine.

Finally, in connection with skin disorders, the salicylates are considered to be one of the safest sunscreens, even when used in high concentrations. The most widely used salicylates are homosalate and octyl salicylate.

The following is taken from **the British Pharmaceutical Codex**: "Salicylic acid, $C_6H_4OHCOOH$, may be obtained from the oils of wintergreen and sweet birch, or by the action of carbon dioxide on sodium phenate, the commercial varieties being distinguished as "natural" and "artificial", according as they are produced from the natural salicylates or prepared synthetically. It is also official in the U.S.P. It occurs in white prisms, or as white, light, silky crystals, the natural acid being usually less white than the artificial, and possessing a slight odour indicative of its origin. Melting-point, 156° to 157°. The natural acid is free from impurities which formerly were present in the synthetic product, and is still sometimes preferred for internal use. The artificial acid is sold in three varieties, (a) so-called physiologically pure, (b) ordinary crystals, and (c) powder; all three varieties usually comply with the official tests, but the powder is less pure than the crystals and has a slightly lower melting-point.

Soluble in water (1 in 550), boiling water (1 in 9), alcohol (1 in 3.5), ether (1 in 2), glycerin (1 in 200). It forms salicylates when dissolved in solutions of ammonium citrate, ammonium acetate, sodium phosphate, borax, alkali hydroxides and carbonates.

Action and Uses – Salicylic acid is a powerful antiseptic; it exerts a strong inhibitory influence upon the growth of micro-organisms, and retards the action of unorganised ferments as well as the ferments responsible for alcoholic and acetic fermentation; applied to wounds it is less irritating than phenol, but strong solutions exert a destructive action upon the horny layer of the epidermis, which is softened and may easily be removed. Swallowed in powder or tablets it may cause irritation and corrosion of the mucous membrane of the mouth, throat, and stomach. Salicylic acid is used externally as an antiseptic and antipruritic in the treatment of wounds and parasitic skin diseases; it is also employed as a mouth-wash, and as a local application to diminish sweating, especially when offensive. In concentrated solutions it is employed to remove such epidermal thickenings as corns and warts, and to destroy lupus. For internal use it has been replaced, almost entirely, by sodium salicylate and acetyl-salicylic acid, which resemble it in therapeutic action. A solution of 1 in 1000 is sufficiently strong to preserve alkaloidal and similar solutions. It is employed (½ to 6 in 1000) as a preservative of food and beverages. Salicylic acid is **incompatible** with iron salts and spirit of nitrous ether.

Dose. – 3 to 12 decigrams (5 to 20 grains).

PREPARATIONS
Collodium Salicylicum, B.P.C. – SALICYLIC COLLODION. 1 in 8.
Salicylic collodion is a painless application for warts and corns.
Collodium Salicylicum Compositum, B.P.C. – COMPOUND SALICYLIC COLLODION. *Syn.* – Collodium Callosum; Corn Paint.
Salicylic acid, 12; extract of Indian hemp, 2; acetone, 30; acetone collodion, to 100. Used as a corn and wart "solvent". For use on exposed parts, the colourless Collodium Salicylicum is preferable.
Emplastrum Salicylicum Elasticum, B.P.C. – RUBBER SALICYLIC PLASTER. 1 in 10.
Emplastrum Salicylicum Compositum, B.P.C. – COMPOUND SALICYLIC PLASTER. *Syn.* — Salicylic Acid and Indian Hemp Plaster; Corn Plaster.
Salicylic acid, 20; extract of Indian hemp, 10; rubber adhesive plaster, 70.
Emplastrum Salicylicum Compositum Fortius, B.P.C. – STRONGER COMPOUND SALICYLIC PLASTER. *Syn.* – Stronger Salicylic Acid and Indian Hemp Plaster; Stronger Corn Plaster.
Salicylic acid, 40; extract of Indian hemp, 5; rubber adhesive plaster, 55.
Gossypium Acidi Salicylici, B.P.C. – SALICYLIC ACID WOOL. 4 per cent.
This "wool" should be preserved in air-tight packages, under aseptic conditions, until required for use.
Gossypium Acidi Salicylici Forte, B.P.C. – STRONG SALICYLIC ACID WOOL. 10 per cent.
This "wool" should be preserved in air-tight packages, under aseptic conditions, until required for use.
Linteum Acidi Salicylici, B.P.C. – SALICYLIC ACID LINT, 4 per cent.
This preparation should be preserved in air-tight packages, under aseptic conditions, until required for use.
Parogenum Salicylatum, B.P.C. – SALICYLATED PAROGEN. *Syn.* – Salicylated Vasoliment. 1 in 10.
Pulvis Acidi Salicylici Compositus, B.P.C. – COMPOUND SALICYLIC ACID POWDER. *Syn.*—Pulvis pro Pedibus; Foot Powder,
Salicylic acid, 3; boric acid, 10; French chalk, 87. Used as a dusting powder for the feet when there is tenderness or hyperidrosis. Pulvis Salicylicus cum Talco of the German Pharmacopoeia contains wheat starch in place of boric acid.
Sevum Salicylatum, B.P.C. – SALICYLATED SUET. 1 in 50.
Unguentum Acidi Salicylici, B.P. – SALICYLIC ACID OINTMENT.
Salicylic acid, in powder, 2; paraffin ointment, white, 98. Salicylic acid ointment is used as an application to the skin in chronic eczema, acne, etc.; it is also used, applied thickly on lint, as a dressing for ulcerated wounds.

Chapter Nine

THE ENLIGHTENMENT

Whilst it would come as no surprise to realise that no-one in ancient times had thought to ask the question as to how aspirin (or salicin, its natural precursor) worked, it does seem a little odd that nearly a century after its manufacture, curiosity as to its mode of action was restricted to very few people. Perhaps this was because it was perceived as an old pain-killing drug, which was becoming obsolete with the introduction of paracetamol (acetaminophen in the USA), and the non-steroidal anti-inflammatory drugs (NSAIDs), of which early examples were indomethacin (Indocid), ibuprofen (Brufen, Nurofen), naproxen (Naprosyn). Aspirin had a strong reputation within the medical and nursing professions, as a drug which caused gastro-intestinal bleeding, manifesting dramatically as vomiting blood (haematemesis), or passing black tarry coloured motions (melaena). Yet despite this, it continued to enjoy regular over the counter sales in chemist shops. There was no doubt of its effectiveness as a pain killer, nor of its ability to lower temperature in patients with fever. Strange perhaps that it did not lower temperature below normal in people without fever. But that sort of question was not asked, though perhaps it offered a clue as to its mode of action. Put another way, why was it necessary to have a fever in the first place, for its effect on body temperature to be revealed? Answer – it required the presence of inflammation! As Celsus had pointed out in the first century AD, the features of inflammation included redness and swelling with heat and pain (rubor, tumor, calor, dolor). And there was ample everyday evidence of aspirin's ability to act on two of the signs of Celsus – what about the other signs, namely swelling and redness?

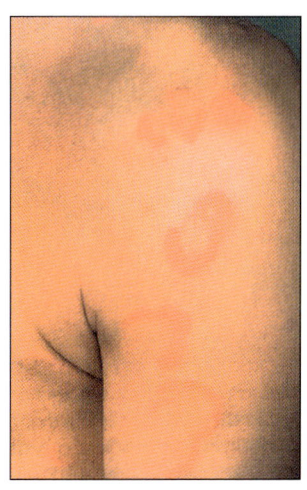

Figure 9.1. Erythema marginatum. (From 'Clinical Medicine' by Forbes and Jackson, 2nd Edition 1997, Mosby-Wolfe. Reproduced with permission from Elsevier).

Rheumatic fever is a disease that is now rare in Western Europe, but was quite common until the 1960s. It started in children following a sore throat due to a bacterium called *Streptococcus pyogenes*. About 2 to 3 weeks later, the child would develop a swollen joint, lasting a few days. There would also be a fever, and sometimes a rash, called *erythema marginatum* (redness with margins), see figure 9.1.

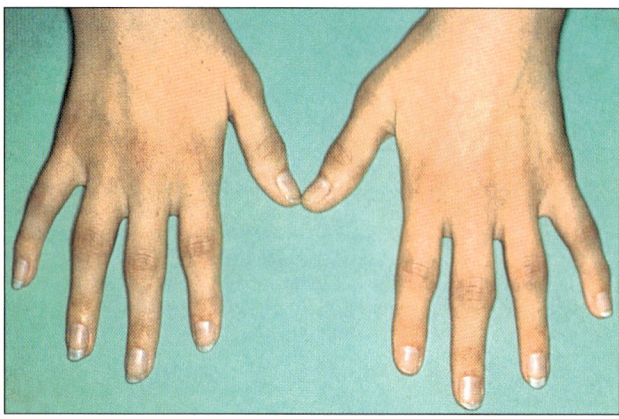

Figure 9.2. Early rheumatoid arthritis.

The arthritis would typically be flitting, and eventually settle within a few months, without any permanent damage. Occasionally, there would be evidence of heart involvement, revealed by murmurs (rheumatic carditis). More often, there would be no evident heart disease until many years later, when patients developed valve problems, usually the mitral valve which would become scarred and narrowed (mitral stenosis). During the early phase in childhood, the fever would respond well to aspirin, though it offered no protection to the eventual development of heart valve damage. Also, the joint pains would be relieved. The doses given were large, and often taken to the point where the drug resulted in ringing in the ears (tinnitus). Those patients with evidence of carditis would instead of aspirin, be given steroids. It was believed by Maclagan of Dundee that this would prevent the late appearance of cardiac complications, but he was wrong. Although patients were symptomatically relieved from the symptoms of acute rheumatic fever, the underlying inflammation around the heart valves continued insidiously for years, with the body's natural response to chronic inflammation, namely fibrosis (scarring) resulting in either narrowing of the heart valve orifice ('stenosis'), or inability to close properly when required ('incompetence', or 'regurgitation').

Rheumatoid arthritis, though similar sounding, is an altogether different disease. There is inflammation of many joints, see figure 9.2.

If the disease is not controlled by disease modifying drugs, it can lead to permanent damage of joints, see figure 9.3.

There is usually no fever, except in severe cases. The joint swelling, as well as the pain and stiffness experienced by the patient, will usually respond well to aspirin.

So we have clinical evidence of aspirin's ability to ameliorate signs of inflammation in patients. Nowadays, the research into new drugs requires testing of these drugs in

Chapter Nine – The Enlightenment

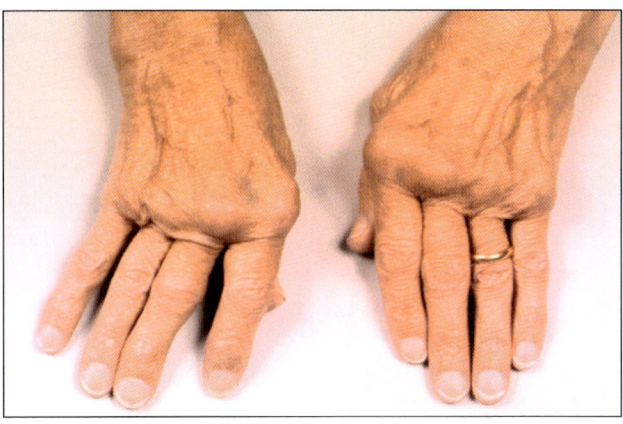

Figure 9.3. Advanced rheumatoid arthritis showing deviation of the fingers, and dislocation of the knuckle joints after several years.

animal models. For over half a century, there have been methods developed of inducing arthritis in animals, and then it has been possible to test the effect of new drugs on them. One such is experimental arthritis in the rat, see figure 9.4. The effect of treating the rat with aspirin is shown in figure 9.5. It can quite clearly be seen that there is less swelling in the aspirin-treated rat. But how is this brought about?

The answer, if indeed we have the answer, is slowly being elucidated. Great prizes are at stake, both in terms of honours such as Nobel prizes, and commercial rewards eagerly pursued by the pharmaceutical industry. As a practising physician it has been truly amazing, and at times comical, to recall the extent to which representatives of the latter industry have gone to make clear the efficacy of their products, only some time later, sheepishly to apologise as they were withdrawn from the market on account of side-effects. Yet, if we had been possessed of all knowledge regarding its precise mode of action, we might well have been in a position to predict its side effects, and furthermore, to predict other extremely beneficial properties. As Collier (1963) has stated,

"It has always been easier to catalogue the wide application of aspirin to man's commonest ills than to explain its mode of action. – "

An early theory was that acetylsalicylic acid (aspirin), released its acidic group at the site in the body where its effects were needed, and that the effective moiety was the salicylic acid. This view has been shown not to be the case – both are effective. In one situation however, it was shown that only the intact aspirin was effective. This was the experiment in which an irritant called thurfyl nicotinate was rubbed into the skin. A rash comprising reddening and wealing would result. Truelove and Duthie, working at the Northern General Hospital in Edinburgh in 1959 showed that in volunteers, 650 milligrams of aspirin would delay the reddening and abolish the swelling. At a salicylate symposium in 1962, Adams and Cobb of the Boots company used the same skin test and showed that whilst aspirin was effective, sodium salicylate was not.

One of the main researchers in the field at that time was H.O.J. Collier, working for Parke Davis and Co. in Hounslow, Middlesex. He pointed out that the main effect of aspirin therapy was to inhibit excess of body defensive reactions such as fever, pain and inflammation. He used the term "anti-defensive drug." But the crucial elucidation of the mode of action of aspirin in inflammation was elucidated in the laboratory of Professor John Vane, see figure 9.6, working at the Royal College of Surgeons, in Lincoln's Inn Fields, London, together with Priscilla Piper, who previously had worked for H.O.J. Collier.

Again, the use of experimental animals has served to clarify our views on the mode of action of aspirin. The guinea pig is well known to researchers as being a creature poised on the brink of an allergic death should it encounter something to which it had become allergic earlier on. This can be brought about experimentally by exposing it to an allergy provoking substance, for example the albumin derived from egg white. It will make antibodies, because its immune system recognises differences in chicken albumin to guinea pig albumin. These antibodies are attached to some very important cells called **mast cells**, which line the respiratory and gastro-intestinal tracts. Mast cells contain several powerful substances which, if released, can have extremely potent effects on the host animal, the most dramatic being **anaphylactic shock** followed by death. The signal which causes release of these substances, (or 'mediators'), is the attachment of the allergen (in this case egg albumin), to the antibody (known as IgE i.e. immunoglobulin of class E) itself attached to the mast cell surface. This triggers mediator release. The effective mediators include histamine, and serotonin, plus a family of substances called **prostaglandins**. These are also released by other cells as a consequence of damage, either physical or after infection, and result from cell membrane phospholipids being enzymically digested (by phospholipase A2) to produce **arachidonic acid**. This is further acted upon by enzymes called **cyclo-oxygenases** resulting in prostaglandins, (and lipoxygenases, which we will not discuss further). Prostaglandins are involved in protecting the stomach lining from gastric acid, promoting normal kidney metabolism, normal blood platelet function, and making nerve endings aware of inflammation, by rendering them more sensitive. But what about the guinea pig?

Healthy guinea pigs were injected into their abdominal cavity and under the skin with a small amount of egg albumin. They remained perfectly well. 14–28 days later, in the interest of medical science, they were humanely killed. Their lungs were removed intact, and connected up to an apparatus which permitted nutritious fluid to circulate through them carrying essential salts plus oxygen. The effluent from the lungs was collected in a small chamber. It will be seen therefore, that one could now mimic the production of anaphylactic shock by including egg albumin in the perfusing liquid. The

Chapter Nine – The Enlightenment

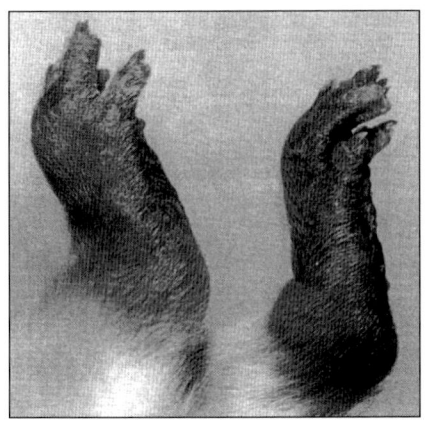
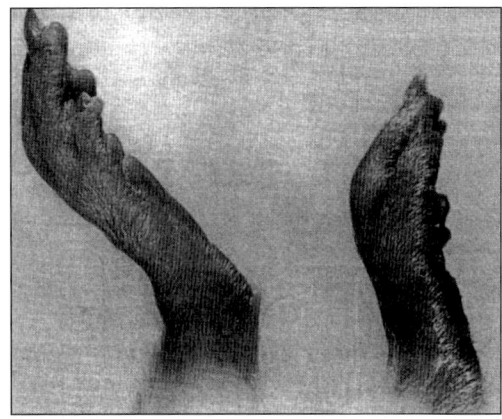

*Left: Figure 9.4. Inflamed rat paw in experimental arthritis.
(With permission from Scientific American. 1963; 209: 100. Author H.Collier).
Right: Figure 9.5. Effect of aspirin treatment in experimental arthritis.
(With permission from Scientific American. 1963; 209: 100. Author H.Collier).*

design of Piper and Vane's pivotal experiments can be tabulated as follows, (assuming the tissue contraction detects the presence of histamine), see table 9.1. By analysing the effluent, one could deduce which mediators were being produced. By adding known 'antagonistic' (i.e. neutralising) substances either to the perfusate, or to the effluent, one could further localise what was happening, where it was happening and also study the effect of various drugs. For instance, if histamine was produced in the lung during anaphylaxis, and detected by an observed phenomenon on a chosen test tissue, then one should be able to prevent this effect being manifest by incorporating an anti-histamine in the effluent before it could react on the chosen test tissue.

If this was found not to prevent the effect, one would deduce that something else, not histamine, was able to mimic the histamine effect. On the other hand, if one wished to know whether the histamine was formed in the lung in the course of the anaphylactic reaction, one could incorporate an antagonist in the perfusate. If this resulted in neutralisation of the histamine effect of the effluent, one could deduce that the histamine had arisen as a result of the anaphylactic reaction.

Now let us assume that instead of histamine, we are studying the effect of aspirin, and that contraction of the rat thoracic aorta (abbreviated RTA), reveals the presence of prostaglandin, see table 9.2.

Here we see that for the aspirin to prevent contraction of rat thoracic aorta, it has to be present in the perfusate, not the effluent. This proves its effect is occurring in the lung where the prostaglandins are being synthesised in the course of the anaphylactic reaction, and not by any direct effect on the RTA.

Addition to perfusate		Addition to effluent	Target tissue contraction
Allergen	+	Nil	+
Histamine	−		
Allergen	−	Nil	−
Histamine	−		
Allergen	+	Anti-histamine	−
Histamine	−		
Allergen	−	Nil	+
Histamine	+		
Allergen	+	Nil	−
Histamine antagonist	+		
e.g. mepyramine			

Table 9.1. Piper and Vane's experiment. Simplified scheme detecting histamine.

Addition to perfusate		Addition to effluent	RTA contraction
Allergen	+	Nil	+
Allergen	+	Aspirin	+
Allergen	+	Nil	−
Aspirin	+		

Table 9.2. Piper and Vane's experiment. Simplified scheme detecting prostaglandin.

The same logic could be applied for various suspected mediators. One such was prostaglandin, the test tissue in this case being a strip of male rabbit thoracic aorta (RTA). In the presence of prostaglandin, its muscle component would contract, even when blitzed with antagonists to histamine, serotonin and sympathetic nervous system metabolites.

This substance, which contracted male rabbit thoracic aorta, was named 'rabbit (aorta) contracting substance – or RCS – which coincided with the initials associated with the place where these experiments took place – the Royal College of Surgeons, in Lincoln's Inn Fields, London. It had not previously been detected in

Chapter Nine – The Enlightenment

this way. But now came the crucial experiment. What effect if any, would anti-inflammatory drugs have on RCS? See the figure below. First, the effect of incorporating aspirin in the effluent bathing the male rabbit thoracic aorta under the afore-mentioned experimental condition was studied. The result was as shown in table 9.2 i.e. no preventive effect on the detection of RCS. ***And now, the definitive test. When aspirin was applied to the perfusate, and the appropriate time elapsed for the repeated experiment to complete – no RCS was detected***. The conclusion was that aspirin prevented the synthesis of prostaglandin in the guinea-pig lung undergoing anaphylactic shock.

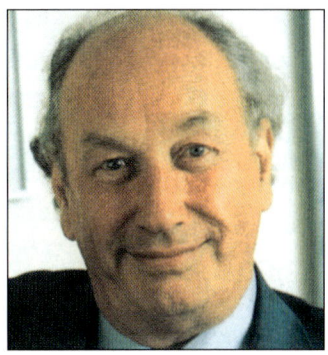

Figure 9.6. Portrait of the late Sir John Vane. (1927–2004).

Further experiments showed that indomethacin, another non-steroidal anti-inflammatory drug had similar effects.

The demonstration that aspirin inhibited prostaglandin synthesis was then applied to explain its anti-inflammatory effects. As mentioned above, during inflammation, tissue damage affects membrane phospholipids, resulting in the involvement of cyclo-oygenase-mediated prostaglandin synthesis.

Below is shown a portion of the crucial experiment reproduced from the original paper which demonstrated the effect of aspirin on prostaglandin synthesis, using the aforementioned guinea pig model, see figure 9.7.

The actual description of their findings, which included other test substances as well, but which have been omitted for clarity, was as follows:

"The perfusate from sensitized lungs was used to superfuse a guinea-pig trachea (GPT), rabbit aorta strip (RbA), guinea-pig ileum (GPI), rat stomach strip (RSS), rat colon (RC) and chick rectum (CR), all treated with combined antagonists. Anaphylaxis was induced in the lungs by ovalbumen (ovalb 10 mg IA) while sodium aspirin (5 microgram/ml, DIR) was being infused over the assay tissues. RCS was released. The sodium aspirin infusion was then made so that it also passed through the lungs and the shock was repeated. No RCS was released after this shock, or during the third, even though the aspirin infusion was stopped. Note that the tissues measuring SRS-A release (GPT and GPI) still contract, showing that the RCS release has been selectively abolished. – "

Prostaglandin (to be precise, PGE_1), when injected into the third ventricle of the cat brain, induces fever. Thus, one may explain fever reduction by putative reduction of PGE_1 (Vane 1971). Nowadays, PGE_2 is considered more likely to be relevant, if less potent at inducing fever than PGE_1. The control centre for body temperature is in the brain in the region of the hypothalamus. This does not explain why paracetamol is equally effective as an anti-pyretic, even though when injected into the cat brain, there is no temperature lowering effect. Nevertheless, the perceived wisdom is that inflammatory cytokines (see chapter on inflammation) result in PGE_2 release, and that this arrives at the hypothalamus, there to be hindered by administered aspirin.

It is interesting to observe that whilst there is a mountain of knowledge about the chemistry and synthesis of salicylates, and a huge body of knowledge about their adverse effects, relatively little progress has been made in explaining the mode of action in temperature lowering.

Not surprisingly, some of the foregoing is contentious. The author recalls the euphoria when the holy grail of aspirin (its mode of action), was apparently revealed in 1969. However, Professor Gerald Weissman of New York, studying the molecular biology of inflammation voiced a note of caution about accepting Vane's work as the full elucidation of aspirin's mode of action (Weissman 1991). He made the following points:

1. The dose of aspirin needed to reduce pain is far lower than that required to reduce inflammation. This would not be the case if the same mechanism was invoked in both. It could be explained if at a higher concentration, the anti-inflammatory effect of aspirin was being brought about by some other mechanism.
2. Reduction in pain and inflammation can easily be produced by paracetamol (acetaminophen) despite it not having an anti-prostaglandin effect.
3. The effects of non-steroidal anti-inflammatory drugs (NSAIDs) as a whole, probably are due to their physical effects on biological membranes. These contain lipids which attract these drugs (they are said to be lipophilic – lipid loving).

In his laboratory, he demonstrated that, at therapeutic concentrations, salicylates and NSAIDs inhibit cell-cell adhesion of neutrophils to other neutrophils, and to endothelium. Furthermore, the degree of interference by sodium salicylate was similar to that of aspirin, though the former does not and the latter does inhibit prostaglandin synthesis. Finally, he showed that NSAIDs were able to hinder the adhesion of marine sponge cells to each other. Given that this is relevant (and he claimed it was), then it is of great interest to learn that these cells are incapable of making prostaglandins, and even when prostaglandins are artificially added into the cell suspensions, there is no observed change in the NSAID effects on their adhesion. However his data derived as a result of work on cell-cell adhesion, though doubtless interesting, and possibly relevant, does not really undermine the prostaglandin hypothesis. Whilst cell adhesion is of considerable interest, these observations in no way materially detract from Vane's original observations. But that is not to say that all is well in the cyclo-oxygenase garden, as will now be described.

The (simplified) perceived wisdom is that there are at least two cyclo-oxygenases, cyclo-oxygenase 1 and 2 (Cox 1 and Cox 2). Cox 1 is involved in ensuring adequate

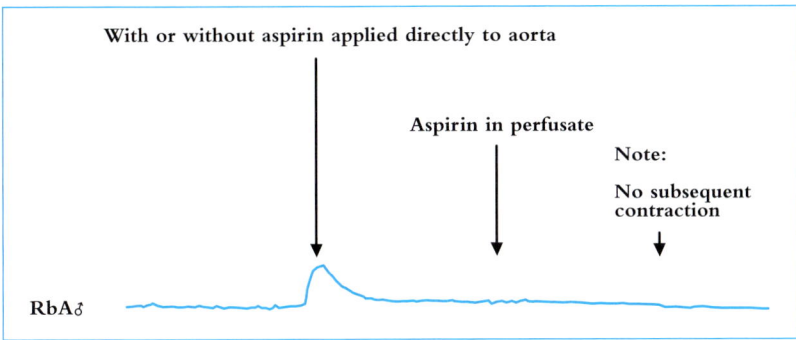

Figure 9.7. Prostaglandin inhibition by aspirin. Contraction of male rabbit thoracic aorta. (Modified from Piper & Vane, Nature 1969; 223: 29).

gastric protection from gastric acid, failure of which might result in stomach ulcer or bleeding. It is also present in the kidney and blood platelets. It is present during normal health and its presence is spoken of as *"constitutive"*. It is also known as a "housekeeping" enzyme, i.e. it is involved in everyday normal healthy protective functions of the body. By contrast, Cox 2 is present in low concentration in health, but is *induced* at sites of inflammation, and sensitises nerve cells, thus leading to the perception of pain at such sites. There are certain laboratory tests which can assess the degree to which a given substance, or drug, can affect Cox 1 or Cox 2 production. It has been shown that aspirin inhibits production of both. This has been seized upon as the explanation of its best known side effect, stomach ulceration and bleeding. By inhibiting Cox 1, there is less protection in the patient against the harmful effect of gastric acid. Also, it affects platelets, and these, as has been explained, play a pivotal role in staunching bleeding. Armed with these (simplified) facts, the pharmaceutical industry endeavoured to find a way in which a drug could be made that inhibited Cox 2 without inhibiting Cox 1. Such a drug would be the answer to the maiden's prayer – a drug which relieved pain, fever and inflammation, yet was safer than aspirin, and would by inference not cause stomach ulceration or bleeding. All that was needed was a simple test, and off they would go. Unfortunately life is not that simple. Tests could be carried out using whole blood, or using genetically engineered (and therefore pure) cyclo-oxygenases. When both were performed, the results of Cox selectivity did not show a strong correlation. The drugs which were designed to be selective, the so-called "selective Cox 2 inhibitors" were rapidly put through the necessary drug trials, and when shown to satisfy the basic safety tests, were advertised to the medical profession, and prescribed on the NHS and in the USA and Europe. The first two were celecoxib (Celebrex), made by Searle, and rofecoxib (Vioxx), made by Merck Sharp and Dohme. Below is shown an abbreviated list of Cox selectivity using assays of their effect against genetically engineered pure cyclo-oxygenases and on cyclo-oxygenase activity in whole blood. If the selectivity of aspirin is taken as 1, figures greater than 1 imply selectivity i.e. selectively inhibits Cox 2 more than does aspirin, figures less than 1 imply the drug works less selectively than does aspirin.

It was a great surprise to find that two fairly long in the tooth NSAIDs (etodolac and meloxicam) were apparently also selective, and not far behind the designer drugs. Clinical studies including endoscopic examination of the stomach and duodenum confirmed the superiority of the selective Cox 2 inhibitors over aspirin. So far, entirely as anticipated. The National Institute of Clinical Excellence (NICE), went so far as to recommend use of selective Cox 2 drugs in the over 60s, because generally speaking, gastro-intestinal haemorrhage from NSAIDs is particularly likely in this age group. In addition to the afore-mentioned selective inhibitors ("coxibs"), along came valdecoxib (Bextra), etoricoxib (Arcoxia), and lumiracoxib (Prexige).

However, the problems arose following a randomised double blind clinical trial, published in 2002, in which rofecoxib (Vioxx) was compared with a traditional NSAID, naproxen (the VIGOR study). 8076 rheumatoid arthritis patients aged over 40 years received either 50 milligrams of test drug, or 500 milligrams naproxen. The purpose of the trial was to let patients continue until they experienced perforation or obstruction of the gastro-intestinal tract, bleeding from the upper gut, or indigestion ("dyspepsia"), due to stomach or duodenal ulceration. Then by unmasking the treatment, the relative risk of these GI events could be compared with the treatments used. The anti-inflammatory effects against the arthritis were also recorded.

At the end of the trial, efficacy against arthritis was equal, and there were half as many gastro-intestinal side effects with rofecoxib. This was just what the

Drug	Genetically engineered cyclo-oxygenases	Whole human blood assay
Aspirin	1	1
Celecoxib (Celebrex)★	571	127
Rofecoxib (Vioxx)★	275	744
Ibuprofen (Brufen)	0.5	4
Naproxen (Naprosyn)	0.25	4
Diclofenac (Voltarol)	5	47
Etodolac (Lodine)★★	4353	90
Meloxicam (Mobic)★★	118	69

★ = Designer Cox 2 selective drug
★★ = 'Incidental' Cox 2 selective

Table 9.3. Relative Cox-2 selectivity.

manufacturers had hoped for. But unfortunately there was a sting in the tail. There were 4 times as many heart attacks (myocardial infarctions) in the rofecoxib treated group, though fortunately there were no more cardiac deaths. The manufacturers were satisfied as to the GI safety profile, and explained the adverse effect on the heart on a proposed, but not actually proved, beneficial effect of the naproxen! (Bombardier et al 2000). I recall prescribing this drug to my patients with rheumatoid arthritis, aware of the advice given by the manufacturer not to prescribe it in high dosage to patients with a history of cardiovascular disease. In April 2002, Merck warned against an increased risk of cardiovascular events (heart attack and stroke). The conclusion drawn from this study was that Vioxx carried with it nearly four times the risk of developing a heart attack or stroke in high risk patients (i.e. with a previous history of this), but no increased risk in patients with a normal pre-trial risk.

The next year, another trial involving rofecoxib was published. It was called the APPROVe study, in which Merck hoped to emulate their rivals, Searle, who had earlier gained approval for their product, celecoxib, for prevention of pre-cancerous colo-rectal polyps. Unfortunately, the trial had to be terminated early, because 18 months into the trial, data accrued showing a doubling of risk of heart attack and stroke in the rofecoxib group. Prior to 18 months, this effect was not detected. The Federal Drugs Administration, the American regulatory authority, estimated that rofecoxib had caused between 88,000 and 139,000 heart attacks, of which 30–40% were fatal. On September 30th, 2004, Merck withdrew the drug. It was not unexpected therefore that litigation soon followed – and it did. On August 19th 2005, a jury in Texas awarded the widow of a 59 year old man who had died allegedly of a rofecoxib induced irregularity of heart beat, over 250 million US dollars!

At present, the most vexing question is whether the coxibs as a whole are more risk to the heart, or whether this is something peculiar to rofecoxib. For many patients there is no doubt rofecoxib was regarded very highly, especially by those with a history of stomach ulcers, and who had been very chary of NSAIDs. With the advent of rofecoxib, they had enjoyed considerable pain relief.

So now we have been enlightened as to the mode whereby aspirin reduces inflammation, but with this knowledge has come an awareness of the requirement for Cox-2 – that it is not purely an induced cyclooxygenase, but that it is also constitutive, albeit at low concentration, and that it is involved in preventing coagulation of blood, interference with which has been shown convincingly in the case of Vioxx, to lead to an increased risk of heart attacks. So by refining the effects of aspirin in order to prevent gastro-intestinal bleeding, we now have the situation of an increased risk of heart attacks. By turning the argument on its head, we may state that perhaps the bleeding tendency of aspirin and non-selective Cox-2 inhibitors could be advantageous in actually preventing heart attacks. This aspect will be explored in the next chapter.

Chapter Ten

THE RISE OF ASPIRIN

Coagulation (blood clotting), and bleeding

Why is this subject of relevance in a book about aspirin? Aspirin as everyone knows, has been a mainstay in treatment for common types of pain for over a century. It is still one of the most commonly purchased over the counter drugs for this purpose. Yet, as we have seen, its heritage, from salicylic acid, came with gastric irritant properties, which in many people, over the years, has led to stomach bleeding, rarely but occasionally fatal. This is believed to occur because of a local corrosive effect on the stomach lining. On the other hand, many people now take aspirin to prevent blood clots. So it will behove us to examine in further detail just where aspirin intervenes in these situations.

First of all it is essential to point out that the process of blood coagulation is extremely complicated, and way beyond the remit of this book. But if it is possible to present in a clear way what is by no means clear, then the author will feel that some good will have been served.

What is a clot? Anyone who has eaten black pudding will perhaps know that it consists of clotted pigs' blood to which seasoning and herbs have been added. A clot has the texture of jelly, but with time becomes harder and blacker. Eventually, by another process the reverse of that which caused it, the clot may liquefy. Amazing!

Evolution has required that animals which commonly fight in order to establish the fittest and strongest to carry on the germ line, and in so doing frequently get injured, and bleed, should have a mechanism whereby the flow of blood would be staunched. Common everyday traumatic events will also cause bleeding, and so the process is again invoked. The initial process of clotting (coagulation) is also termed **haemostasis**, and the opposite, i.e. the liquefaction of a clot, **fibrinolysis**.

Next we need to picture the blood vessel, be it an **artery** (large vessel carrying oxygenated blood under considerable pressure, towards the tissues and away from the heart), arterioles (smaller versions of arteries), capillaries (the smallest vessels – the end of the line before they again become larger), then leading to venules, which move blood, by now depleted of oxygen, at low pressure towards the heart. As these vessels get nearer to the heart they become larger, being known as **veins**, and the largest are known as the great veins. That coming from the abdomen, and including veins originating in the legs, is known as the **inferior vena cava**, and the largest veins draining the head are known as the **jugulars** which, after joining the **innominate** veins from the arms, drain into the **superior vena cava**.

Chapter Ten – The Rise of Aspirin

The inner lining of all these blood vessels consists of a smooth surface, called **endothelium**. Whilst the endothelium is smooth, blood rushing past will have streamlined flow, like a river along a smooth bank. If however the endothelium is roughened, or by some means rendered sticky, the formed elements of the blood (which will be described), will strike against the roughened surface, and the little pebble like fragments, called **platelets**, will adhere. This of course makes the roughened surface project more. To add to the traffic jam caused by these events, the platelets, the endothelium, and some of the proteins circulating in the blood (the non-cellular portion of unclotted blood is called **plasma**), will commence a most complicated series of events perhaps somewhat reminiscent of the dancing at a ceilidh, where people circulate in complex paths, then re-join, only to part in a well choreographed fashion. Similarly with these proteins, which include many clotting factors given numbers 1 to 13. The climax of the clotting reel is to form the substance of the clot, called **fibrin**. This has originated from a precursor substance called **fibrinogen**. The conversion is brought about by a protein called **thrombin**, which has been formed by the action of certain controlling substances upon its precursor, known as **prothrombin**. The complicated part concerns the interplay of the various factors 1–13, which will not be described.

The formed elements of the blood will now be introduced. They are the red blood cells, also known as **erythrocytes**, which give blood its colour, and which contain the pigment **haemoglobin**, whose job is to combine with oxygen in the lungs, and which incidentally give arterial blood its bright red colour, which can immediately be differentiated from the dark colour of venous blood, and for the reason that people with failing lungs often appear to have a bluish tinge around their lips, spoken of as 'cyanosis.' It also combines with carbon dioxide in the tissues, and returns via the veins, to the heart, and thence to the lungs to release carbon dioxide and take up oxygen. The red blood cells are the main constituents of blood clots. Then there are the white blood cells, of which there are several types. Most numerous are the **neutrophils**, which are designed to swallow (phagocytose) and kill bacteria, as well as foreign particles. Less frequent are **lymphocytes**, which are involved in conferring immunity, and killing viruses. Least common are **eosinophils** and **basophils**. These are involved in killing parasites including worms, but also come into play in allergies. **Monocytes** are important cells which work together with lymphocytes in conferring immunity, but they can also phagocytose. Lastly, but by no means least, are some peculiar particles, much smaller than the aforementioned cells. These are the platelets, as already mentioned, which have a central role in stopping bleeding from wounds, and in promoting the clotting process. Next to the red blood cells, they are the most numerous flowing structures in blood.

The process of coagulation is usually the consequence of a cut. This exposes damaged cells, including those lining capillaries, which interact with platelets. The platelets act as a sort of makeshift plug, see figure 10.1. But the process does not end there. The platelets release substances called **prostaglandins**, of which one, called **thromboxane A$_2$**, causes the local blood vessels to constrict, thus reducing the escape of blood. The platelets release another substance, called ADP, which acts as a kind of glue, thus sticking platelets together. Substances now released from the capillary lining, called the **endothelium**, and from the plug of platelets, stimulate the conversion of fibrinogen (the immediate clot precursor), to fibrin, the chief constituent of the clot itself. Factor 13 present in the blood, now acts as a sort of ball of twine, and winds around the clot, strengthening it. This of course is important, both in stopping the bleeding at the site of the clot, and to prevent fragments breaking away. Should this happen, they could travel on, and wreak havoc further along. This for instance, can happen when a piece of clot disengages from a clot in a calf vein, and travels along the veins, until it reaches the heart, from which it is pumped out to the lungs. Up to this point, every blood vessel has been getting progressively larger as it moves towards the heart. This situation continues as it enters the large artery leading out from the heart towards the lungs. This is the pulmonary artery. But from now on, as they go deep into the lungs, the blood vessels get smaller and smaller. The detached clot may now seriously block an artery in the lung. This is called a **pulmonary embolism**, and can cause immediate death, or if not, then severe shortness of breath, chest pain, and

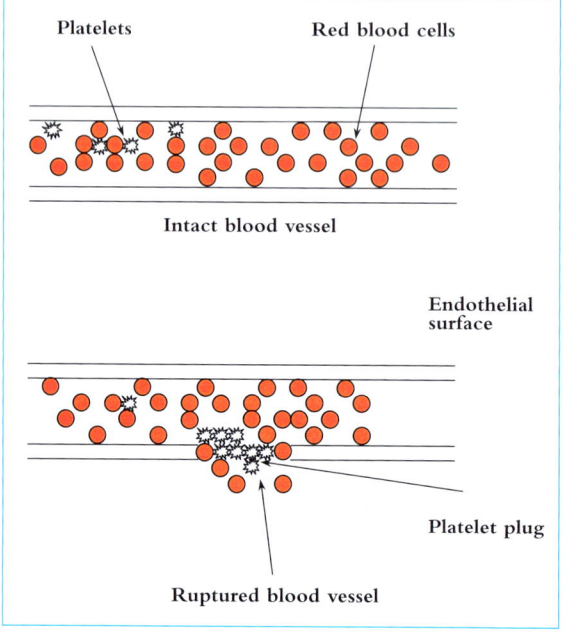

Figure 10.1. Platelets form a plug to stop bleeding.

Chapter Ten – The Rise of Aspirin

occasionally the coughing up of blood. It should be made clear that the blood flow along arteries is far quicker than that along veins. Platelets are particularly important in stopping bleeding in arteries, as they are capable of working in high speed turbulent conditions. By contrast, the flow of blood along the veins is more reminiscent of a slow moving stream, as compared to a gushing torrent. In the slow moving conditions found in the veins, conditions for the coagulation process are more concerned with the coagulation cascade of proteins, and less with the involvement of the blood platelets. This will be seen to be of importance in the treatment of venous thrombosis by anti-coagulants, like **warfarin**, as apart from arterial thrombosis, where a drug is needed to prevent the development of stickiness of the platelets. By now you may have guessed what is being driven at.

In February 1950, several momentous events were taking place. Top nuclear scientist Klaus Fuchs was charged with supplying Russian agents with information about how to construct an atom bomb. He had worked at Harwell as well as top secret American bases. On the other side of the world, Vietnam effectively became two nations, with Emperor Bao Dai recognised as its leader, by Britain and the United States, whereas Russia and its allies recognised Ho Chi Minh. At home, Clement Attlee for Labour won the general election with the closest result for 100 years. The interpretation was that the nation, whilst pleased with the Welfare State created in 1945, was not feeling enthusiastic about further Socialist experimentation.

Meanwhile in Glendale, California, a **Dr. Lawrence L. Craven** submitted an interesting letter to the editor of a journal called the Annals of Western Medicine and Surgery (Craven 1950). It read as follows:

"For several years, I have observed that hemorrhage following tonsillectomy occurs with noteworthy frequency when acetylsalicylic acid (aspirin) is administered for the relief of pain.

When Aspergum became available several years ago, I began the practice of routinely supplying each patient with a package of this product after a tonsillectomy. The patients were instructed to chew one stick, containing 3.5gr. of acetylsalicylic acid, one half hour before each meal and at bedtime in order to enable them to eat and sleep well. Although pain was usually materially relieved, in the following months, several of my patients had serious postoperative hemorrhages which were difficult to control. The bleeding was sometimes so severe that hospitalisation was necessary. In each instance the laboratory reported a prolonged coagulation time. Almost all of the hemorrhages occurred between the fifth and the eighth day postoperatively. After investigation, I discovered that in every instance of severe hemorrhage the patient had not only chewed the four sticks of Aspergum per day as ordered but had purchased an additional supply, consuming up to 20 sticks (70gr. of acetylsalicylic acid) daily. Although these doses do not seem inordinate when compared with the massive amounts administered to patients with rheumatic fever, rheumatic iritis and rheumatic heart disease, such large quantities of salicylates may be dangerous in the presence of a recent wound. This experience caused me to suspect that following operations including dental extractions, acetylsalicylic acid should perhaps be considered a dangerous drug unless its anticoagulant effect is counteracted by adequate amounts of vitamin K. For the past three years I have continued to prescribe aspirin for the relief of post-tonsillectomy pain but patients are also given not less than 2mg of Menadione (2-methyl-naphthoquinone) daily. No serious postoperative hemorrhages have occurred on this regimen. Similarly, in 9 instances of troublesome nosebleed, it was found that the patients had for various reasons been taking large doses of aspirin over long periods of time. None of these patients has had recurrences since discontinuing the use of salicylates.

Medical literature contains many reports concerning the anticoagulant effect of acetylsalicylic acid. –

An editorial in the *Journal of the American Medical Association* stated that aspirin is not only a dangerous drug when used postoperatively but is also contraindicated in the presence of peptic ulcer and may lead to massive hemorrhage in patients with rheumatic fever. Govan studied the effects of salicylates in 24 children and found that the prothrombin time was definitely prolonged in the majority but returned to normal after the medication was discontinued. –"

Craven went on to make some extremely controversial remarks:

"That the coagulation time of the blood may become shorter as certain individuals grow older is suggested by the progressive decrease in nosebleeds as well as in bleeding from shaving wounds which I, and no doubt other men, have experienced between youth and middle age. The apparently lower incidence of coronary disease and thrombosis in undernourished nations and lower income groups suggests that this change in coagulation time is to some extent due to over consumption of rich foods. However, only a small percentage of the many overweight middle aged and elderly women in the American population die of coronary thrombosis. A possible explanation of this apparently contradictory evidence is that women frequently use aspirin to relieve minor discomforts while men hesitate to employ such allegedly effeminate methods. Of course, other factors are also involved in thrombosis and coronary disease." (This is an astonishingly sexist allegation, yet such views were commonly held at the time, and the male gender could get away with remarks then which would create howls of protest nowadays).

"If further study confirms the impression that acetylsalicylic acid prolongs coagulation time, it would appear that the drug might be of value as a preventative of vascular thrombotic conditions, including coronary thrombosis –

During the past two years, I have advised all of my male patients between the ages of 40 and 65 to take from 10 to 30 grains of acetylsalicylic acid daily as a possible preventative of coronary thrombosis. More than 400 have done so, and of these, none has suffered a coronary thrombosis. From past experience, I should have expected at least a few thrombotic episodes among this group.

There would appear to be enough evidence of the antithrombotic action of acetylsalicylic acid to warrant further study under more carefully controlled conditions". (Bold italics by the author).

Of course Craven's claims would not convince any modern day designer of drug trials, or hard-headed statistician. Of his 400 volunteers, did they all inform him after 2 years of taking aspirin, that (a) they had taken the drug religiously, and (b), that they had definitely not had a heart attack, and (c) where was the electrocardiographic evidence to support this, and (e), most important of all, was there a control group of closely matched volunteers who promised not to take any aspirin for a similar period?

Craven's observations were inspired, but left certain questions unanswered. In a subsequent paper in 1953, he pointed out that many people at autopsy were found to have severe arteriosclerosis of their blood vessels, yet no evidence of local blood clot. This he attempted to explain by suggesting that perhaps there were methods of rapid dissolution of blood clots, so that by the time the autopsy was performed, they would have disappeared. There could be no doubt aspirin caused bleeding.

In his third-prize winning essay, he went on to describe an experiment he had performed on himself. He ingested 12 aspirin tablets daily for 5 days, and suffered a nosebleed. He repeated this twice more, and on each occasion suffered a profuse bleed. Prior to this, he had not had nosebleeds for 50 years. He admitted that there was no consensus of opinion of the effect of aspirin on the prothrombin level. But at that point, with the medical world well aware of the existence and value of anti-coagulants in medical practice, attention was focused on one particular test of blood coagulability, namely the **prothrombin time**. Patient's plasma was added to a mixture containing all the essentials for clotting to occur, (**thromboplastin**, prepared from the brain), except prothrombin. This is known as **Quick's** method.

---

38   MISSISSIPPI VALLEY MEDICAL JOURNAL

EXPERIENCES WITH ASPIRIN (ACETYLSALICYLIC ACID) IN THE NONSPECIFIC PROPHYLAXIS OF CORONARY THROMBOSIS*

Lawrence L. Craven, M.D.
Glendale, California

Figure 10.2. Craven's paper which won third prize in the 1952 Mississippi Valley Medical Society's essay contest.

The stop-watch was started as the constituents were reacted, the tube shaken gently, and the stop-watch clicked as soon as a clot appeared. Subsequently it was discovered that aspirin (and sulphonamides), caused an increase in the prothrombin time i.e. effectively caused a relative lack of prothrombin termed "hypoprothrombinaemia." To achieve this required aspirin in considerable dosage, more than is used nowadays to prevent thrombosis. Nevertheless, Craven stated that for the past 7 years, presumably 1946–1953, he had advised all male patients between the ages of 45 and 65, especially if overweight, or with a tendency to over eat and to lead a sedentary life with little or no physical exercise, to take 10 to 30 grains (600 to 1800 milligrams, or about 2 to 6 tablets of standard strength i.e. 300 milligrams each, per week), but in the course of time he found 5 to 10 grains to be sufficiently effective. Some patients managed with only 5 tablets per week, but many preferred 7, so that the same regimen was followed every day. In all, this treatment had been recommended to 1465 patients who were attending his practise for problems unrelated to the heart. During the time span studied, not one suffered a heart attack. He concluded:

"Aspirin (acetylsalicylic acid), taken consistently in small daily doses, has proved valuable in the non-specific prophylaxis of coronary thrombosis, before the first attack, as well as in the prevention of recurrences. The series is too small to be statistically significant, and observations were not carried out under scientific conditions. However, the anti-coagulative properties of aspirin cannot be doubted, and others have reported earlier that acetylsalicylic acid is a valuable adjunct to dicumarol" – (a drug similar to warfarin) – "in long-term anticoagulative therapy. The observations presented will have to be confirmed by clinical research. But they suggest strongly that aspirin medication for non-specific prophylaxis of coronary thrombosis is an inexpensive and innocuous procedure whose possible benefits should not be overlooked by the general practitioner."

His remarks concerning the usefulness of aspirin in the prevention of heart attacks was inspired, and largely ignored. His explanations, i.e. that it was working via an effect on the prothrombin level in the blood was wrong. There was another reason, which had eluded him.

What had not been appreciated was that other things than clots could obstruct narrowed blood vessels. In 1961, two scientists at Oxford came up with the idea that blood platelets might be responsible.

Medical students are taught the difference between the **clotting time**, and the **bleeding time**. (One recalls the immortal moment in the Doctor series film, when the pompous surgeon Sir Lancelot Spratt asks the hapless medical student Simon Sparrow, 'What is the bleeding time?' to which Sparrow replies 'A quarter to nine Sir').

The bleeding time is the time it takes for bleeding to stop after a standard cut is made in the skin of the forearm, using a lancet. First a cuff is placed over the upper

Chapter Ten – The Rise of Aspirin

arm, as for taking the blood pressure. It is inflated to 40 millimeters of mercury pressure (just enough to compress the veins, but not enough to stop arterial flow). This is the method described by **Ivy**. The cut is made, the stop-watch started. Blotting paper is applied every 30 seconds. Initially, the blood continues oozing, but after a short time, ceases. At this point the stop-watch is again pressed. The normal value for this test is 3 to 10 minutes. It is prolonged in patients who have an abnormality of their blood platelets, or have insufficient platelets. In the latter case, this would be detected earlier by counting them, nowadays using automated apparatus. The bleeding time test should not be carried out if there are too few platelets, as the result would be misleading. Drugs known to interfere with this test, by their effect on blood platelets, include aspirin (and, interestingly, cocaine).

The clotting time is a more complicated procedure, as described above. It is the test routinely carried out in anti-coagulant clinics, for the millions of patients on drugs such as warfarin, to prevent venous thrombosis, and also thrombus formation on heart valves in cases with atrial fibrillation (a state in which the smaller chambers of the heart beat fail to contract, but merely quiver, thus increasing the likelihood of clots to form). This used to be common in patients with narrowing of the mitral valve, due to previous rheumatic fever. Rheumatic fever is uncommon in the western world nowadays, but atrial fibrillation commonly occurs in patients with coronary artery disease, high blood pressure, and overactivity of the thyroid gland.

In 1962, a haematologist from Portsmouth, **John O'Brien**, was fascinated by these platelets. The author has also worked with them and what is special is that if you place a drop of blood from which the red cells have been removed, onto a glass slide, they are very abundant and actually twinkle at you. O'Brien showed that these platelets would spontaneously adhere to glass, regardless of temperature, and that this adherence was increased by a substance called adenosine diphosphate (ADP), but not by adenosine mono-or triphosphate. He postulated that platelets interacted with a surface activator. Incidentally, he showed that cocaine would also do this, both at 37°C and 0°C.

In 1968, **Harvey Weiss** in New York, took some volunteers, and measured their bleeding time. He compared the effect of aspirin (acetylsalicylic acid), 1.5 grams daily, against sodium salicylate or placebo taken for several days. 2 hours after ingestion, the bleeding time was estimated. Only aspirin affected it. It was felt that it did so by preventing the release of ADP by the platelets.

So now there was evidence that aspirin could affect both the coagulation process, using fairly high doses, with demonstrable reduction in prothrombin activity, whereas at low doses, it exhibited an effect on the adherence, or stickiness, of platelets. The time was fast approaching to see whether aspirin use among the general public, where its use was extremely common, was having an effect on the pattern of admissions to hospital.

So it was that in March 1974, one week after Conservative leader Edward Heath sought to form a coalition government with Jeremy Thorpe of the Liberal party, and

11 days before Princess Anne and her then husband, Mark Phillips, escaped a kidnap attempt, a paper appeared in the British Medical Journal summarising the findings of the **Boston Collaborative drug surveillance group**. Hospitals from the United States, Canada, New Zealand, Israel and Scotland participated. The method of investigation consisted of taking a drug history from patients, aged between 40 and 69 years, admitted to hospital with an acute heart attack ('acute myocardial infarction'), and comparing it with patients hospitalised for other diseases. Excluded under other diseases, were conditions likely to have resulted in aspirin ingestion, for example, chronic headaches, or arthritis. The non-myocardial infarction group were termed the "control" group, and included patients with chest, stomach or kidney diseases. The details were extracted by specially trained nurse monitors, who asked a variety of questions without hinting at the true purpose of the study, in order to prevent bias. Over 9,000 patients were targeted. After excluding patients who, for one reason or another failed to satisfy the criteria for inclusion, they were left with 325 myocardial infarct patients, and 3,807 controls. A second study was undertaken in the Boston area alone, and involved 451 myocardial infarct patients, and 10,091 controls. The results of both these studies are shown in the table.

From the data it could be calculated that in the first study, patients with heart attacks were nearly five and a half times less likely to be taking aspirin than patients admitted with the other diseases. In the second study, the figure indicated that they were twice less likely to be taking aspirin. Of course there were weaknesses in the study e.g. those patients too unfit to be interviewed, and those discharged within 72 hours of admission, and who therefore couldn't be interviewed. The authors of this paper even considered whether the findings could have arisen purely by chance. Statistics, as the reader knows, can be misleading. Nevertheless, the authors stated:

"Hence the available data, while suggestive, fall far short of establishing that aspirin prevents myocardial infarction. Thus these data should not preclude the conduct of controlled trials on ethical grounds. Such trials are vital before the use of aspirin for preventing myocardial infarction can be recommended with complete confidence –"

	Acute infarction and taking aspirin	*Other conditions and taking aspirin*
International study	0.9% (325 cases)	4.9% (3,807 cases)
National study	3.5% (451 cases)	7% (10,091 cases)

Table 10.1. Usage of aspirin among patients admitted for heart attacks ('acute infarction'), or for other reasons.

Chapter Ten – The Rise of Aspirin

In 1979, **Elwood** and **Sweetnam** of the Medical Research Council Epidemiology Unit, based in Cardiff, published the results of a randomised placebo controlled double-blind trial of aspirin in 1682 patients who had had a myocardial infarct. After one year, of 832 aspirin treated patients, 102 died (12.3%), and of 850 placebo treated patients, 126 died (14.8%). Although these results (a 17% reduction in deaths from all causes), were consistent with hitherto published evidence, they were not conclusive.

The case for using aspirin to prevent re-infarction was beginning to look a little shaky. And matters were not helped by the publication of another trial in February 1980. Whilst in Britain we were suffering the economic damage of a seven weeks long national steel strike, costing £2 million each day, sparked by the proposed closure of the Llanwern and Port Talbot plants in Wales, the aspirin myocardial infarction study research group (AMIS) sponsored by the National Heart, Lung, and Blood Institute of Bethesda, Maryland, published its results in the Journal of the American Medical Association on February 15th. The major objective of this study, was to see whether the administration of aspirin to men and women who had suffered at least one previous heart attack, would lower their overall mortality over a three years period. It was a double blind placebo controlled study. It also sought to establish whether it reduced death from coronary heart disease specifically. 4,524 people aged between 30 and 69 years were randomised to receive either one gram of aspirin or placebo daily. 2,267 people got aspirin, 2,257 placebo. At 3 years, the all-cause mortality of the aspirin group was 10.8%, and 9.7% in the placebo group. When mortality from coronary heart disease was lumped together with non-fatal myocardial infarction, the figure for aspirin was 14.1%, and for placebo 14.8%. This was just a hint of a beneficial effect of aspirin. When however, non-fatal myocardial infarction alone was considered, the figure for aspirin was 6.3%, and for placebo 8.1%. When they compared strokes, they also found a similar effect, namely that aspirin treatment appeared protective. But because overall, there was no significant protection from death by any cause e.g. being run over by a bus, they concluded that aspirin should not be recommended for routine use in patients who had survived one myocardial infarction.

In 1985, the Physicians' Health Study Research Group published their findings following a randomised trial of aspirin and beta-carotene among United States physicians. It was a somewhat unusual study in that it was using 'reliable' patients i.e. physicians, who had never had a heart attack, stroke, mini-stroke (also called a transient ischaemic attack, or TIA), cancer, current liver or kidney disease, peptic ulcer, or gout. The aspirin was used to hopefully prevent heart attacks and strokes, and the beta carotene, cancer. The study comprised male physicians 40 to 85 years of age, resident in the USA at the start of the study in 1982. After suitable weeding out from the original 59,285 willing subjects, 33,223 doctors were enrolled. For 18 weeks, they all received both aspirin 'Bufferin', 325 milligrams, to be taken on alternate days, plus

End Point	Aspirin	Placebo	Degree of protection
Fatal heart attack	5	18	75%
Non-fatal heart attack	99	171	44%
Total	104	189	47%

Table 10.2. The Physicians' Health Study (see Preventive Medicine 1985. Volume 14, pages 165–168). 325 milligrams aspirin on alternate days, versus placebo.

50 milligrams of beta carotene, also to be taken on an alternate day basis. About 11,000 dropped out for various reasons, leaving a hard core of 22,071 eager and willing participants. Half continued on the aforementioned therapy, the other half were given placebo tablets. The trial was intended to run for several years. However, in 1988, on January 28th the New England Journal of Medicine published a Special Report. It stated that, at a special meeting on December 18th 1987, the Data Monitoring Board of the Physicians' Health Study, took the unusual step of recommending that the trial be stopped, at least from the point of view of aspirin, because one group was showing far less non-fatal and fatal myocardial infarctions. It was therefore essential to break the code in case the aspirin was, in effect, killing people. But, amazingly, it transpired that the aspirin group were being protected from heart attacks. Some of the numbers are shown in table 10.2.

The above findings were statistically highly significant, with P values of 0.006 or less (anything less than 0.05 is significant 95% of the time. These figures therefore were highly significant).

The same could not be said for the figures concerning strokes. Fatal strokes were 3 times more likely in the aspirin group, and combining fatal and non-fatal strokes, the increase was 15%, but because the range of figures was very great, they failed to reach significance. Nevertheless, there was a trend, and considering that aspirin reduces clot formation (by whatever means), the price that was paid was a slightly increased risk of a bleed into the brain. (It should be made clear that no effect on heart attack or stroke was found as a result of taking beta carotene). There were a small number of cases of severe or fatal stroke, 10 out of over 11,000 participants on aspirin, versus 2 on placebo. This difference was significant, P value 0.02. So the experts then had to work out whether the swings (heart attacks prevented) outweighed the roundabouts (strokes). When all events were combined, i.e. fatal plus non-fatal heart attacks, plus fatal and non-fatal strokes, the overall protection given by aspirin was 23%, P value 0.006. It must be remembered that some participants died of other causes than those mentioned. When these were compared, there was no difference in people on or off aspirin.

Chapter Ten – The Rise of Aspirin

Almost simultaneously, the British Medical Journal, on January 30th 1988, published the outcome of a randomised trial of daily aspirin, 500 milligrams, in 5139 apparently healthy male doctors.(Randomised trial of prophylactic daily aspirin in British male doctors. **Peto R** et al). It was argued that by the late 1970s, it had been established that taking aspirin following a heart attack would prevent further attacks. It seemed likely therefore that giving aspirin to people who had never had an attack might also be preventive. This trial was not as homogeneous as the American, in that some doctors received 500 milligrams of aspirin, others 300 milligrams of enteric coated tablets. There was no placebo tablet. For pain relief, paracetamol was allowed. Twice as many participants received aspirin compared to no aspirin. Unfortunately, some of the doctors taking aspirin stopped it on account of stomach related problems, which was circumvented in some cases by switching to the enteric coated preparation. Some of the doctors allocated no aspirin started taking it when they developed heart or arterial disease. So what did the results show?

The results were expressed as deaths per 10,000 man years. For the aspirin treated group the figure was 63.2, and for the controls, (no aspirin), 62.3. Very disappointing! Even when they compared all sorts of other events, no significant differences emerged, except for migraine and musculo-skeletal disorders where, surprise surprise, the aspirin group fared significantly better. Paradoxically, the United Kingdom trial suffered from there being too few myocardial infarctions to allow any trend, if indeed there was one, to emerge. The authors rather sadly concluded that no benefit from the administration of aspirin to healthy British doctors had been demonstrated.

In the same journal, following on the same page, appeared the findings of the United Kingdom aspirin trial in cases of transient ischaemic attack (abbreviated 'TIA'), or minor stroke. An ischaemic attack is a mini-stroke evidenced by a sudden paralysis of one side, or loss of speech, lasting for a short period, often minutes or hours, but not longer than 24 hours. A minor stroke can last up to one week. Between 1979 and 1985, 2,435 patients thought to have had a TIA or a minor stroke were randomly allocated either aspirin 600 milligrams twice daily, 300 milligrams once daily, or placebo. There were over 800 patients in each group. The hope of the statistically biased observer in such a trial, is that the number of relevant events encountered will be high, so that an effect of the treatment will be made more obvious. Alas, this is often not the case. Perhaps this is just as well for the patient, but it makes life difficult for the epidemiologist. In the event, by 1986, about 700 patients were still alive from each group. No obvious difference. Deaths in the groups were 15% (placebo), 13.4% (aspirin 300 milligrams), and 13.6% (aspirin 1200 milligrams). However, overall among the patients who survived the study, the effects of aspirin on the numbers of non-fatal vascular (i.e. related to blood vessels) events were to reduce the number of non-fatal strokes and non-fatal heart attacks. Interestingly in this study, though aspirin didn't protect against vascular death, it did seem to offer some protection against death from other causes, including cancer.

A third paper in the same issue (Secondary prevention of vascular disease by prolonged antiplatelet treatment, authored by the Antiplatelet Trialists' Collaboration, of the Clinical Trial Service Unit of the Nuffield department of Clinical Medicine, Radcliffe Infirmary, Oxford) related to the combined findings from 25 randomised trials of antiplatelet treatment for patients with minor and major strokes, and unstable angina or heart attacks. 29,000 patients were involved, of whom 3,000 had died. (Sad though this sounds, it plays into the hands of the epidemiologists, because without deaths there would be no end-point, no results, and no statistics. At least in this regard, death is of use!). Treatment had no effect on non-vascular mortality, but reduced vascular mortality by 15%, and non-fatal strokes or heart attacks by 30%. There was no difference in dose of aspirin (or other antiplatelet drugs – sulphinpyrazone and dipyridamole). The final point made was that this was a secondary prevention trial of patients at pre-determined higher risk because they had already manifested vascular disease. In the case of primary prevention ("let's give aspirin to everyone"), the findings might well be different, because it might cause as many brain haemorrhages as thromboses prevented.

In 1989, the final report of the Physicians' Health study (see above) appeared in the New England Journal of Medicine (volume 321, part 3, pages 129–135), from Harvard Medical School in Boston, USA. It will be recalled that it was a randomised, double blind, placebo-controlled trial, to see whether aspirin in a dose of 325 milligrams daily (approximately equivalent to one adult strength tablet) decreased cardiovascular mortality (and whether beta carotene reduced the incidence of cancer). Because early on the data appeared to show a marked difference in one of the groups in cardiovascular mortality, the study had to be unblinded. This was because the group that was surviving better might have been taking placebo, and we might have been seeing aspirin causing excess deaths. Only by breaking the code would we know. Among 22,071 participants, followed for an average time period of 5 years, there appeared to be a 44% reduction in the risk of myocardial infarction ('heart attack'), with a P value (anything below 0.05 being statistically significant), of less than 0.00001 in one of the treatment groups. Nail biting until the code was broken. Breathe again! The result indicated a beneficial effect of the group receiving aspirin. Sweet relief! There was however, a slight increase in haemorrhagic stroke ('brain haemorrhage'), but statistically it did not reach significance. It could therefore be argued quite reasonably, that this was purely due to chance. Interestingly, when they looked at the various age groups, it was seen that this benefit was only present in the over 50s. The price paid was an insignificant increase in the risk of a stomach ulcer. Although this trial demonstrated a reduction in heart attacks, there was no reduction in mortality from all cardiovascular causes. One might express this by saying that aspirin reduced the number of non-fatal heart attacks in the over 50s. Overall, whilst reducing the risk of myocardial infarction, its effect on stroke and total cardiovascular deaths remained inconclusive because of an inadequate number of participants.

The Physicians' Health study, (1994) looked at the effect on the incidence of myocardial infarction of different frequencies of aspirin administration in 22,071 male physicians from the United States. They had no previous history of cardiovascular or cerebrovascular disease ('primary prevention') and were prescribed aspirin on alternate days. It was carried out in double-blind placebo controlled fashion. The average duration of follow up was 5 years. Interestingly, they also studied the effect of how good the participants were at taking their aspirin. This was done by a questionnaire which included checking on the previous medical history. This could be subsequently verified by a perusal of their medical records. They found that poor adherence ('not taking the aspirin properly', i.e. taking less than 50% of the tablets), was found among cigarette smokers, the obese, those not prone to taking exercise, and with a history of angina. Therefore they weeded out those with poor compliance, and looked at the others. Those on aspirin had a 51% reduction in myocardial infarction compared to the good compliers in the placebo group. Amongst the poor compliers, those on aspirin still had a reduction (of 17%), but this was found not to be statistically significant. Tantalisingly, the compliant placebo group had a lower risk overall of death compared to their non-compliant colleagues, but no decrease in the incidence of myocardial infarction.

The fear of aspirin causing death by haemorrhage in the brain is a very real one. This was addressed in a study published in the Journal of the American Medical association ('JAMA'), in 1998. This report was based on the data accrued from analysing several trials ('meta-analysis'). All trials published in the English language before July 1997 in which participants were randomised to receive aspirin or placebo for at least one month, and in which the type of stroke (haemorrhagic or thrombotic) was reported. In all, 16 trials involving 55,462 participants were analysed. 108 cases of haemorrhagic stroke were identified. The average dose of aspirin equated to just under one adult type tablet daily for 3 years. Among 10,000 persons, 12 more haemorrhagic strokes occurred in the aspirin as compared to the placebo treated group. But there were 137 fewer myocardial infarcts, and 39 fewer thrombotic strokes. The conclusion reached was that the overall benefit of aspirin on the prevention of myocardial infarction and ischaemic stroke ('cerebral thrombosis') outweighed its adverse effects, namely increased risk of haemorrhagic stroke in most populations. A subsequent review (Gorelick 2005) concluded that the benefits of aspirin significantly outweigh the risk of major haemorrhage. A reasonable estimate of the risk of haemorrhagic stroke with use of aspirin in primary prevention was 1 event in 5000 patient years.

In 2000, Peter Elwood, Controller for Applied Public Health Medicine at the University of Wales College of Medicine in Cardiff, wrote in the Cardiovascular Journal of South Africa that although aspirin was of undoubted value in secondary prevention of myocardial infarction, and that there was only limited evidence that it was of value in primary prevention, nevertheless, where infarction seemed likely on the basis of a risk estimate, aspirin should be administered by a doctor, nurse or paramedic on first contact with a patient experiencing sudden severe chest pain. Patients already known to be at risk should be advised to carry aspirin tablets on their person at all times, and to chew or swallow one or two as soon as the typical symptoms strike.

In the same year, from Oslo appeared a paper looking at the effect of careful blood pressure control and aspirin taking on the incidence of heart attacks and strokes. In addition, they wanted to compare the effects on men and women. The author was **Dr. S.E. Kjeldsen** from the Department of Cardiology. They found that careful control of blood pressure alone was protective in women, and that aspirin conferred no significant additional benefit, whereas in men, with well controlled blood pressure, the addition of aspirin did significantly reduce the risk of heart attacks.

Based on previous observations that warfarin, an anti-coagulant, conferred a protective effect against re-infarction, as did aspirin, an anti-platelet agent, the question arose as to whether a combination of the two would have an even better effect. In the warfarin aspirin reinfarction study ('WARIS II'), the end point was death, reinfarction or thromboembolic stroke, whichever came first over a four year period. (An embolus is a portion of blood clot which becomes detached from wherever it arose, and travels along with the flow of blood. Eventually it may cause a blockage which can range from trivial without any symptoms, to catastrophic and fatal. In the venous system, it can cause chest pain, breathlessness and sudden death if the main arteries to the lungs are affected. This is known as a pulmonary embolism, or 'PE'. In the arterial system, a clot may detach from the wall of the heart where the heart muscle has been damaged as a result of an infarct, and travel through the carotid arteries to the brain, causing a stroke). After a first heart attack, taking aspirin (160mg) was 19% inferior to taking warfarin, and 29% inferior to taking both (aspirin 75mg). However, the benefits conferred by warfarin were outweighed by the risks of bleeding. Out of 3,630 patients, major bleeds occurred in 8 patients on aspirin, 33 taking warfarin, and 28 taking a combination. This paper was by **Dr. S.A. Doggrell** in 2003 from the School of Biomedical Sciences at the University of Queensland.

Strokes frequently occur as a consequence of atrial fibrillation ('AF'). This is a situation in which the two smaller chambers of the heart, called the atria (as apart from the larger chambers which are called the ventricles), instead of contracting at a rate of 50 to 160 per minute, quiver at a rate of about 400 per minute. This quivering, or fibrillation, is ineffective at moving the blood along. Stagnation ensues, and this predisposes to formation of a clot. AF occurs after heart attacks, in high blood pressure ('hypertension'), rheumatic heart disease, overactive thyroid, and sometimes in viral infections of the heart muscle ('myocarditis'). The clot may be harmless at its site of origin, but if it detaches, severe consequences may follow, as already described above. Anti-coagulation with warfarin is the most common form of treatment but has the disadvantage of requiring careful control by measuring the coagulability (or clottability) of the blood. If too much warfarin is given, there will be a risk of haemorrhage, if too little, then emboli may form. In some people, it is very difficult to find the correct dose of warfarin, and this in turn can be affected by certain other drugs which the patient may be taking, e.g. non-steroidal anti-inflammatories ('NSAIDs'). In 2003, **Dr. S.J. Connolly**, from Hamilton Health Sciences in Canada, presented an overview of several trials, which compared the effectiveness of warfarin as compared to aspirin in prevention of strokes. Warfarin reduced strokes by 67%, whereas aspirin only by 22%. But 70–100% more major haemorrhages occurred with warfarin. The perceived message therefore is that warfarin should be given to patients with AF, unless they already have a high risk of bleeding e.g. active peptic ulcer. In the absence of increased bleeding risk, but where control of coagulation status on warfarin is difficult, or presents problems e.g. living in remote areas with logistical difficulties in having the necessary regular blood tests carried out, then aspirin may be used instead.

In regard to the thorny question of the value of aspirin in the primary prevention of cardiovascular disease i.e. protective effects when given to a population who have

Title of trial	*No. participants*	
Physicians Health Study		22,071
British Doctors Trial		5,139
Thrombosis Prevention Trial		5,085
hypertension optimal treatment study		18,790
primary prevention project		4,495
Total		55,580
OVERALL	**32% REDUCTION IN RISK OF FIRST MYOCARDIAL INFARCT**	
	15% REDUCTION ALL IMPORTANT VASCULAR EVENTS, no significant effects on non-fatal stroke or vascular death	

Table 10.3. Aspirin in the prevention of a first heart attack – an overview of several clinical trials (Eidelmans 2003).

not already been diagnosed with cardiovascular disease, predominantly heart attacks, an overview of several studies by **R.S. Eidelmans** in 2003 provided strong support that aspirin reduces the risk of a first heart attack, as shown in the table below. A computerised search of trials published in English was instigated.

The authors concluded: **"The current totality of evidence provides strong support for the initial finding from the Physician's Health study that aspirin reduces the risk of a first myocardial infarct. For apparently healthy individuals whose 10 year risk of a first coronary event is 10% or greater, according to the US Preventive Services Task Force and the American Heart Association, the benefits of long-term aspirin are likely to outweigh any risks."**

Despite all the accumulated data, the authors noted that there was under-utilisation of aspirin and mis-medication. By this was meant the fact that some people were taking what they thought was aspirin, when in fact they were taking paracetamol (acetaminophen), or non-steroidal anti-inflammatory drugs (e.g. diclofenac – 'Voltarol' or 'Voltaren'). For a list of virtually all aspirin or aspirin containing preparations, see end of chapter 11.

There can be little doubt that aspirin sales are strong, that the general public are aware of its potential benefit in preventing heart attacks, and strokes, and are still taking the drug as a pain killer. They are still poorly aware of its risks regarding bleeding from the gut, though this is always explained in the accompanying leaflet present within every box. The revelation of how aspirin works in relieving pain, by its effect on prostaglandin synthesis (Chapter 9) was followed by the production of selective Cox 2 inhibitors. The fact that one in particular, namely rofecoxib (Vioxx), was associated with an increased and unexpected risk of heart attacks and strokes, led to an urgent re-evaluation of this group of drugs, and the withdrawal of rofecoxib. The complex effects of these drugs on blood platelets and kidneys, as well as cyclooxygenases involved in prostaglandin synthesis, has in effect brought us round full circle to examine the other effect of aspirin, and perhaps its most valuable one so far – namely prevention of clotting through its effect on blood platelets. The major killers remain heart attacks and cancer, and, as we shall see, aspirin may under certain circumstances also be of value in preventing the latter!

Chapter Eleven

THE FUTURE

1. Colon polyps and colon cancer

The writings as far back as the hieratics of the Eber's papyrus to the present day, span over 4000 years, in which salicylates, whether as bark extract, meadowsweet, wintergreen or tablets of aspirin or its several variants, have been found beneficial variously for relief of fevers, pains, inflammatory swellings, or corns. In more recent times, aspirin has been found to be of immense value in the prevention of heart attacks and strokes, as described in the previous chapter. Discoveries of these properties have come about serendipitously, and not necessarily as a consequence of the reasoning of the time e.g. the doctrine of signatures which was the thought in the mind of the Reverend Edward Stone in the 18th century, leading to the historic letter to the Royal Society describing the use of the willow bark for the treatment of agues (fevers), whereas serendipity and an astute mind permitted the observation of Lawrence Craven in the 1950s, in his post-tonsillectomy patients given aspirin-containing chewing gum, and who then went on to manifest a bleeding tendency. This was accompanied by his recommendation to all his physician colleagues to take aspirin in order to prevent the thrombotic accompaniment of heart attacks. The methodical elucidation of the mysteries of Cox-1 and Cox-2, with the target of selective inhibition of the latter, was followed by the anticipated reduction in adverse events relating to the gastro-intestinal tract. Applied science! But what was unexpected, was the increased risk of heart attacks, as revealed by experience gained using Vioxx. However, chance findings have then been followed by epidemiological and laboratory research, which has proved fruitful. It is likely that chance observation will continue to reveal avenues worthy of exploration. This has been the case with what will follow in this chapter. By way of background, the reader is reminded that colorectal cancer is one of the most common cancers in the industrialised world. It is the third most common cancer and third most lethal in the USA, with an anticipated annual incidence in the USA in 1996 of 133,500 new cases, with 55,300 deaths (Berkel 1996).

In 1976, scientists at the National Heart and Lung Institute in Maryland, USA were taking further the observation that salicylates including aspirin would inhibit growth of bacteria, and also DNA and protein synthesis in dividing immune cells. They wondered whether this could have any application in cancer. Quite justifiably therefore, they chose to use mice which had been injected with tumour cells, in order to detect any changes in the rate at which these tumours progressed, either in the presence of aspirin, or another non-steroidal anti-inflammatory drug called indomethacin, or without either

(Hial 1976). Their experiments showed that daily administration by mouth of these drugs reduced growth of these tumours by about 40%–50% (they used two types of tumour). In 1973, aspirin and indomethacin had been shown to inhibit bone tumour deposits in rats (Powles 1973). The concept of the use of indomethacin in treating a tumour was taken forward in 1980, when workers at the University of Colorado Medical School in Denver, described 3 cases of human desmoid tumours which responded (Waddell 1980). (A desmoid tumour is not malignant, but can cause damage by local invasion. It typically arises in the abdominal wall muscles, but can affect the chest, as in the first case, to be described). This was a 38 year old engineer, found to have a large swelling behind the breastbone, and growing backwards into the membrane surrounding his heart. Surgeons were only able to cut part of it away, and it promptly grew back. Several anti-tumour drugs and radiotherapy were tried. The tumour shrank down to 8.5cm by 7.5 cm, by 1 cm. By now a lot of fluid appeared around the heart, and for this, the patient received 100 milligrams of indomethacin daily (the sort of dose commonly used today to treat rheumatoid arthritis). Over the next 2 months, the tumour disappeared.

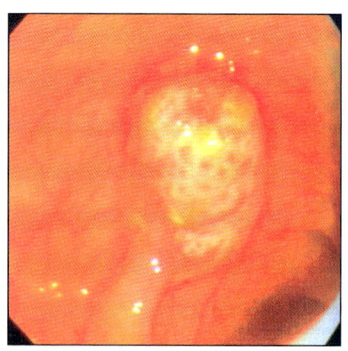

Figure 11.1. A large polyp, in the lower left portion, as seen through a colonoscope. (Reprinted from 'Clinical Medicine', Gastro-intestinal disease, page 274 by Kumar P & Clark M, 5th Edition, 2002, with permission from Elsevier).

Familial polyposis of the colon is a serious disease with a known mutation on the 5th human chromosome. It is inherited and dominant i.e. everyone with the gene gets the disease. The disease consists of a variable number of polyps (excrescences) ranging from a few to thousands, in the colon. The appearance of a colonic polyp is shown in figure 11.1.

It invariably leads eventually to cancer of the colon, average age 39 years. The gene is present in 1 in a million people. The development of the cancer is prevented by removing the entire colon, and the rectum with the contents of the bowel being drained through a pouch of gut, called ileum, through the abdominal wall, covered by an ileostomy bag. A variant of this condition is called Gardner's syndrome, in which case, these patients also have benign bony tumours called osteomas, and skin cysts, plus various other features including a predisposition to desmoid tumours. Families with affected members are urged to undergo screening for the gene, and when found, these unfortunate people are advised to have this operation as soon as possible. This naturally is devastating news to anyone, but especially youngsters. Waddell and Loughry (1983) described four members of a Gardner's syndrome family who had rectal and colonic polyps treated with a non-steroidal anti-

Chapter Eleven – The Future

inflammatory drug called sulindac (also known as Clinoril). The polyps almost completely disappeared.

Having read this paper, some doctors in Portugal came across a 19 year old patient with familial polyposis, with multiple polyps throughout colon, rectum and stomach. Total removal of the colon and rectum was proposed, but these doctors knew that this procedure was likely to have psychosocial effects, including the possibility of impotence. In addition, this particular man would also need a total removal of his stomach (gastrectomy). The consequences of this would be a permanent malnourished state, with associated unpleasant symptoms such as dumping syndrome, plus chronic anaemia due to a combination of iron, vitamin B12 and folic acid deficiency. Not much of a prospect! These surgeons published their (and the patient's) dilemma (Gonzaga 1984). Luckily Dr. Waddell read the article, and wrote to Dr. Gonzaga suggesting a trial of a non-steroidal anti-inflammatory drug, based on his previous findings. Accordingly, this was explained to the patient, who gave informed consent to try such a drug (sulindac). Prior to commencing treatment he had thousands of colorectal adenomatous polyps. After a year's treatment with sulindac, he was left with only six small rectal polyps (Gonzaga 1985). The hope would remain that by removing these benign adenomatous polyps, the eventual cancers would also be prevented. This however has not been proved – in other words, we do not know whether colon cancer when it appears, has necessarily arisen from an adenomatous polyp, or whether it has arisen *de novo* independently of the polyps. Were this to be the case, there would be no point in treating or observing the polyps. On the other hand, if it were the case, then by using drugs which encouraged the disappearance of polyps, the colon cancer would hopefully be prevented, and without recourse to mutilating surgery.

In 1988, some Australian workers, using a questionnaire, reported their findings based on a retrospective survey of 715 cases of colorectal cancer, and 715 age and sex matched people who did not have colorectal cancer, to see whether there were any differences in their previous medical history, reported symptoms, and previous medications (Kune 1988). Patients with colorectal cancer were less likely to have hypertension, heart disease, stroke, chronic chest disease, and chronic arthritis. "Haemorrhoids" were commoner among the colorectal cancer cases. (The lay meaning for "haemorrhoids" may hide a more sinister cause, or it could indicate that constipation – a recognised common cause of rectal bleeding – was more common among the colorectal cancer cases). No differences were found between groups, for asthma, diabetes, diverticular disease, nervous breakdowns, or allergies. The answers to questions regarding medications were very interesting, see table 11.1. No significant differences were found for non-steroidal anti-inflammatory drug (NSAID) usage, steroids, oral contraceptives, tranquillizers and sedatives, or sleeping pills. This was when colon and rectal cancer cases combined were studied. When colon and rectal cancer cases separately were analysed,

Previous Medication	Males		Females	
	With Cancer	Without Cancer	With Cancer	Without Cancer
Aspirin alone, or in Combination	10.5%	16.8%	11.9%	20.2%
Vitamin A	2%	7%	1.7%	7.2%
Vitamin C	5.2%	11.6%	4.5%	12.7%

Table 11.1. Effect of prior aspirin, vitamin A and Vitamin C on cancer (unclassified) showing significant differences between cases and controls (P<0.001 for females, and males plus females combined. For males, P=0.02) (388 male cases, 398 controls; 713 female cases, 727 controls) (from Kune et al 1988).

there was a significant reduction in NSAID use among colon cancer cases. Other risk factors they found were low intake of dietary fibre vegetables, cruciferous vegetables (e.g. cabbage), dietary Vitamin C, pork, fish, other meats, vitamin supplements, low or high intake of milk drinks, high fat intake, high beef intake (males only).

The important take home message from the authors was that there was a statistically significant deficit of the use of aspirin and aspirin-containing compounds among cases of colorectal cancer, and this significant difference remained regardless of hypertension, heart disease, chronic arthritis, or diet. They felt that aspirin may have an important role in prevention of colorectal cancer.

In 1994, another 'case-control' study was carried out, this time in Atlanta, Georgia (Peleg 1994). It differed from the previously described one, in that for each 'case' (of colorectal cancer), there were four age and sex-matched controls. Patients were asked about their previous consumption of aspirin, NSAIDs, and acetaminophen (paracetamol). This study differed from previous ones, in that it sought to record in a reliable fashion the cumulative dose of previous medication, based on replies to specially constructed questions e.g over a 208 period of observation, taking a named drug 0 days a week, meant 0 tablet days of exposure, less than 1 day a week, equated to 0–208 tablet days, 1–3 days a week, 208–624 tablet days, and more than 3 days a week, to 624 tablet days or more during the observation period. The next step was to calculate the mean dose of these drugs as ascertained from the pharmacy records of the hospital concerned. The duration of drug history was 4 years, i.e. a record of what drugs these patients had been taking in the 4 years prior to the diagnosis of colorectal cancer. The results are shown in table 11.2. What is not shown, is the effect of paracetamol. This drug which was also studied, showed no effect in regard to risk

Chapter Eleven – The Future

reduction. This is a shame from the point of view of patients who might experience indigestion or bleeding as a consequence of having to take aspirin, or NSAIDs, but represents another possible advantage of aspirin, not shared by its arch analgesic rival, paracetamol. The authors of this paper were self-critical, and pointed out that some patients taking aspirin or NSAIDs for whatever reason, would develop bleeding, which would have brought them to the attention of a doctor. If ultimately, after investigation, they were found to have a polyp, then its treatment would likely have reduced the risk of subsequent colorectal cancer.

If these drugs do indeed offer protection, then we might expect to find a reduced frequency in patients with diseases for which aspirin or NSAID therapy would be likely, e.g. rheumatoid arthritis. In 1996, Kauppi and colleagues in Finland looked at the records of 9,469 patients with rheumatoid arthritis who were hospitalised between 1970 and 1991. The total patient-years observed was 65,400. The combined incidence of all malignancies was greater for rheumatoid patients than for the general population (increase, 16%), but that for colorectal cancer was reduced by 38%. They did not actually check whether the rheumatoid patients were in fact taking aspirin or NSAIDs, but it is very likely they were.

Exposure to aspirin (days)	*Reduction of colorectal cancers*
Less than 208 days	48% (range 9–70%)
208–624 days	68% (range 6–88%)
More than 624 days	92% (range 41–99%)

Exposure to non-aspirin NSAIDs	
Less than 350 days	33% (range 52–123%)★
More than 350 days	66% (range 23–85%)

Cumulative aspirin dose (grams)	*Reduction of colorectal cancers*
Less than 66 grams	59% (range 19–79%)
66–313 grams	54% (range 5–77%)
More than 313 grams	75% (range 7–91%)

Cumulative nonaspirin NSAID dose (units)	*Reduction of colorectal cancers*
Less than 325	20% (range 50–129%)★
More than 325	62% (range 22–82%)

★ Not statistically significant

Table 11.2. Effect of exposure to aspirin and non-aspirin NSAIDs during the study period on the appearance of colorectal cancer (from Peleg et al 1994).

The method(s) by which these drugs work against colorectal (and hopefully, other cancers), may be by 3 different ways:

1. By boosting the response of immune cells.
Whereas under normal circumstances, immune cells only respond to substances *(antigens)* for which they have memory, *mitogens* are substances capable of non-specifically stimulating huge swathes of immune cells without the need for triggering their specific antigen receptors. It has been found that in cancer, the response to mitogens may be weak, but salicylates can restore it. Indomethacin has been shown to enhance immune cell responses from patients with various forms of cancer.

2. By inhibition of prostaglandins.
Prostaglandin E2 has been shown to stimulate the growth of some tumour cell lines, which can be inhibited by the presence of prostaglandin inhibitors. It will be recalled from chapter 9 that aspirin and NSAIDs work by inhibiting cyclooxygenase, which is a step in the formation of prostaglandins. Prostaglandin E2 is a kind of sleep inducing drug for the immune system, and these drugs may help keep it awake. In some types of cancer, the tumour cells themselves produce these prostaglandins e.g colon tumours. Some workers have shown that the greater the colonic tumour size the larger the production of prostaglandin E2 (Narisawa 1990).

There is good evidence that mechanisms involved in malignant change of cells and their growth are affected by prostaglandin production, and this may well be an avenue for exploration in preventing formation and subsequent proliferation of tumours.

3. Induction of apoptosis
Mortality is a subject not exactly known for producing a sense of good cheer around the dinner table, but the reader is invited to ponder on what would happen if the cells of the body, most of which are occasionally dividing, never died. In fact it is most important that old cells are from time to time removed and replaced. Nature has designed this beautifully, and the process is known as *apoptosis,* or 'programmed cell death'. It is a basic rule for all cells, though they can also die by being subjected to physical, chemical, or biological trauma e.g. by germs. This form of cell death, is known as *necrosis*. An example of the latter, is the pus which discharges from an abscess. It is made up of dead cells, including tissue cells, immune cells, and dead bacteria. Cancer cells on the other hand, do not generally undergo apoptosis, and may be regarded as immortal. In fact, this is the reason that cancer cell lines can so easily be preserved and kept in continuous culture. By contrast, non-cancer cells will always die after a certain number of divisions. So another strategy for dealing with cancer would be to induce apoptosis in them. Laboratory studies using colorectal cancer cell lines, and following their growth cycles, have demonstrated arrest of growth at certain stages when exposed to sulindac or

salicylate. Interestingly, a precursor of sulindac called sulindac sulphone, which does not inhibit prostaglandin synthesis, nevertheless inhibits tumour formation without significant reduction in prostaglandin E2 levels. This is therefore evidence of a separate way in which these drugs may be of use in combating cancer.

With the realisation that most NSAIDs inhibit both cyclooxygenase 1 and 2, and that this non-selectivity was likely to cause the gastro-intestinal side effects so well characterised, it became clear that we needed to know whether a Cox-2 selective drug would still have the ability to prevent colorectal cancer, or whether this property required Cox-1 inhibition as well. Accordingly, a multi-centre study was designed which included doctors at the University of Texas, the Imperial Cancer Research Fund at St. Mark's Hospital in London, the National Cancer Institute in Maryland, USA, and the manufacturers (Searle) of the Cox-2 selective drug, Celecoxib (Celebrex) (Steinbach 2000). 77 patients with familial adenomatous polyposis were randomly assigned to receive dummy (placebo), or Celebrex 100 milligrams twice daily, or 400 milligrams twice daily. The trial was carried out double-blind, i.e. neither the patients nor the doctors knew which treatment the patients had received, until after the trial when the results were analysed. The observations were made by endoscopy, and the number of polyps, and their diameters were charted (the 'polyp burden'). After 6 months, the patients on the higher dose of Celebrex had 28% reduction in number of polyps, (4.5% reduction for placebo), which was statistically significant (P=0.003). There was a 30.7% reduction in the polyp burden (4.9% for placebo). This too was statistically significant, (P=0.001).

This therefore was evidence that tumour regression was likely to involve Cox-2, though it did not exclude the possibility that Cox-1 was also involved. Interestingly, it should be realised that Celebrex is by no means the most selective of the so-called Coxibs, which somewhat weakens the assertion. Unfortunately there is still a cloud hanging over this group of drugs, since the withdrawal of the more selective Vioxx, which had led to an increased number of heart attacks.

So far, only colon and rectal cancer have been addressed. What about others?

A study from Birmingham, England, using the general practice research database, looked at 12,174 cases of cancer, with 34,934 controls who were age and sex-matched, the ratio being 1:3 (Langman 2000). The database included prescriptions of aspirin and NSAIDs, as well as smoking. The results showed trends towards a reduced incidence of colorectal cancer in patients taking NSAIDs or aspirin, with the greatest reductions in those taking the most prescriptions. There was also protection against cancer of the oesophagus and stomach. Unexpectedly, there appeared to be a significant increase in prostate and pancreatic cancer in those on aspirin or NSAIDs. The authors commented: "The increased risks of pancreatic and prostatic cancer could be due to chance or to undetected biases and warrant further investigations."

Colon cancer is believed to occur as a result of a sequence of changes, going from normal lining cells of the colon, through adenomatous polyps, to cancer. One third of the population at age 50 years have these polyps, and one half by age 70 years. The cancer cells arise as a result of genetic changes, which determine the transitional stages mentioned. 90% of sporadic colon cancers and 40% of adenomas over-express Cox-2, but the normal colonic lining (epithelium) does not over express. Raised Cox-2 is also found in familial polyposis. Experimental rats with intestinal adenomas treated with sulindac (which inhibits Cox-1 and Cox-2), show a 90% reduction in the number of intestinal adenomas, and 52% reduction in the total volume of colon tumours (Janne 2000). Selective Cox-2 inhibition will also reduce polyp formation, as can deletion of the gene responsible for Cox-2. (This can be shown by selectively breeding mice without the gene for Cox-2 – so called 'knock-out' mice – and then comparing their susceptibility to tumour formation with genetically intact mice). Cox-2 inhibition may also increase apoptosis, and reduce new blood vessel formation, which in turn could influence the development of these tumours. Before getting carried away by the possible use of these drugs, one should bear in mind the observation that their effect may be transient. 3 months after discontinuing sulindac, the number and size of polyps increased in patients (Giardello 1993).

In August 1993, in the Journal of the National Cancer Institute, Gann and colleagues from Harvard Medical School, Boston USA, reported their results of the Physicians Health Study, which included 22,071 male physicians from the USA. The study ended in 1988, after a follow-up period of 5 years. The relative risk among aspirin takers for the development of colorectal cancer was 115% i.e. it appeared to *increase* the risk. Yet for *in situ* cancers (cancers which remained within the epithelial layer of the intestinal wall, and had not spread deeper into or through the wall), and polyps, it appeared to offer protection of the order of 14%. The authors concluded:

"Regular aspirin use, at a dose adequate for preventing myocardial infarction, was not associated with a substantial reduction in the incidence of colorectal cancer during 5 years of randomised treatment and follow-up. A small decrease in polyps in the aspirin group could not be reliably distinguished from a chance association. Our results suggest that among low-dose aspirin users (a) colorectal cancer mortality is not likely to be reduced by earlier detection and (b) incidence is not likely to be increased due to aspirin-induced gastro-intestinal bleeding. *Implications*: The potential for a benefit from higher doses of aspirin or longer duration of use should be addressed by more detailed observational epidemiologic studies and prevention trials with longer follow-up of randomised participants."

So now we have the suggestion that perhaps aspirin's other uses do not all occur with the same low dose associated with prevention of cardiovascular disease,

Chapter Eleven – The Future

but may require something more closely approximating its dose in its traditional role as an analgesic.

In 2003, Sandler and colleagues published results of a randomised double-blind trial to determine the effects of aspirin on the incidence of colorectal adenomas among patients all of whom had previously had a colorectal cancer. These patients were chosen to ensure that they were observing a very high risk group of patients, for whom a smaller number would be needed to answer the question.

All had a preliminary examination of the lower bowel by colonoscopy and removal of any visible polyps within 4 months of entry into the study. This study excluded any patients with familial polyposis, i.e. it utilised patients with sporadic colon cancer. Clearly it was desirable to know whether participants were able to tolerate aspirin medication, so all took aspirin for a 3 month run-in period, prior to the study itself though they did not know whether they were on aspirin or placebo, but the doctors did (single blind). Staff members then decided, on the basis of self-reported adherence, motivation, and toxic effects at 6 weeks and 10 weeks, whether they were suitable to enter the trial proper. To do so, they needed to have taken an average of at least 5 tablets per week during the run-in period.

615 patients satisfied the run-in schedule and were randomly assigned either aspirin 325 milligrams or placebo each day. (A further 20 did not start for various reasons). Trials all start out with great enthusiasm, shared both by investigators and (generally) participants. Then, one by one, the numbers fall – would be participants fall ill, move away, die, retract their initial consent, or fail to obey the ground rules, and are excluded from further study on account of failure to comply. Colonoscopy was performed prior to the study, as mentioned above, and at exit after 3 or 4 years. Additionally, it was performed as clinically determined during the interim period, e.g. if the patient had a rectal bleed, and it was considered clinically appropriate to investigate and treat. At endoscopy, all polyps were enumerated, and examined microscopically. Unfortunately, during the course of the study involving the 615 patients, there were 35 deaths. It will immediately be apparent to the reader that it would be necessary to unblind the treatment for these cases, in case they all turned out to have one treatment rather than the other, in which case it would be unethical to continue. For example, say all 35 cases were in the aspirin and none in the placebo group. The trial would have indicated that aspirin was very dangerous. Or alternatively, suppose all 35 deaths occurred in the placebo group. That would suggest that aspirin was a tremendous life-saver, and this conclusion should have been reached before so many died. Of course, clinical trials are not that straightforward, as the figures indicate. In fact it was revealed that 18 deaths had occurred among patients receiving aspirin, and 17 placebo. Obviously no significant difference, but at least they were not killing their patients. What a relief! Anyway, the outcome was as seen in table 11.3.

Number of polyps	Aspirin	Placebo
0★	83%	73%
1★	10%	14%
2★	3%	7%
3★	3%	5%

*$P<0.003$ i.e. all these results were statistically significant.
Fewer polyps in the aspirin treated group*

Table 11.3. Results showing number of polyps during the period of observation in the patients previously diagnosed with colorectal cancer and receiving either aspirin or placebo. (From Sandler et al 2003).

In the same issue of the New England Journal of Medicine, March 6th 2003, Baron and colleagues from New Hampshire published their results of a randomised double blind trial of aspirin against colorectal adenomas (note, these patients, unlike Sandler's, did not have a preceding history of colorectal carcinoma). They investigated 327 patients who received placebo, versus 377 who received 81 milligrams aspirin, and 372 who received 325 milligrams of aspirin daily. Follow-up endoscopies were performed at least 1 year after entry into the trial. The summary of results is shown in table 11.4.

Treatment	1 or more adenomas	Advanced tumours including cancer
Placebo (372 cases)	47%	12.9%
Aspirin 81mg (377 cases)	38%	7.7%
Aspirin 325 mg (372 cases)	45%	10.7%

Table 11.4. Aspirin at 2 doses v. placebo. Incidence of adenomas and advanced tumours appearing in patients previously diagnosed with colorectal adenoma. (From Baron et al 2003).

The conclusion was that low-dose aspirin has a moderate protective effect on large bowel adenomas.

The accompanying editorial (Imperiale 2003) sought to put into perspective the value of treating large numbers of patients with aspirin in order to secure meaningful protection against colorectal cancer, and compared this with its now accepted benefits in the prevention of cardiovascular disease. In order to illustrate this, figures were given for the numbers needed to treat (NNT). This means, "How many people do we need to treat and for how long, in order to achieve a defined effect?" The defined

Chapter Eleven – The Future

effect can either be a desired effect, or a harmful effect, see table below taken from this paper. Primary prevention means in people who have never knowingly had the disease in question. Secondary prevention, means in people known to have had the disease in the past, see table 11.5.

The figures show quite clearly, that primary prevention (which means treating the whole population including those people without known disease), is clearly a huge task involving possibly thousands of people treated for up to 20 or more years, in order to save just one life. Hardly cost effective when there are so many other demands on the Health Service. On the other hand, targeting efforts where there is clearly an increased risk i.e. cases with a previous history of colonic adenomatous polyps, is more likely to be fruitful. The author concludes:

"Although aspirin may be of some benefit in preventing colorectal cancer, it cannot yet be recommended for this indication and is not a substitute for screening and surveillance. Nevertheless, the well-conducted trials – provide proof of the principle that aspirin moderately reduces the risk of recurrent colorectal neoplasia" – (i.e. cancer) – "and provide support for the assumptions and probabilities that have been used in published analyses of cost effectiveness. Determination of whether aspirin has a role in preventing colorectal cancer must await the results of clinical trials designed to determine whether it can be used to decrease the required frequency or intensity of screening or surveillance."

Effect	*NNT*	*Duration*
Secondary prevention:		
Adenoma prevention	10	31 months
Advanced colon cancer	19	33 months
Primary prevention:		
Coronary heart disease event	50–250	60 months
Colorectal cancer	471–962	More than 60 months
Death from colorectal cancer	1250	12–20 years or more
Adverse events:		
Gastro-intestinal haemorrhage	100	26–28 months
Major gastro-intestinal haemorrhage	300–800	4–6 years
Haemorrhagic stroke	800	4–6 years

Table 11.5. Estimates of numbers needed to treat (NNT) for some benefits and harms from aspirin. (From Imperiale 2003).

A study from Paris (Benamouzig 2003), looked at 272 patients aged 18–75 years, with a history of colorectal adenomas. They either had at least 3 adenomas at outset, or 1 which was more than 5 millimetres in diameter. They were assigned 160 or 300 milligrams of lysine aspirin daily, or placebo in double-blind fashion. (Lysine aspirin was shown to be more soluble than standard aspirin, and to reach its peak concentration more rapidly. It was hoped that this form of drug would cause less tendency to bleeding than standard aspirin though they did not actually measure this). They were to be studied at 1 and 4 years. The 1 year results are presented. 238 completed the study at this stage. Of the 126 aspirin patients, at least 1 adenoma was found in 30%, compared to 41% of the placebo group. This result was not statistically significant, though the trend was clear ($P=0.08$). Considering the incidence of adenomas more than 5 millimetres diameter, the figures were 10% in the aspirin group, and 23% in placebo. This result was statistically significant, ($P=0.01$). For adenomas more than 10 millimetres diameter, the percentages were 1 and 6 respectively, $P=0.05$. Differences between the two different dosages of aspirin insofar as adenoma occurrence were not significant. The conclusion of this interim evaluation was that daily soluble aspirin was associated with a reduction in the risk for recurrent adenomas shown by colonoscopy at 1 year.

A large study of nurses in Boston USA (Chan 2004), involved 121,701 nurses aged 30 to 55 years, who completed a questionnaire on risk factors for cancer and coronary heart disease starting in 1976. They were mailed every 2 years. From 1980, additional questions were included, enquiring about diet, aspirin use, and whether or not anyone had required a colonoscopy or sigmoidoscopy (sigmoidoscopy is less extensive and informative than colonoscopy, because it only looks at the last part of the colon – called the sigmoid colon – which leads on to the rectum). The design of the study was to assess whether or not they took aspirin, and if so, how much. This was the critical purpose of the study. How much aspirin and over how many years were they taking it? From the replies, it emerged that 27,077 women had adenomas. This was good news, because it allowed every chance for the breakdown of aspirin use to yield some meaningful results. They were able to determine the effects of

Groups of women			Aspirin tablets per week		
	0	*0.5–1.5*	*2–5*	*6–14*	*more than 14*
All	0	6%	18%	24%	43%
Less than 5 years	0	6%	19%	9%	57%
More than 5 years	0	5%	18%	32%	39%

Table 11.6. Risk reduction for development of colorectal adenoma, looking at duration and number of aspirin tablets taken weekly. (From Benamouzig 2003).

anything from 0 to more than 14 tablets of aspirin weekly, on the relative risk of developing a colorectal adenoma. A simplification of their findings is shown in table 11.6. Instead of relative risk, is shown the percentage reduction in risk.

The authors concluded:

"Regular, short-term use of aspirin is inversely associated with risk for colorectal adenoma. However, the greatest protective effect is evident at substantially higher doses (more than 14 tablets per week) than those recommended for the prevention of cardiovascular disease. Before aspirin can be recommended for chemoprevention in the general adult population, these results suggest the need for a more thorough evaluation of the risks and benefits of routine aspirin use at doses not previously considered."

But of course, this study was only looking at adenomas (benign tumours), and not at carcinoma of the colon – the killer. The assumption, fairly widely held, is that carcinoma is preceded by adenoma, but this is by no means certain. In an attempt to answer this question, the same group of nurses received twice yearly questionnaires (Chan 2005). The medical records of women who reported a diagnosis of colorectal cancer were obtained and studied. In general, those women who reported aspirin use were older, less likely to exercise regularly, more likely to smoke and take multivitamins, hormone replacement therapy and non-steroidal anti-inflammatory drugs. They also drank slightly more alcohol and ate slightly more folate containing ingredients. All these confounding variables were taken into account in the final analysis. 82,911 women were eligible for the study, for an average 19.2 years, making a total of 1,592,017 person years. 962 cases of colorectal cancer were documented.

In regard to duration of aspirin use, where regular aspirin use meant at least 2 tablets daily, they found a reduction in development of colorectal cancer, see table 11.7.

Taking all variables into account, over a 20 years period, regular users of aspirin had a 23% reduction in colorectal cancer compared to non-regular users. But this did not become apparent until after 10 years of use. It also appeared to be dose dependent, the most beneficial being more than 14 tablets weekly. Interestingly, the drug history revealed that non-steroidal anti-inflammatory drugs conferred the same benefit. By contrast with risk reduction for colon cancer, there was no reduction for rectal cancer,

Years of regular aspirin use (396 cases)

0	1–5	6–10	11–20	more than 20 years	% Reduction in risk
0%	-4%	11%	33%	32%	(Risk reduction; minus sign – signifies increase in risk)

Table 11.7. Showing reduction in risk of colorectal cancer with years of consuming aspirin. (From Chan et al 2005).

both for aspirin and non-steroidals. There was also no reduction in either for acetaminophen (paracetamol). The flip side of aspirin benefit, was that there was an, as expected, increased incidence of gastro-intestinal bleeding, which not surprisingly was dose dependent. Surprisingly, the same problem with bleeding applied to non-steroidal use. Whether selective Cox-2 inhibitors, such as celecoxib reduce colon cancer whilst not causing gastro-intestinal bleeding remains to be seen. With the Cox-2 inhibitors, however, whilst they may be less prone to causing gastro-intestinal bleeding, nevertheless, they may result in a greater incidence of heart attacks, as was found with Vioxx.

The authors concluded:

"Regular, long-term aspirin use reduces risk of colorectal cancer. Non-aspirin NSAIDs appear to have a similar effect. However, a significant benefit of aspirin is not apparent until more than a decade of use, with maximal risk reduction at doses greater than 14 tablets per week. These results suggest that optimal chemoprevention for colorectal cancer requires long-term use of aspirin doses substantially higher than those recommended for the prevention of cardiovascular disease, but the dose-related risk of gastro-intestinal bleeding must also be considered."

So, to conclude, aspirin appears to reduce the appearance of colonic polyps, and when taken in doses averaging 2 tablets or more daily, for years, the appearance of colon though not rectal cancer. But it also causes bleeds, and is not yet sufficiently established to be regarded as a standard chemopreventive agent for colon cancer. Perhaps the combined administration of aspirin and a stomach protective agent, on a long term basis would be worthy of consideration in attempting to answer this question.

2. Alzheimer's disease

In 1901, a 51 year old lady, named Auguste D, was admitted to the state asylum in Frankfurt. She had difficulty in remembering everyday things, and her speech had suffered in that she could not remember words. More worryingly, she was hearing voices, was imagining things, felt that people were plotting against her, and was becoming aggressive. Dr. Alois Alzheimer, see figure 11.2. was assigned to study her case. (The word 'study' is appropriate, because there was not much else that could be done). Dr. Alzheimer then moved to Munich in order to work with Germany's currently most eminent psychiatrist, Dr. Emil Kraepelin. Unfortunately they could do nothing for poor Auguste, and in 1906, she died. Alzheimer presented her case at a psychiatric meeting. It is important to understand that he did not intend to give the impression that he was the first person to describe this clinical picture, which was clearly that of a lady of 56 years who had become demented and died. The interesting feature, because demented elderly people were two a penny, was that she was relatively young when her symptoms started. He described how, at post-mortem, viewing slices of her brain under the microscope, he had found plaques, arteriosclerotic changes, and 'tangles', see figure 11.3.

Chapter Eleven – The Future

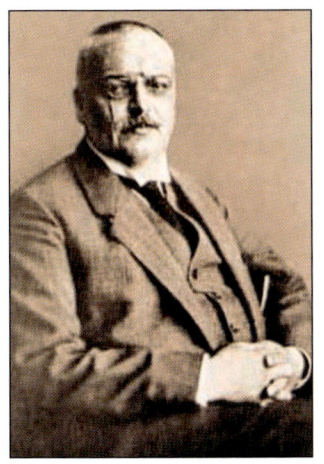
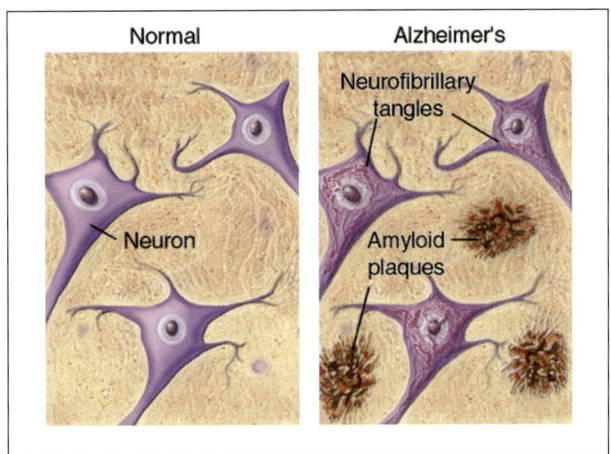

Left: Figure 11.2. Alois Alzheimer (1864–1915).
Right: Figure 11.3. Histology of Alzheimer's disease.

However, the great Kraepelin called the dementia 'Alzheimer's disease' thereby implying that a new disease had been discovered in his institute. Now, one wonders why he would have done that. The answer almost certainly was that by so doing, the impression would be given that great work and discoveries were continuing to emanate from the institute, and thus it would receive grants to continue its work. In Kraepelin's description he omitted to mention the arteriosclerosis (narrowed arteries with thickened walls), the hallucinations, delusions and other psychiatric symptoms. There followed some controversy as to whether this was in any way different from senile dementia, either in some specific way, or whether it was the same process albeit occurring earlier. The appearances noted by Alzheimer had in fact been reported months earlier by an American called Fuller.

What is the position today? There are several forms of dementia, and the name Alzheimers is given to the condition characterised by dementia, insidious in onset, coming on in middle life or earlier, though more usually in later life. It progresses to death within about 10 years. Often there is a family history, or a history of head injury, or the patient has Down's syndrome (the medical term for mongolism). The hallmark of the disease is the finding on microscopic brain sections, of **neurofibrillary tangles, loss of nerve cells (neurones), and accumulation of an abnormal protein called amyloid**. Genetic studies have revealed abnormalities on chromosome 1, 14, or 21, 50% of cases of pre-senile dementia being associated with a change in chromosome 14. There is also an association with an apolipoprotein called ε4.

The other form of dementia considered a separate entity to Alzheimer's disease, is **multi-infarct dementia**. This, as its name implies, is preceded by little strokes, and is due to arterial blockages. Functionally, the effect on the brain may be the same as that in Alzheimers, the difference being that in the former, there is insufficient blood, in the latter the blood supply is not significantly compromised, but some other process causes breakdown and loss of neurones, with accumulation of amyloid protein, and the neurofibrillary tangles.

In Alzheimers, neurochemical changes have been described, particularly a reduction in the amount of choline acetyltransferase, or in acetylcholine, or other chemicals involved in the transmission and control of nerve impulses.

The potential exists to try the effect of salicylate or non-steroidal anti-inflammatory drug therapy in both types of dementia. The rationale in Alzheimers is that we know that these cases have evidence of inflammation in affected sites within the brain. Increased levels of Cox-2 have been detected at these sites, together with the anticipated increase in prostaglandin concentration. Thus there would appear to be a logical target for drug therapy. Interestingly, increased levels of Cox-1 have also been detected. If Cox-1 is important in Alzheimers, then aspirin, but not selective Cox-2 inhibitors might be expected to prove beneficial.

Studies of twins are often used in medicine to find out more about disease causation. This is because it can reasonably be supposed that the effect of the environment will in most cases be the same for both twins (except of cause where for some reason they have been separated early in life and brought up in different environments). However, for the most part, they provide a valuable tool for studying the effect of environment. As an example, if we wished to know whether rheumatoid arthritis was a purely genetic disease, and one had access to identical twins, it would be most informative to see in all instances where one twin was known to have the disease, whether the other twin also had it. In fact, twin studies have shown that although there are cases where both have the disease, there are also cases where this is not the case. Thus it is inferred that the disease is not purely genetic, and there are environmental factors also at play. Interestingly, where both twins have a given disease, they do not all get it at the same time. This could of course be due to a number of factors, such as diet, environment, and the presence of other diseases which may accelerate or retard the time of onset. Another factor could be previous drug therapy. This has been applied in Alzheimer's disease. Breitner and colleagues in North Carolina in 1993 published the results of such a study.

They found 50 pairs of twins who had both got Alzheimer's disease, but with at least 3 years' difference in the age at onset. 23 male pairs were found in the list of World War II veterans. The others, mostly female, had responded to advertisements or were referred from Alzheimer's disease clinics. 26 pairs were identical twins. They found that a previous history of steroid therapy reduced the chance of getting Alzheimers by 75%, and by 76% if both steroids and anti-inflammatory drugs had been taken. However, by past steroid treatment they included patients who recalled a single steroid injection. What was more likely was that these patients had arthritis, for which these treatments had been prescribed. Perhaps the arthritis itself, with or without its treatment, made Alzheimers less likely.

McGeer and colleagues in the Lancet in 1970, looked at the hospital discharges of 7,490 elderly patients with a diagnosis of both rheumatoid arthritis and Alzheimer's disease in the same patient. They found 29. But the expected result, knowing the prevalence of Alzheimers in the age-matched general population, and that of rheumatoid arthritis, should have been anything between 175 to 350. The authors postulated that this might have been due to the drugs prescribed for the rheumatoid arthritis – i.e. anti-inflammatory drugs, which would have comprised mainly non-steroidal anti-inflammatories, but also steroids, and methotrexate (the latter is currently the most used second-line – also known as disease-modifying anti-rheumatic drug – in rheumatoid arthritis). And there is evidence of various molecules associated with inflammation being present within various parts of the brain affected in Alzheimer's disease. Steroids, though potently anti-inflammatory, are not particularly so-endowed by dint of their anti-Cox activity, so the postulated benefit of non-steroidal anti-inflammatory drugs is very likely to be as a consequence of specific activity against Cox. These drugs though are not without their side-effects, particularly in patients over the age of 60 years. In these cases, it is generally considered preferable to prescribe a selective Cox-2 inhibitor, but would such a drug work in Alzheimers?

An initial study of this kind was carried out by Aisen and colleagues in Washington DC, and published in Neurology in 2002. It was a pilot study, designed primarily to monitor safety. For 12 weeks, 20 patients received nimesulide, a selective Cox-2 inhibitor, and 20 received placebo. After 12 weeks, all 40 received nimesulide, and were followed up for over 2 years. In the short term, they were not able to detect any significant improvement in their Alzheimers, but we await the results of larger long-term studies. Encouragingly, the drug was well tolerated. One problem was that all the participants were already receiving therapy for their disease (choline-esterase inhibitors – which help a bit), so any difference from placebo would be the result of an additional effect, and for such an effect to become detectable, would have required much larger numbers of patients.

It will be recalled that deposition of amyloid in the brain substance is also a feature of Alzheimer's disease. It is possible to breed mice with a gene causing Alzheimer's disease, a so-called transgenic mouse. By 10 months of age, they have the characteristic brain changes. Mice then fed a non-steroidal anti-inflammatory drug (ibuprofen), showed a reduction in various markers of inflammation in the brain, as well as a reduction in the number of amyloid deposits (Lim 2000).

In the dementia that may follow small strokes, alluded to above as multi-infarct dementia, it would seem reasonable to try out the effect of aspirin, for its well-characterised anti-platelet effect. In 4 out of 6 studies, it was found that aspirin resulted in an improvement in cognitive function i.e. mental function (van Kooten 1998). Other studies are still ongoing.

Conclusion
For thousands of years, medicaments including salicin have been prescribed by herbalists. For one hundred years, aspirin, and for over 50 years, NSAIDs have been prescribed by physicians. In more recent times they have been obtainable by the general public using over the counter purchases. Initially their intended use was as a febrifuge, or analgesic. Later, they were used to counteract chronic inflammation, as in rheumatoid arthritis. The potential of aspirin for preventing coronary thrombosis was recognised in the 1950s, and confirmed towards the end of the century. Unfortunately both aspirin and NSAIDs possess a very prominent Achilles' heel – gastro-intestinal intolerance. This led to the development of the selective Cox-2 inhibitors, and with that, the awareness of a trade off for gastric comfort, namely increased risk of heart attack. More recently it has received attention as a possible preventative for colon cancer, and tentatively for the amelioration of Alzheimer's disease. Prior to the advent of the pharmaceutical industry, and designer drugs, together with current strict controls over drug trials, Man was forced to look to Nature to provide cures. Nature had preceded Man in evolving complex, and not so complex molecules which clearly had some properties which serendipitously worked in human disease. The quest for new drugs continues apace, whilst that of herbalism has stood still. Therapeutic adventures by the latter could provide more remedies, but today's medicine makes this a difficult area into which to venture. Litigation in the event of harm would put anyone off. Yet aspirin has fallen and risen, and appears set to continue as one of the most widely taken preparations.

The British National Formulary (as in September 2005) listed the following aspirin, or aspirin-containing preparations, under the section on analgesics:

Aspirin, Caprin, Nu-seals Aspirin, Co-codaprin (includes codeine), Aspav (contains papaveretum).

Preparations on sale to the public include:

Alka-Seltzer, Alka-Seltzer XS (aspirin, caffeine, paracetamol), Anadin (aspirin, caffeine), Anadin Extra, Anadin Extra Soluble (aspirin, caffeine, paracetamol), Angettes 75 (aspirin), Askit (aspirin, aloxiprin, caffeine), Aspro-Clear (aspirin), Beechams Lemon tablets (aspirin), Beechams Powders (aspirin, caffeine), Boots Seltzer (aspirin), Codis 500 (aspirin, codeine), Mrs. Cullens (aspirin, caffeine), Disprin, and Disprin Direct (aspirin), Disprin Extra (aspirin, paracetamol), Doans Bachache Pills (paracetamol, sodium salicylate), Maximum strength Aspro Clear (aspirin), Nurse Sykes Powders (aspirin, caffeine, paracetamol), see figure 11.4. Phensic (aspirin, caffeine).

Chapter Eleven – The Future

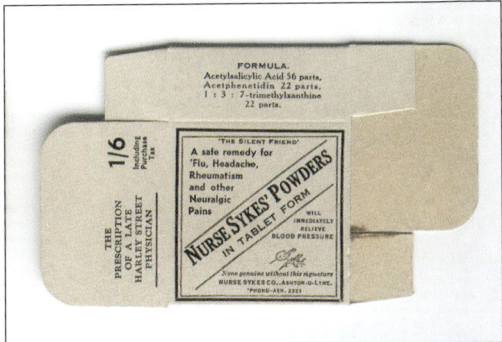
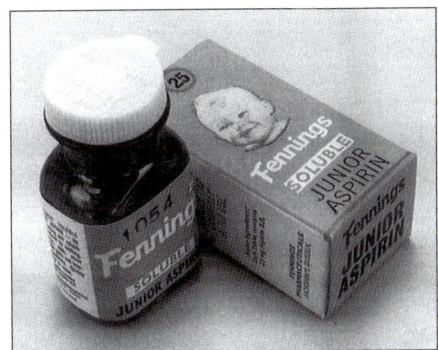
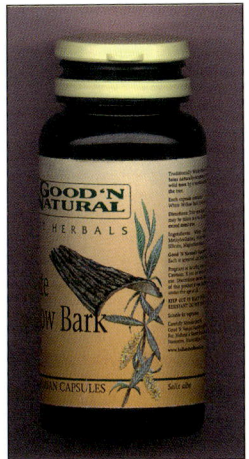
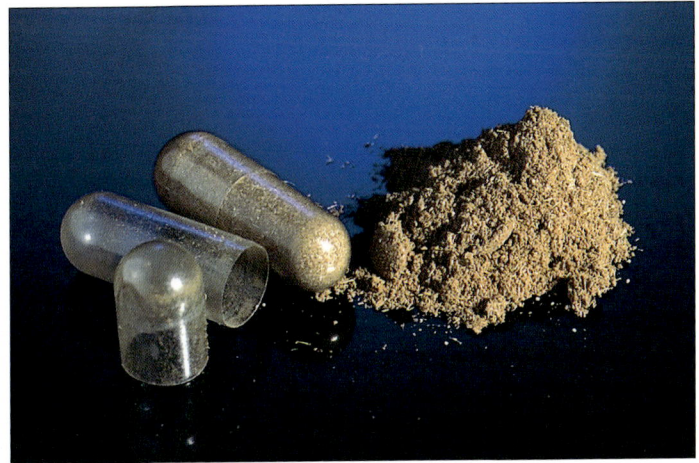

*Top Left: Figure 11.4. Nurse Sykes' powders advertisements c.1960.
(With kind permission of Anglian-Pharma).
Top Right: Figure 11.5. Fennings Junior Aspirin. (With kind permission of Anglian-Pharma).
Bottom Left: Figure 11.6. Proprietary brand of willow bark extract.
(Reproduced with permission of Good 'N' Natural, USA, and Holland & Barrett, UK).
Bottom Right: Figure 11.7. Willow bark extract, 2006.
(With permission of Good 'N' Natural, USA, and Holland & Barrett, UK).*

Some examples of advertising are shown above. Junior aspirin is no longer on sale, since the recognition of Reye's syndrome. One proprietary preparation was Fennings, see figure 11.5. Health food shops still sell willow bark extract to the public, see figures 11.6, and 11.7.

The Reverend Edward Stone would have expressed his approval!

Bibliography (in chronological order)

1633   Gerard G. The Herball or Generall Historie of Plantes. London. Thomas Johnson, (Botanical drawings of the shrub meadowsweet, and of the white willow – Salix alba).

1757   An Essay on Fevers 3rd Edition by John Huxham. London. Printed for J. Hinton, in Newgate-Street.

1763   The Entire Works of Dr. Thomas Sydenham. 4th Edition by John Swan M.D. London: Printed by R.Cave, at St. John's Gate.

1772   Lettsom WC. Reflections on the General treatment and Cure of Fevers. London: Printed by JD Cornish.

1792   Observations on the bark of a particular species of willow showing its superiority to the Peruvian, and its singular efficacy in the cure of agues, intermittent fevers, fluor albus, abscesses, haemorrhages, &c. Illustrated by cases. By Samuel James, of the Corporation of Surgeons. London: Printed for J. Johnson, St. Paul's Church Yard.

1798   Observations and experiments on the Broad-leaved Willow Bark Illustrated with cases. By W. White, Member of the Corporation of Surgeons, and Apothecary to the Bath City Infirmary and Dispensary Bath: Printed and Sold by S. Hazard Sold also by Vernor and Hood, Poultry, London.

1803   Wilkinson G. Experiments and Observations on the Cortex *Salicis latifoliae* or broad-leafed Willow bark. Newcastle-upon-Tyne: Walker.

1818   An Arrangement of British Plants according to the Latest Improvements of the Linnaean System, by William Withering M.D. F.R.S. 6th Edition by William Withering Esq., F.L.S. Printed for Cadell and Davies, Cuthell and Co., Longman and Co., Rivingtons, Baldwin and Co., Lackington and Co., Sherwood and Co., I. Richardson, S. Bagster, Mawman P.W. and G. Wynne, R. Fenner, Harding, Ogles, Whitmore and Fenn, T. Hamilton, Black and Son, J. Richardson, Taylor and Hessey, J. Walker, G. Robinson, W. Reid, R. Saunders, C. Brown, and Robert Scholey.

1824   Culpepper's Family Physician. The English Physician Enlarged. Revised, Corrected, and Enlarged by James Scammon. Exeter: Published by James Scammon.

1875   Papyrus Ebers, the Hermetic Book of Medicine of the Ancient Egyptians, in Hieratic writing. Published, with Synopsis of Contents and Introduction, by George Ebers. With a Hieroglyphic-Latin Glossary by Ludwig Stern.

Bibliography

	Under the Patronage of the Royal Bureau of Education in Saxony, Leipzig: William Engelman, 2 vols, folio.
1884	Papyrus Ebers. The earliest medical work extant by Professor H. Carrington Bolton PhD. Reprinted from Weekly Drug News, Vol. IX, No. 15. New York. Weekly Drug News Press.
1892	The Principles and Practice of Medicine. Author William Osler. 1st Edition New York. D. Appleton and Company.
1912	Herbals Their Origin and Evolution Author Agnes Arber. Published by Cambridge University Press.
1930	Bryan CP The Papyrus Ebers. Translated from the German version by Cyril P. Bryan M.B. B.CH. B.A.O. Demonstrator in Anatomy, University College, London. With an introduction by Professor G. Elliot Smith M.D. D. SC. Litt. D F.R.C.P. F.R.S. Professor of Anatomy, University College, London. Published by Geoffrey Bles, 22 Suffolk Street, Pall Mall, London, S.W.1.
1934	The Greek Herbal of Dioscorides. Illustrated by a Byzantine AD 512. Englished by John Goodyer AD 1655. Edited and first printed AD 1933, by Robert T. Gunther. Oxford University Press.
1946	The Herbal of Rufinus. Edited from the Unique Manuscript by Lynn Thorndike. University of Cambridge Press.
1948	The Salicylates: A critical bibliographic review, New Haven, Conn. Hillhouse Press: 1–8 (citing Gunzius (1772), van Geuns (1778).
1959	A Textbook of Medicine Authors Cecil R.L. and Loeb R.F. 10th Edition. Published by W.B. Saunders Company. Philadelphia and London.
1959	Hutchison's Clinical Methods. Authors Donald Hunter, and R.R. Bomford. 13th Edition Cassell London.
1963	Keele, Kenneth D. "The evolution of Clinical Methods in Medicine." Fitzpatrick Lecture delivered to the Royal College of Physicians in 1960–1961. London. Pitman Medical Publishing Co. Ltd.
1975	An historical account of pharmacology to the 20th century, by Chauncey D. Leake. Published by Charles C. Thomas, Springfield, Illinois, USA.
1978	Davidson's Principles and Practice of Medicine. Edited by John Macleod. 12th Edition. Churchill Livingstone, Edinburgh, London and New York.
1978	Schindler PE Aspirin therapy New York NY. Walker & Co.. 1–134 (derivation of the term 'aspirin' in Jan. 1899 by Dreser).
1983	Oxford Textbook of Medicine. Edited by D.J. Weatherall, J.G.G. Ledingham, and D.A. Warrell. 1st Edition. Oxford University Press.
1984	Aspirin, the medicine of the century. R. Alstaedter (ed). Germany: Bayer AG.
1985	Dioscorides on Pharmacy and Medicine. John M. Riddle. University of Texas Press, Austin.
1985	Sneader W Drug Discovery. Chichester. John Wiley and Sons.

1987	Papyros Ebers. Das Hermetische Buch Uber Die Arzenmittel Der Alten Agypter. In Hieratischer Schrift. Biblio Verlag. Osnabruck.
1988	Milestones: the Bayer story 1863–1988. E. Verg, P. Gottfried, and H. Scultheis. Leverkusen: Bayer AG.
1992	Brune K, Fenner H, Kurolski M, Lanz R and members of the SPALA group Adverse reactions to NSAIDs: Consecutive evaluation of 30,000 patients in rheumatology. In: KD Rainford and GP Velo (eds), Side effects of Anti-inflammatory Drugs 3, pp 33–42, Dordrecht: Kluwer Academic Publishers.
1992	Murder, Magic and Medicine. John Mann, Oxford University Press.
1994	Henry Wellcome. Author Robert Rhodes James. Published by Hodder & Stoughton.
1997	The herbal in history. John M. Riddle. Notes accompanying *Medicina Magica*, by Hans Biedermann, commissioned by the Editors of The Classics of Medicine Library. 1986, revised.
2002	Clinical Medicine. Parveen Kumar and Michael Clark 5th Edition W.B. Saunders.
2003	Edward Stone and the Discovery of Aspirin. By Ralph Mann. Copyright. Monograph.
2001	The fever trail. In search of the cure for malaria. Mark Honigsbaum. Pan Books.
2004	Aspirin and related drugs. K.D. Rainsford. London: Taylor & Francis.
2004	Aspirin the story of a wonder drug. Diarmuid Jeffreys. Bloomsbury.

References (in chronological order)

Stone E. **(1763)** Phil Trans Roy Soc XXXII An account of the success of the willow in the cure of agues 195–200.

Leroux **(1829)** J Chimie Medicale **6**: 341.

Piria R. **(1838)** "CHIMIE ORGANIQUE Sur la composition de la Salicine et sur quelques-unes de ses reactions;" par M. RAFAEL PIRIA. (Commissaires, M.M. Dumas, Pelouze) Comptes Rendues de l'Academie des Sciences, Paris **6**: 338.

Gerhardt C.F. **(1853)** "Untersuchungen uber die wasserfreien organischen Sauren." Liebig's Annalen **87**: 149.

Stricker S. Berl.klin.Wschr. **(1876) 13**: 15, 99.

Kolbe H. and Lautemann, E. Justus **(1860)** Liebigs. Ann. Chem. **115**: 157.

Maclagan T.J. **(1867)** Thermometrical Observations Edin Med J **XIII** 601–625.

Riess L. **(1876)** Berl. Klin. Wschr. **13**: 86.

Myers ABR **(1876)** Salicin in acute rheumatism Lancet, November 11th 676–677.

Riess L. **(1876)** Berl klin. Wschr. **13**, 86.

Stricker S. **(1876)** Berl. Klin. Wschr. **13**, 15, 99.

See G. **(1877)** Bull. Acad. Med. (Paris), **26**, 689.

Maclagan T.J. **(1879)** The treatment of acute rheumatism by salicin and salicylic acid. Lancet, June 21st 875–877.

Dreser H. **(1899)** Pharmacologisches uber aspirin (acetylsalicylsaure) Archiv fur die Gesammte Physiologie Pflugers Arch **76**: 306–318.

Douthwaite A. & Lintott G **(1938)** Gastroscopic observation of the effect of aspirin and certain other substances on the stomach. Lancet November 26th 1222–1225.

Lehmann J. **(1946)** *Para*-aminosalicylic acid in the treatment of tuberculosis. Preliminary communication. Lancet **1**: 15–16.

Westergren A. **(1946)** Kemoterapi vid tuberkulos med para-aminosalicylsyra. Nord. Med **33**: 55.

Lester D. & Greenberg L.A. **(1947)** The metabolic fate of acetanilide and other aniline derivatives: II. Major metabolites of acetanilide appearing in the blood. Journal of Pharmacology and Experimental Therapeutics **90**: 68–75.

Carstensen B. & Sjolin S. **(1948)** Para-aminosalicylsyra (PAS) vid lungtuberkulos med sekundar tarmtuberkulos Svenska Lakaartidn. **45**: 729–743.

Streptomycin treatment of tuberculous meningitis. Streptomycin in tuberculosis trials committee. Medical Research Council. Lancet **(1948) 1**: 582–596.

Flinn F.B. & Brodie B.B. **(1948)** The effect on the pain threshold of N-acetyl-p-aminophenol, a product derived in the body from acetanilide. Journal of Pharmacology and Experimental Therapeutics **94**: 76–77.

Svartz N. **(1948)** The treatment of rheumatic polyarthritis with acid azo compounds Rheumatism **4**: 56–60.

Sinclair R.J.G. & Duthie J.J. **(1949)** Effect of aspirin on Salazopyrin in treatment of rheumatoid arthritis. Ann Rheum Dis **8**: 226–231.

Brodie B.B. & Axelrod J. **(1949)** The fate of acetophenetin (phenacetin) in man and methods for the estimation of acetophenetidin and its metabolites in biological material. Journal of Pharmacology and Experimental Therapeutics **97**: 58–67.

Dunner E. Brown W.B. & Wallace J. **(1949)** Effect of combined streptomycin and PAS on emergence of resistance. In: *Minutes of the seventh streptomycin conference, April 21–24, 1949, Denver, Colorado.* Veterans Administration, Washington, 25–28.

Therapeutic trials committee of the Swedish national association against tuberculosis **(1950)** Para-aminosalicylic acid treatment in pulmonary tuberculosis. Amer. Rev. Tuberc. **61**: 597–612.

Treatment of pulmonary tuberculosis with streptomycin and para-amino-salicylic acid. A Medical Research Council Investigation **(1950)** British Medical Journal **2**: 1073–1085.

Craven L.L. **(1950)** Acetyl Salicylic acid, possible prevention of coronary thrombosis. Ann West Med & Surg **4**: 95–99.

Kuzell W.C. & Gardner G.M. **(1950)** Salicylazosulfapyridine (salazopyrin or azopyrin) in rheumatoid arthritis and experimental polyarthritis California Medicine **73**: 476–480.

Craven L.L. **(1953)** Experiences with aspirin (acetylsalicylic acid) in the nonspecific prophylaxis of coronary thrombosis. Miss Vall Med J **75**: 38–44.

Various combinations of isoniazid with streptomycin or with P.A.S. in the treatment of pulmonary tuberculosis **(1955)**. Seventh Report to the Medical research Council by their Tuberculosis Chemotherapy Trials Committee. British Medical Journal **1**: 435–444.

Winder C.V. **(1959)** Nature (London) **184**: 494 (nociceptive properties).

Truelove L.H. & Duthie J.J. **(1959)** Effect of aspirin on cutaneous response to the local application of an ester of nicotinic acid. Ann Rheum Dis **18**: 137–141.

O'Brien J. **(1962)** Platelet aggregation: some results from a new method of study. J Clin Path **15**: 446–455.

Collier H.O.J. **(1963)** Aspirin. Sci Am **209**: 97–108.

Reye R.D.K. Morgan G. & Baral J. **(1963)** Encephalopathy and fatty degeneration of the viscera. A disease entity in childhood. Lancet **2**: 749–752.

Chamberlain E.N. **(1964)** James Currie – His Life and Times Proc Roy Soc Med **57**: 908.

References

Weiss H.J. **(1968)** The effects of the salicylates in the hemostatic properties of platelets in man. J Clin Investigations **47** Abstract 300.

Birath Gosta **(1969)** Introduction of Para-amino-salicylic acid and streptomycin in the treatment of tuberculosis. Scandinavian Journal of Respiratory Medicine **50**: 204–209.

Piper P.J. & Vane J.R. **(1969)** Release of additional factors in anaphylaxis and its antagonism by anti-inflammatory drugs. Nature **223**: 29–35.

Vane J.R. **(1971)** Inhibition of prostaglandin synthesis as a mechanism of action for aspirin-like drugs. Nature New Biology **231**: 232–239.

Powles T.J. Clark S.A. Easty DM **(1973)** The inhibition by aspirin and indomethacin of osteolytic tumour deposits and hypercalcaemia in rats with Walker tumour, and its possible application to human breast cancer. Br J Cancer **28**: 316–321.

Regular aspirin intake and acute myocardial infarction. **(1974)** Boston Collaborative drug surveillance group. British Medical Journal 9th March. **1**: 440–3.

Lanza F.L. Royer G, & Nelson R. **(1975)** An endoscopic evaluation of the effects of non-steroidal anti-inflammatory drugs on the gastric mucosa. Gastrointestinal Endoscopy, **21**: 103–105.

Hial V. Horakova Z. Shaff R.E. & Beaven M. **(1976)** Alteration of tumor growth by aspirin and indomethacin: studies with two transplantable tumors in mouse. European Journal of Pharmacology **37**: 367–376.

Azad Khan A.K. Piris J. & Truelove S.C. **(1977)** An experiment to determine the active therapeutic moiety of sulphasalazine. Lancet **(ii)**: 892–895.

McConkey B. Amos R.S. Butler E.P. Crockson R.A. Crockson A.P. Walsh L. **(1978)** Salazopyrin in rheumatoid arthritis Agents & Actions **8(4)**: 438–441.

Elwood P.C. & Sweetnam P.M. **(1979)** Aspirin and secondary mortality after myocardial infarction. Lancet December 22nd. 1313–5.

A randomized, controlled trial of aspirin in persons recovered from myocardial infarction **(1980)** Aspirin myocardial infarction study research group. Journal of the American Medical Association February 15th. **243**: 661–9.

Rees W.D.N. & Turnberg L.A. **(1980)** Reappraisal of the effects of aspirin on the stomach. Lancet **2**: 410–413.

Starko K.M. Ray G. Dominguez L.B. Stromberg W.L. & Woodall D.F. **(1980)**. Reye's syndrome and salicylate use. Pediatrics **66**, no. 6:859–864.

Waddell W.R. & Gerner R.E. **(1980)** Indomethacin and ascorbate inhibit desmoid tumors. Journal of Surgical Oncology **15**: 85–90.

Dew M.J. Hughes P.J. et al **(1982)** Maintenance of remission in ulcerative colitis with oral preparation of 5-aminosalicylic acid. British Medical Journal **285**: 1012.

Neumann V.C. Grindulis K.A. Hubball S. McConkey B. & Wright V. **(1983)** Comparison between penicillamine and sulphasalazine in rheumatoid arthritis: Leeds-Birmingham trial Brit Med Journal Clin Res Edition **287(6399)**: 1099–1102.

Pullar T. Hunter J.A. & Capell H.A. **(1983)** Sulphasalazine in rheumatoid arthritis: a double-blind comparison of sulphasalazine with placebo and sodium aurothiomalate Br Med Journal Clin Res Edition **287(6399)**: 1102–1104.

Waddell W.R. & Loughry R.W. **(1983)** Sulindac for polyposis of the colon. Journal of Surgical Oncology **24**: 83–87.

Gonzaga R. Amarante Junior M. & Reis Lima F. **(1984)** Familial polyposis coli: the difficult choice. Lancet, February 18th, page 402–403.

Gonzaga R. Reis Lima F. Carneiro S. Maciel J. & Amarante Junior M. **(1985)** Sulindac treatment for familial polyposis coli. Lancet, March 30th, page 751.

The Physicians' Health Study **(1985)** Preventive Medicine **14**: 165–168.

Pinals R.S. Kaplan S.B. Lawson J.G. Hepburn B. **(1986)** Sulfasalazine in rheumatoid arthritis. A double-blind placebo-controlled trial. Arthritis & Rheumatism **29(12)**: 1427–1434.

Arrowsmith J.B. Kennedy D.L. Kuritsky J.N. & Faich G.A. **(1987)** National patterns of aspirin use and Reye syndrome reporting, United States, 1980–1985 Pediatrics **79** no.6: 858–863.

Stewart W.K. & Fleming L.W. **(1987)** Perthshire pioneer of anti-inflammatory agents. Scottish Medical Journal; **37**: 141–146.

Kune G.A. Kune S. & Watson L.F. **(1988)** Colorectal cancer risk, chronic illnesses, operations, and medications: case control results from the Melbourne colorectal cancer study. Cancer Research **48**: 4399–4404.

Dubovsky H. **(1988)** The history of para-aminosalicylic acid(pas), the first tuberculosis anti-microbial agent, and streptomycin (sm): a comparative study. Adler Museum Bulletin **14**: 7–11.

Peto R. Gray R. Collins R. Wheatley K. Hennekens C. Jamrozik K. Warlow C. Hafner B. Thompson E. Norton S. Gilliland J. Doll R. **(1988)** Randomised trial of prophylactic daily aspirin in British male doctors. British Medical Journal 30th January. **296**: 313–316.

United Kingdom transient ischaemic attack (UK-TIA) aspirin interim results **(1988)** British Medical Journal 30th January **296**: 316–331.

Special report. Preliminary report: Findings from the aspirin component of the ongoing Physicians' health study. **(1988)** The New England Journal of Medicine January 28th. **318**: 262–264.

Secondary prevention of vascular disease by prolonged antiplatelet treatment. Antiplatelet Trialists' Collaboration. **(1988)** British Medical Journal. 30th March **296**: 320–331.

Carroll G.J. Will R.K. Breidahl P.D. Tinsley L.M. **(1989)** Sulphasalazine versus penicillamine in the treatment of rheumatoid arthritis Rheumatology International **8(6)**: 251–255.

Belanger C. Buring J.E. Cook N. Eberlein K. Goldhaber S.Z. Gordon D. Hennekens C.H. Mayrent S.L. Peto R. Rosner B. Stamfer M.J. Stubblefield F. Willett W.C. **(1989)** Final report on the aspirin component of the ongoing physicians' health study. The Steering Committee for the Physicians' Health Study Research Group New England Journal of Medicine **321** (3): 129–135.

Vane J.R. Flower R.J. & Botting R.M. **(1990)** History of aspirin and its mechanism of action Stroke; **21** (suppl IV, 12–23).

Schadewalt H. **(1990)** Historic aspects of pharmacological research at Bayer. Stroke 1990; **21**: (Suppl IV): 5–8.

Narisawa T. Kusaka H. Yamazaki Y. **(1990)** Relationship between blood plasma prostaglandin E2 and liver and lung metastases in colorectal cancer. Dis Colon Rectum **33**: 840–845.

Dubovsky H. **(1991)** Correspondence with a pioneer, Jurgen Lehmann (1898–1989), producer of the first effective antituberculosis specific. South African Medical Journal, **79**: 48–50.

Weissman G. **(1991)** Aspirin. Sci Am; **264**: 84–90.

Gann P.H. Manson J.E. Glynn R.J. Buring J.E. & Hennekins C.H. **(1993)** Low-dose aspirin and incidence of colorectal tumours in a randomized trial. Journal of the National Cancer Institute; **85**: 1220–1224.

Giardello F.M. Hamilton S.R. Krush A.J. Piantadosi S. Hylind L.M. Celano P. Booker S.V. Robinson C.R. & Offerhaus G.J. **(1993)** Treatment of colonic and rectal adenomas with sulindac in familial polyposis. New Eng J Med **328** (18): 1313–1316.

Breitner J.C. Gatz M. Bergem A.L. Christian J.C. Mortimer J.A. McClearn G.E. Hestan L.L. Welsh K.A. Anthony J.C. Folstein M.F. & Radebaugh T.S. **(1993)** Use of twin cohorts for research in Alzheimer's disease. Neurology **43** (2): 261–267.

The Physicians' Health study **(1994)** Archives of Internal Medicine **154** (23), 2649–2657.

Peleg I I, Maibach H. T. Brown S.H. & Mel Wilcox C. **(1994)** Aspirin and nonsteroidal anti-inflammatory drug use and the risk of subsequent colorectal cancer. Arch Intern Med **154**: 394–399.

Smedegard G. & Bjork J. **(1995)** Sulphasalazine: mechanism of action in rheumatoid arthritis Brit J. Rheumatol **34** (Suppl 2): 7–15.

Berkel H.J. Holcombe R.F. Middlebrooks M. & Kannan K. **(1996)** Nonsteroidal anti-inflammatory drugs and colorectal cancer. Epidemiologic Reviews **18**(2): 205–217.

Kauppi M. Pukkala E. & Isomaki H. **(1996)** Low incidence of colorectal cancer in patients with rheumatoid arthritis Clin & Exp Rheum **14**: 551–553.

Singh G. & Ramey D. **(1997)** NSAID induced gastro-intestinal complications: the ARAMIS perspective. Journal of Rheumatology **26(suppl.51)**: 8–16.

Sturmer T. Glynn R.J. Lee I-Min, Manson J.E. Buring J.E. & Hennekens C.H. **(1998)** Aspirin use and colorectal cancer: post-trial follow-up data from the Physician's Health Study. Ann Intern Med **128**: 713–720.

The Medical Research Council's General Practice Research Framework. Thrombosis Prevention Trial: randomized trial of low-intensity oral anti-coagulation with warfarin and low-dose aspirin in the primary prevention of ischemic heart disease in men at increased risk. **(1998)** Lancet **351**: 233–241.

Van Kooten F. Ciabattoni G. Patrono C. & Koudstaal P. **(1998)** Role of platelet activation in dementia. Haemostasis **28**: 202–208.

Aspirin and risk of haemorrhagic stroke. A meta-analysis of randomized controlled trials. **(1998)** He J. Whelton P.K. Vu B. & Klag M.J. Journal of the American Medical Association **280** (22): 1930–1935.

Van Kooten F. Ciabattoni G. Patrono C. & Koudstaal P.J. **(1998)** Role of platelet activation in dementia. Haemostasis; **28**: 202–208.

Lim G. Yang F. Chu T. Chen P. Beech W. Teter B. Tran T. Ubeda O. Ashe K. Frautschy S. & Cole G. **(2000)** Ibuprofen suppresses plaque pathology and inflammation in a mouse model for Alzheimer's disease. Journal of Neuroscience **20**: 5709–5714.

The discovery of aspirin: a reappraisal. **(2000)** Walter Sneader. British Medical Journal December 23rd.

Bombardier C. Laine L. Reicin A. Shapiro D. Dr. P.H. Burgos-Vargas R. Davis B. Day R. Bosi Ferraz M. Hawkey C.J. Hochberg M.D. Kvien T.K. Schnitzer T.J. for the VIGOR study group (Vioxx Gastrointestinal Outcomes Research study) **(2000)**. Comparison of upper gastro-intestinal toxicity of Rofecoxib and Naproxen in patients with Rheumatoid Arthritis. N Engl J Med **343**: 1520–1528.

Influence of gender and age on preventing cardiovascular disease by anti-hypertensive treatment and acetylsalicylic acid: the Hypertension Optimal Treatment (HOT) study. **(2000)** J. Hypertens **18**: 629–642.

Elwood P.C. Stillings M.R. Use of aspirin in cardiovascular prophylaxis. **(2000)** Cardiovascular Journal of Southern Africa **11** (3): 155–160.

Kjeldsen S.E. Kolloch R.E. Leonetti G. Mallion J-M, Zanchetti A. Elmfeldt D. Warnold I. Hansson L. **(2000)** Influence of gender and age on preventing cardiovascular disease by anti-hypertensive treatment and acetylsalicylic acid. The HOT study. Journal of Hypertension **18** (5): 629–642.

G, Lynch P.M. Phillips R.K. Wallace M.H. Hawk E. Gordon G.B. Wakabayashi N. Saunders B. Shen Y. Fujimura T. Su L.K. & Levin B. **(2000)** The effect of celecoxib, a cyclooxygenase-2 inhibitor, in familial adenomatous polyposis. N Eng J Med **342** (26): 1946–1952.

Langman M.J. Cheng K.K. Gilman E.A. & Lancashire R.J. **(2000)** Effect of anti-inflammatory drugs on overall risk of common cancer: case-control study in general practice research database. BMJ; **320**: 1642–1646.

Janne P.A. & Mayer R.J. **(2000)** Chemoprevention of colorectal cancer. N Eng J Med **342**(26): 1960–1968.

Breuer-Katschinski B. Nemes K. Rump B. Leiendecker B. Marr A. Breuer N. & Goebell H. **(2000)** Long-term use of nonsteroidal anti-inflammatory drugs and the risk of colorectal adenomas. Digestion **61**: 129–134.

Prasad K.N. Hovland A.R. Cole W.C. Prasad K.C. Bahreini P. Edwards-Prasad J. & Andreatta C.P. **(2000)** Multiple antioxidants in the prevention and treatment of Alzheimer's disease: analysis of biological rationale. Clinical Neuropharmacology **23**: 2–13.

Steinbach G. Lynch P.M. Phillips R.K. Wallace M.H. Hawk E. Gordon G.B. Wakabayashi N. Saunders B. Shen Y. Fujimura T. Su L.K. & Levin B. **(2000)** The effect of celecoxib, a cyclooxygenase 2 inhibitor, in familial adenomatous polyposis N Engl J Med **342**: 1946–1952.

Collaborative Group of the Primary Prevention Project. Low dose aspirin and vitamin E in people at cardiovascular risk: a randomized trial in General Practice **(2001)**. Lancet **357**: 89–95.

Aisen P.S. Schmeidler J. & Pasinetti G.M. **(2002)** Randomized pilot study of nimesulide treatment in Alzheimer's disease. Neurology **59** (8): 1293.

Sandler R.S. Halabi S. Baron J.A. Budinger S. Paskett E. Keresztes R. Petrelli N. Marc Pipas J. Karp D.D. Loprinzi C.L. Steinbach G. & Schilsky R. **(2003)** A randomized trial of aspirin to prevent colorectal adenomas in patients with previous colorectal cancer (2003) N Eng J Med **348** (10): 883–890.

Ruuhola T. Julkunen-Tiitto R. Vainiotalo P. **(2003)** *In vitro* Degradation of Willow Salicylates. Journal of Chemical Ecology **29** (5): 1083–1097.

Imperiale TF **(2003)** Aspirin and the prevention of colorectal cancer N Eng J Med **348** (10): 879–880.

Baron J.A. Cole B.F. Sandler R.S. Haile R.W. Ahnen D. Bresalier R. McKeown-Eyssen G. Summers R.W. Rothstein R. Burke C.A. Snover D.C. Church T.R. Allen J.I. Beach M. Beck G.J. Bond J.H. Byers T. Greenberg E.R. Mandel J.S. Marcon N. Mott L.A. Pearson L. Saibil F. & van Stolk R.U. **(2003)** A randomized trial of aspirin to prevent colorectal adenomas N Eng J Med **348** (10): 891–899.

Benamouzig R. Deyra J. Martin A. Girard B. Jullian E. Piednoir B. Couturier D. Coste T. Little J. Chaussade S. for The Association pour la prevention par l'aspirine du cancer colorectal study group **(2003)** Daily soluble aspirin and prevention of colorectal adenoma recurrence: one-year results of the APACC trial Gastroenterology **125**: 328–336.

Sandler R.S. Halabi S. Baron J.A. Budinger S. Paskett E. Keresztes R. Petrelli N. Pipas J.M. Karp D.D. Loprinzi C.L. Steinbach G. Schilsky R. **(2003)** A randomized trial of aspirin to prevent colorectal adenomas in patients with previous colorectal cancer. New Engl J Med **348 (10)**: 883–890.

Doggrell S.A. Warfarin and aspirin give more benefit than aspirin alone but also more bleeding after myocardial infarction. **(2003)** Expert Opinion on Pharmacotherapy **4** (4): 587–590.

Connolly S.J. Prevention of vascular events in patients with atrial fibrillation. **(2003)** Journal of Cardiovascular Electrophysiology **14** (9 Supplement): S52–S55.

Eidelmans R.S, Hebert P.R. Weisman S.M. Hennekens C.H. An update on aspirin in the primary prevention of cardiovascular disease **(2003)** Archives of Internal Medicine **163** (17): 2006–2010.

Chan A.T. Giovannucci E.L. Schernhammer E.S. Colditz G.A. Hunter D.J. Willett W.C. & Fuchs C.S. **(2004)** A prospective study of aspirin use and the risk for colorectal adenoma. Ann Intern Med **140**: 157–166.

Chan A.T. Giovannucci E.L. Meyerhardt J.A. Schernhammer E.S. Curhan G.C. & Fuchs C.S. **(2005)** Long-term use of aspirin and nonsteroidal anti-inflammatory drugs and risk of colorectal cancer. JAMA **294** (8): 914–923.

Gorelick P.B. and Weisman S.M. Risk of haemorrhagic stroke with aspirin use: An update **(2005)** Stroke **36** (8): 1801–1807.

Bresalier R.S. Sandler R.S. Quan Hui, Bolognese J.A. Oxenius B. Horgan K. Lines C. Riddell R. Morton D. Lanas A. Konstam M.A. Baron J.A. for the Adenomatous Polyp Prevention on Vioxx (APPROVe) Trial Investigation **(2005)** Cardiovascular events associated with Rofecoxib in a Colorectal Adenoma Chemoprevention Trial N Engl J Med **352**: 1092–1102.

References

A Bibliography of material available on agricultural practices in the Middle ages. Source: Medieval Herbals and plant books

Aelfric Abbot of Eynsham Colloquy Nominum Herbarum 995.

Angelicus, Barthlomaeus. De Proprietatibus Rerum. 1399. ed. M. C. Seymour, Claredon Press, 1975, 2 vols. John Trevisa On the Properties of Things.

Bald and Cild. "Leechbook of Bald and Cild" M.S. Royal 12 D., British Museum. in Leechdoms, Wortcunning, and Starcraft of Early England, Being a Collection of Documents…illustrating the history of science in this country before the Norman conquest. Vol II, collected and ed. by Oswald Cockayne, London, Rolls series 35, 1864.

Banckes, Richard. Banckes's Herbal. 1525. ed & transcribed into modern English with an introduction by Sanford V. Larkey & Thomas Pyles: New York, NY: Scholars' Facsimilies & Reprints 1941.

Barbarus, Apuleius. "Herbarium Apuleii, British Museum ms. 5294." in Leechdoms, Wortcunning, and Starcraft of Early England, Being a Collection of Documents… illustrating the history of science in this country before the Norman conquest. Vol I. collected and ed. by Oswald Cockayne, London, Rolls series 35, 1864.

Bassus, Cassianus. Geoponia. Translated by T. Owen, London Printed by the author 1805–0806. Geoponia, a collection of agricultural literature, was compiled by Cassianus Bassus, at the end of the 6th or beginning of the 7th century. This compilation was revised about 950 by as unknown writer.

Book of Simples. 1650.

Cole, William. Adam in Eden, or Nature's Paradise. London: J. Streater for Nathanial Brooke, 1657.

Cole, William. The Art of Simples. London: J. G for Nath, 1656.

Crescentius. Opus Ruralim Commodorum, Italian Edition, dell' Agricultura, Venice, 1495.

Crescenzi, Pietro de. De Agrievltvra. Venice: Matteo Capcass (di Codeca), 31, May 1495.

Culpeper, Nicholas. The English Physican Or an Astrologo-physical discourse of the Vulgar Herbs of this nation. Foulsham 1652, 1820.

Didaxeon, Peri "Peri Didaxeon" of Schools of Medicine' British Museum Harleian, ms 6258" in Leechdoms, Wortcunning, and Starcraft of Early England, Being a Collection of Documents… illustrating the history of science in this country before the Norman conquest. Vol III. collected and ed. by Oswald Cockayne, London, Rolls series 35, 1864.

Digby, Kenelm. The Closet of Sir Kenelm Digby Kt. Opened. 1650.

Dioscorides. The Greek Herbal of Dioscorides. Trans. John Goodyear 1655. Robert T. Gunther 1933, New York, NY: Hafner 1968.

Dodoens, Rembert. Medecijn van der stadt van Mechelen. Ghedruckt Tantwerpen by Jan vander Loe. translated by Henery Lyte London: G. Dewes 1578.

Firenzuola, Girolamo .??. 16th cent.

Fitz-Herbert, John. FitzHerberts booke of Husbandrie. London Edward White 1598. (rpt) ed Skeat, W. W. Englosh Dialect Society, 1882.

Gardner, Ion "The Feate of Gardeninge" 1440–1450. in "A Fifteenth Century Treatise on Gardening" Archaeologia, 54 (1844) 160–167.

Gerarde, John. The Herball or Generall Historie of Plantse. 1597. rpt 1633 edition Dover Press, 1975.

Googe, Barnaby. Foure bookes of husbandry, collected by M. Conradus Geresbachius, … conteyning the whole arte and trade of husbandry, with the antiquitie, and commendation thereof. Newly Englished and increased by Barnabe Googe esquire, London: Richard Watkins 1577. (Translation of Rei Rusticae Libri Quatuor by Conrad Heresbach, 1570).

Grosseteste, Robert. The Rules of Saint Robert, Walter of Henley's Husbandry together with an anonymous Husbandry, Seneschaucie, and Robert Grosseteste's Rules. the Transcripts and translations and glossary by Elizabeth Lamond, with an introduction by W. Cunningham. London and New York, NY: Longmans, Green & Co. 1890.

Guilbert, Philbert. The Charitable Physitian. Paris 1639.

Henley, Walter de. The Mannor Farm by Francis Henry Cripps-Day, to which are added reprint facsimilies of the Boke of husbandry and English translation of the XIIIth century tract on husbandry by Walter of Henley, ascribed to Robert Grosseteste and printed by Wynkyn de Word, c. 1510, and the Booke of thrift, containing English translation of the same tract and of the anonymous XIIIth century tract Hosebonderie, by James Bellot, printed 1589. London, B. Quartich Ltd 1931.

Henley, Walter de. Walter of Henley's Husbandry together with an anonymous Husbandry, Seneschaucie, and Robert Grosseteste's Rules. the Transcripts and translations and glossary by Elizabeth Lamond…with an introduction by W. Cunningham. London and New York, NY: Longmans, Green & Co. 1890.

Hieronymus, Brunschwig. The vertuose boke of distyllacyon of the waters of all maner of herbes, with fygures of the styllatoryes, fyrst made and compyled by the thyrte yeres study and labor of… Master Jerom Bruynswyke and now newly translated out of Duyche into Englyssche. Imprinted at London by me Laurens Andrew 1527.

Hildegard of Bingen. Causae et Curae., ed Paul Kaiser Leipzig: Teubner, 1903. (Also called Liber Composiae Medicinae).

Hildegard of Bingen. Liber Simplicus Medicinae. (Also called Physica).

Hill, Thomas. The Gardeners Labyrinth. London: H Ballard, 1577. rpt Oxford University Press, 1987.

Hill, Thomas. The Proffitable Arte of Gardeninge. 1568.

Hill, Thomas. A Tryeatyse Teaching Howe to Dress, Sowe, and Set a Garden. London 1563.

References

James I of Scotland, Kingis Quair, A. Lawson, ed., London, 1910.

John Gardener in Alicia Amherst, "A Fifteenth Century Treatise on Gardening by Mayster Ion Gardener," Archaeologia, LIV, part 1, 1894, 157–172.

Lacnunga "Liber medicinalis de virtutibus herbarum, Recipies from British Museum Harleian. 585" in Leechdoms, Wortcunning, and Starcraft of Early England, Being a Collection of Documents… illustrating the history of science in this country before the Norman conquest. collected and ed. by Oswald Cockayne, Vol III. London, Rolls series 35, 1864.

Lyte, Henery. Niew Herball or history of plants, translation of Rembert Dodoens's. Herbal. London: London: G. Dewes, 1578.

Macer, Aemilius Floridus de Viribus Herbarum ed. G. Fisk, A Middle English Translation of Macer Floridus de Viribus Herbarum, Upsala,. 1949.

Macer, Aemilius. Of the Virtues of Herbs. London: 1629.

Magnus, Albert. The boke of Secretes of Albartus Magnus, of the vertues of herbes, stones, and certaine beastes. also a boke of the same author of the maruaylous things of the world and of certaine effectes caused of certayne beastes. London, Wyllyam Copland, 1525. rpt Michael R. Best and Frank H. Brightman ed. Oxford University Press 1974.

Magnus, Albert. The Secrets of Albertus Magnus, of the vertues of herbes, stones, and certaine beastes whereuuto [sic] is newly added a short discourse of the seuen planets gouerning the natiuities of children; also a book of the same author of the maruellous things of the world and of certaine effects caused by certaine beasts. London W. Jaggard 1617.

Neckham, Alexander. De Laudibus Divuviae Sapientiae 12th cent. Rolls Series.

Neckham, Alexander. De Naturis Rerum 12th cent. Rolls Series.

Neckham, Alexander. De Utensilibus 12th cent.

Palladius, Rutilius Taurus. The fourteen books of Palladius, Rutilius Taurus Æmilianus, On agriculture. Translated by T. Owen, London, Printed for J. White 1807.

Palladius, Rutilius Taurus Æmilianus. On husbondrie. from the unique ms. of about 1420 A. D. in Colchester Castle, ed by Barton Lodge… with a ryme index ed. by Sidney J. H. Herrtage London, N Trübner & Co. 1873, 1879. Early English Text Society Original Series 52, 72.

Palladius, Rutilius Taurus. The Middle English translation of Palladius. De re rustica. edited with critical and explanatory notes by Mark Liddell Berlin, E. Ebering 1896.

Parkinson, John. Paridise in sole Paradisus Terristis. London: 1629. rpt Dover Press, 1976.

Parkinson, John. Parkinson's Herbal, during the Reign of Charles I. 1692.

Pichon, Baron Jérôme Le Menagier de Paris: Traité morale et déconomie domestique composé vers 1393 par un bourgeois Parisien. 2 vols. 1846. Reprint Geneva: Slatkin, 1966.

Pichon, Baron Jérôme. The Goodman of Paris (Le Menagier de Paris), A Treatise on Moral and Domestic Economy by a Citizen of Paris, ca. 1393, Eileen Power, trans., and notes, London: Routledge, 1928.

Bayard, Tania. A Medieval home Companion Housekeeping in the Fourteenth Century. (Le Menagier de Paris) Tania Bayard, trans., London, 1991.

Placitus, Sextus. "Medicina de quadrupedibus of Sextus Placitus" in Leechdoms, Wortcunning, and Starcraft of Early England, Being a Collection of Documents… illustrating the history of science in this country before the Norman conquest. Vol I. collected and ed. by Oswald Cockayne, London, Rolls series 35, 1864.

Plat, Sir Hugh. Delights for Ladies. 1594 & 1602.

Pliny the Elder. Natural History. Loeb Classical Library.

Pontano, Giovanni. 16th cent.

Ram, William. Ram's Little Dodoen. London: 1606. Abbreviation of Rembert Dodoens's. Herbal. London: G. Dewes 1578]

Rufinus. The Herbal of Rufinus, thirteenth century, Chicago, Illinois, University of Chicago Press, 1945.

Turner, William. Libellus de herbaria novus. London 1538. rpt. Benjamihn Daydon Jackson, 1877.

Turner, William. Names of Herbs. London, John Day, 1548. rpt. English Dialect Society, 1881.

Turner, William. Theatrum Botanicum. London: 1640.

Turner, William. Herbal. London, 1551, 1568.

Tusser, Thomas. A Hundred Points of Good Husbandrie. London 1557. expanded as Five Hundred Points of Good Husbandrie. London 1571, 1573.

Walahfied-Strabo [807–849]. De Cultura Hortorum, of the little garden; a ninth century poem by Walahfied-Strabo. trans Richard Stanton Lambert, Wembley Hill, Stanton Press 1924. Raef Pay Pittsburgh The Hunt Botanical Linrary, 1966.

Walahfrid Strabo, Hortulus, Raef Payne, trans., commentary by Wilfrid Blunt, The Hunt Botanical Library, Pittsburgh, 1966.

Index

Index Note: *Italicized* page numbers relate to tables and illustrations.

abscesses, 115, 190
Abortus fever, 56-7
Acemetacin, *162*
acetaminophen *see* paracetamol
acetanilide, 161, 163
acetic anhydride, 154
acetylsalicylic acid
    anticoagulant effect of, 229-31
    chemical reaction for producing, *156*
    development of, 135-8, 144-5, 149
    see also aspirin
'Adam in Eden' (Cole), 87
adhesion, 222, 233
advertisements, *149, 152, 154, 261*
Aisen, P.S., 259
Aitken, William, 49, *50*
Alka-Seltzer, 159
alkalis, 121, 147
Allbutt, Thomas Clifford (1836-1925), 49-50, *51*
allergic reaction, 218-21
Alzheimer, Alois (1864-1915), 256, *257*
Alzheimer's disease, 256-60
    histology of, *257*
AMIS (aspirin myocardial infarction study research group), 235
amoeboid movement, 197
amyloid, 259
amyloidosis, 186
anaemia, 185
analgesic nephropathy, 162-3
anaphylactic shock, 218-21
ancient Greek medical practises
    herbalists, 66
    treatment of fevers, 13-15
    Celsus on, 174-81
antibiotics, 57
antibodies, 189, 197-8, 218
Antifebrine, 161
antigens, 189, 190, 197, 198
anti-inflammatory drugs (NSAIDs), 157-8, 161-5, 199, 215
    colorectal cancer research, 245-9, 256
    Cox-2 selective, 223-5
        relative Cox-2 selectivity, *224*
        those prior to, *165*

experiment involving RCS, 221
rank order of gastro-intestinal events, *162*
see also individual drugs' names
Antiplatelet Trialists' Collaboration, 238
antiseptic, 108, 110, 111-12, 134, 213
apoptosis, 248, 250
appendix, normal and inflamed, *182, 193, 194*
Apuleius Platonicus, 70, 71-2
arachidonic acid, 218
Arbor virus, 58-9
Aristotle (384-322 BC), 66, 89
Arrowsmith, J.B., 170
arthritis, 62, 90
    see also rheumatoid arthritis
Asclepiades, 13
Aspergum, 229
aspirin
    action and uses, 147, 201, 215
        in Alzheimer's disease, 256-60
        in colon and colorectal cancer, 243-4, 246-9, *247,* 250-6
        in Rheumatic fever, 216
        on Cox 1 and Cox 2, 223
        on prostaglandin synthesis, 221-2, *223*, 248
    anti-coagulant effects, xi, 229-32
        controlled tests, 233-41, *241*
        gastro-intestinal events, ix-xi, 157, 159, 161, *162,* 256
        stroke risk, 239
    anti-inflammatory effects, 216-22 *223*
        salazopyrin comparison, 211
    chemical formulation and production, *125,* 131, 132-4
        British Pharmaceutical Codex, 146-8
        sources, x, *113*
        synthetic/industrial production, 134-6, *137,* 153-6
    children's, *171,* 171-2, *261*
    commercial exploitation of
        advertisements, *149, 152, 154, 261*
        Bayer's early products, *146, 147, 148*
        early prescription practises, 148
        in America, 143
        in Britain, 143, 151, 152-3
        licencing, 139-40
        patenting, 138, 141-2
        preparations containing aspirin, 160
        trade name, 145, 149-50

Reye's syndrome and, 170-2
solubility, x, 146
usage
    by colorectal cancer patients, *246, 247, 250-6, 253, 254*
    by heart attack patients, *234, 234-9, 236*
    by stroke patients, 237
    purchases by drug stores (USA), *169, 171*
    rates of mention by age groups by year (USA), *168*
    warfarin, combination and comparison with, 240
see also acetylsalicylce acid
Aspro, 149, 151, 152
astrological botany, 82-4
atrial fibrillation, 63, 240-1
atypical mononuclear cells, 60
Australia, 166-7, 170, 245
Azad Khan, 212

bacteria, 189, 200, 203, 215, 243
bacterial infections, 61, 62-3, 64, 188
Bado, Sebastiano, 126
Baker's cyst, 116
Banckes, Rycharde, 72-3
Bang, B., 57
Bartonella quintana, 64
basophils, 227
Bath City Infirmary and Dispensary, 102, 112
Bayer Co. Ltd, (UK), 143
Bayer Company, *x, 135, 136, 136-45*
    Aspirin, official description of, *142*
    Aspirin, powder and tablet, *146, 147, 148*
    advertisements, *149*
    IG Farben cartel, 151-2
    other aniline by-products, 161-3
    Rensselaer factory (USA), *143, 150*
    trade mark renewal application (1909), *144*
Bayer, Friedrich (1825-1880), 135
Beddoes, Dr., 109
Benamouzig, R, 254
Bennett, Dr. Hugh, 54
Benoral, 165
benzene acetic acid derivatives, 165
benzoic acid, 205
Bernheim, Frederick, 203
Blackwater fever, 57-8
bleeding, practise of, 19, 24, 28, 40, 122, 179
    for investigative purposes, 17
bleeding (haemorrhage), 59, 157, 224, 229, 256
    after first heart attack, 240
    postoperative, 229-30
bleeding time, 232-3
blistering, practise of, 28
blood, 190
    acute-phase proteins in, 184-5
    aniline administration, 163
    cell flow, 191
    coagulation, *ix, 187, 193, 200, 226-30*
        defibrination syndrome, 22-3
        emboli, 240-1
        lysosomal products and, 198
        prothrombin time, 231-2
    diapedesis, 196
    formed elements of, 227
    haematological changes, 185-6
    ischaemic damage, 190
    monocytes, 189, 190
    neutrophil flow, 194-6
    platelets, 199, 223, 227-9, *228*
    sedimentation measurement, 206, 211
    vascular permeability and, 192-3
    vomiting of, 159, 215
body temperature, 48-54, 206, 207, 215, 221-2
    effect of para-aminosalicylic acid, *207*
    in acute inflammation, 184
    in typhus, 32-3
    range of, in acute rheumatism, *124*
Boerhaave, Herman (1668-1738), 17, 48-9
bone marrow, 194
Boots of Nottingham, 164, 218
Boston Collaborative drug surveillance group, 234
Bouillaud, Frédéric, 122
bowel disorders, 89-90, 105, 108, 188
    chronic inflammatory (IBD), 112-13, 212-14
    melaena, 159
    see also gastro-intestinal disorders
bradykinin, 200
British Board of Trade, 145
British Doctors Trial, *241*
British Medical Journal, 208, 234, 237
British National Formulary, 171-2
British Pharmaceutical Codex, 146-8, 213-14
Brodie, B.B., 163
Bruce, D, 57
Brucella infection, 56-7
Brugnatelli, L, 131, 132
Brunfels, Otto (1488-1534), 76
Brunton, Lauder, 54
Buchner, J, 132
Bufferin, 235-6

Cahours, Auguste, 131
cancer, 235, 243-56
    primary and secondary prevention, 253-6
    risk reduction looking at aspirin taken, *254,* 255-6
cardiac disorders
    carditis, 62-3, 216, 241
    clotting time and, 233

Index

coronary thrombosis, 230-2
   myocardial infarction, *xi*, 225, 234, 240, 242
      controlled tests into, 234-9, *236, 241*
   through earlier arthritis, 216
cardiovascular mortality, controlled study, 238-9
Carstensen, B., 207
cascara sagrada tree, 89
Castelli, Benedetto, 48
Celebrex (celecoxib), 223, *224*, 225, 249
cells, 218
   adhesion, 222
   immune, 248
   programmed death (apoptosis), 248
cellular exudation, 189, 190, 194
Celus (25BC-50AD), *173*, 173-81, 183-4
cerebral abscess, 190
cerebral thrombosis (ischaemic attack), 237, 239
Chapman, Charles W., 148
chemotaxis of neutrophils, 196-7, 199
chickenpox, *168*
chinchona *see* Peruvian Chinchona tree
chloramphenicol, 65
choline magnesium silicate, 165
chorea, 62, 108
chronic fatigue syndrome, 57
cinchona *see* Peruvian Chinchona tree
ciprofloxacin, 59, 64
clindamycin, 62
clinical aspects of acute inflammation, 183-4
Clinical Trial Service Unit, 238
clotting time, 233
coagulation, *xi*, 187, 193, 200, 226-30, 240-1
   defibrination syndrome, 22-3
   lysosomal products and, 198
   prothrombin time, 231-2
cocaine, 90
Colchicum autumnale, 77
colchicine, 60
colds, 30
Cole, William, 87-8
Collier, H.O.J., 217, 218
colonic disorders, *xi*, 201, 212, 244
   colorectal cancer, 245-9, 251-6
   polyposis and cancer, *224*, 224-5, 250
Columbia University, 163
competitive inhibition, 203
complement system, 189, 197, 199-200
Connolly, Dr. S.J., 241
Cope, Sir Jonathan, 92, 94, 95
Cope family of Bruern, 92-3
coronary thrombosis, 230-2
cortisone, 202, 211
Corynebaceterium diphtheriae, 188
Cox-1, 222-3, 249, 258
Cox-2, and inhibitors, *xi*, 223-5, *224*

Alzheimer's disease, 258, 259
   cancer and polyp prevention, 249, 250, 256
Coxiella burnetti organism, 61
Crateuas, 66
Craven, Dr Lawrence L., *xi*, 229-32
Crohn's disease, 114, 201, 212-13
Cullen, Dr., 99, 110
Culpeper, Nicholas (1616-1654), *82*, 82-3, 85
Currie, Dr. James, 49
cyclo-oxygenases, 218, 222-4
Cyperus papyrus, 1, 1-2

'De Medicina' (Celsus), 174-81
Degesch, 152
delirium, 166
Della Porta, Giambattista (1535-1615), 86-7, 88
Dengue fever, 58-9
Der erste Theyl der Kleynen Teutschen Apotek, Confect
   (Ryff), 78, *78*
diabetes, 104
diaphoretics, 122
diclofenac, *162, 224*
digitalis, 63, 84, 112, 202
Diodes of Carystos (c.300 BC), 66
Dioscorides (40-80 AD), 8, 66-9, 89
diptheria, 188
disease-modifying drugs (DMARDs), 210-11
diseases, 192, 201
   rickettsial diseases, 64
   typhus, 28, 51-3, 59, 121
Disprin, *x*, 151, 152-3, *153, 154*
dissection, 175-4
doctrine of signatures, *viii, x*, 82, 86-9, 116-18
Dodoens, Rembert (1517-1585), 74, 88
Doggrell, Dr. S.A., 240
Douthwaite, A., 157
doxycycline, 57, 59, 62
Dreser, Heinrich, 136-8, *138*
Duckworth, Sir Dyce, 125
Dundee Royal Infirmary, 116
duodenal ulcers, 160, *160*
Duthie, J.J., 217
dyestuffs, synthetic, 135

Ebers, George, *x*, 2-4, 6
Edinburgh Medical Journal, 50
Edinburgh Royal Infirmary, 54
Edinburgh University, 41, 54
Eichengrun, Arthur, 136-8, *138*
Eidelmans, R.S., 242
electuaries, 79
Elwood, Peter, 235, 240
emboli, 240-1
emigration of neutrophils, 195-6, *196*, 199
emodin, 89

empyema, 101
encephalitis, 57, 166-7
endocarditis, 57
endogenous pyrogens, 185
endoscopy, 157, 161
endothelial cells, 190, 193, 194, 195-6
endothelium, 227, 228
Entire Works of Dr. Thomas Sydenham, The, 14
enzymes, 189-90, 201
eosinophilia, 185, 196
eosinophils, 227
epiglottitis, 190
Epstein-Barr virus, 60
Erasistratus, 179
erythrocytes, 227
    sedimentation rate, 185, 211
Essay on fevers (Huxham), *18*, 18-25
etodolac, *224*
'Experiments and observations on the cortex *salicis latifolia*', 108-16
exudation, 188-9, 190, 192-4, 200

Fahrenheit, Daniel, 50
familial polyposis of the colon, *244*, 244-5, 249
Farbenfabriken of Elberfeld Company (USA), 141-2
fenamates, 165
Fennings Junior Aspirin, *161*
fenoprofen, *162*
Ferrosan drug firm, 203
fevers, described
    by Galen, 12-15
    by Heberden, 28-37
        hectic, 32-5
        intermittent, 30-2
    by Huxham, 19-25
        slow nervous fever, 20-2
    by Lettsom, 38-41
    by Rush, 41-8
    by Sydenham, 15-17
fevers, types, 9-11
    Abortus, 56-7
    Blackwater fever, 57-8
    continuous fever, 9, 13, 15, 39
    Dengue fever, 58-9
    depuratory, 5
    disease associated, *55*, 56-7
    epidemic, 15-16
    Epidemic typus fever, 59
    Familial Mediterranean fever, 60
    Glandular fever, 60
    Haverhill fever, 61
    hectic, 15-16, 32-5
    hemitritaion, 13
    intercurrent, 15, 16-17

    intermittent, 10-11, 15-16, 19-20, 30-2, 34-5, 39, 129
    malignant, 15, 20, 22-3, 43
    morbillous, 15
    of unknown origin (FUO), 55
    Pel-Ebstein fever, 61
    pernicious, 12-13, 15
    pestilential, 15, 22
    pleuritic, 15
    puerperal fever, 61
    putrid, 15, 20, 22
    Q fever, 61-2
    quartan, 12, 15, 32, 58
    quotidian, 13, 58
    relapsing, 56
    remittent, 9-10
    Rift Valley Fever, 63-4
    Rocky Mountain Spotted Fever, 64
    scarlet, 15-16
    slow nervous, 20-2
    spotted, 56
    stationary, 15-16
    tertian, 12, 15, 20, 58
    Trench fever, 64
    typhoid (enteric) fever, 64-5
    yellow fever, 41-8, 65
    see also Rheumatic fever
fibrin, 23, 227, 228
fibrinolysis, 226
fibrinous exudation, 189, 193, 200
fibrinous inflammation, *186*, 187, 216
Filendipula ulmaria (meadow sweet), 89, 131, *132*
Finland, studies, 247
5-aminosalicylic acid, 210-12
5-hydroxytryptamine, 199
flavivirus, 63, 65
Flinn, E.B., 163
Flint, Dr., 122-3
flu *see* influenza
fluid exudation, 188-9, 190, 192-4
Fontana, C, 131, 132
4-aminosalicylic acid (PAS), 203-7, *206*
    statistical interpretation of trial results, 208-9
foxglove (*digitalis*), 63, 84, 112, 202
Fuchsius, Leonhart, 77, *78*

Galen (131-201 AD), 11-15, 74
Galileo, 48
gangrene, 188, *188*
gangrenous angina, 25
Gann, P.H., 250
Garcia-Rodriguez, S., 161
Gardner's syndrome, 244-5
Garrod, Archibald E., 125
gastro-intestinal disorders, *ix-x*, 157-61, 224, 256

Index

colonic, *xi*, 201, 212
    polyposis and cancer, *244*, 244-5, 250-6
colorectal cancer, 245-9, 256
rank order of events likelihood, *162*
ulcers, 157-61
    duodenal, 160, *160*
    gastric, *159*, 161, *164*
    VIGOR study of, 224-5
see also bowel disorders
Gaultheria procumbens see wintergreen
Genasprin, 151, *152*
Genatosan Ltd, 151
general practice research data base, 249-50
genetically inherited fevers and disorders, 60, *244*, 244-5, 249
Gerard, John (1534-1612), 74-5
Gerhardt, Charles, 134
Gerland, Henri, 134
GI Toxicity Index, 161
Gillray, James, 77
Glandular fever, 60
glomerulonephritis, 189
gout, 108, 164, *180*
Greenberg, L.A., 163
Greenish, Professor H.G., 143
Griffiths, Samuel P., 44
Gutenberg, Johann, 70
Guy's Hospital, 122-3

haematemesis, 159, 215
haemoglobin, 227
haemorrhage *see* bleeding (haemorrhage)
Harris, James, Earl of Malmesbury (1746-1820), 18
heart attack, *xi*, 225, 234, 240, 242
    controlled tests into, 234-9, *236*
heart murmur, 62-3, 216
Heberden, William (1710-1801), 25-30
hepatitis, 181
herbalism, 260
herbals, manuscript and printed, 66
    Apuleius Platonicus Herbarium, 70, *71*
    Banckes' herbal, 72-3
    Brunfels' herbal, 76
    Bury St. Edmunds herbal, *71*, 72
    Fuchsius' herbal, *77*, 78
    Gerard's herbal, 74-5, *75*
    Grete Herball, The, 73-4
    Herbarius latinus, 70
    Herbarius Sanitatis, 71-2
    Herbarius zu Teutsch, 70-1
    Materia medica, 67-70, *69*
    Physicall Directory, 82-3, 85
    Phytognomonica, 86-7
    Rufinus herbal, The, 81
    Ryff herbal, The, 78-81, *79, 80*
    bibliography of, 273-6
herbs and plants
    dropwort (*filendipula*), 84
    foxglove (*digitalis*), 63, 84, 112, 202
    mandrake, 67
    maidenhair fern, 87
    meadow sweet, 89, 131, *132*
    rosemary, 72-3
    Saint Johns wort, 86, 118
    simples, 70
    waterworte (Mayden), 72
    wintergreen, 79-81, 85, 90, 131, *132*, 134, 213
Herophilus, 175
Heyden Chemical Company, 135, 142
Heyden, Friedrich von, 134, 135
Hill, John, 91
Hippocrates (460-377 BC), 8, 58, 89, *174*, 175
histamine, 193, 194, 199, 219-21
'Historical account of pharmacology to the 20th century, An' (Leake), 89-9
Hodgkin's disease, 61
Hoffman, Felix, *136*, 137-6
    patent announcement, *141*
hormones, 206
Horsenden, Buckinghamshire, *92*, 93, 94
Hulse, Edward, 37
Hutchinson, Dr. J., 42-3
Huxham, John (1692-1868), *17*, 17-25
    on malignant putrid fever, 22-3
    on slow nervous fever, 20-2
hyperaemia, 191
hypersensitive reactions, 183, 189, 190, 199
hypertension optimal treatment study, 241
hypothalamus, 10, 185, 198, 221-2

ibuprofen, *162*, 164, *224*, 259
IG Farben, 151-2
immune response, 189, 203, 248
immunoglobulins, 197
Imperial Cancer Research Fund, London, 249
indole/indene derivatives, 165
indomethacin, 158-9, *162*, 164, 221, 243-4
inflammation, 34, 35, 173
    acute, 181
    of the appendix, *182, 193, 194*
    beneficial effects of, 188-9
    causes, 183
    cellular events, 194
    chemical mediators of, 184, 194, 198-200
    clinical aspects of, 183-4
    clinical indications of, 184-5
    early stages, 190-1, 194-5
    harmful effects of, 189-90
    macroscopic appearance of, 186

response, main functions, 181
  systemic effects of, 185, 188
  vascular component of, 191, 192-4
 as inappropriate response, 190
 catarrhal, 187
 Celsus on ancient Greek practises, 178-81, 183-4
 chronic, 181, 185, 200-1, 216
  amyloidosis and, 186
  bowel disease (IBD), 112-13, 212-14
  rheumatoid arthritis, 209-12
 fibrinous, *186, 187*
 haemorrhagic, 187
 membranous, 188
 necrotising (gangrenous), 188, *188*
 pseudomembranous, 188
 sedimentation rate, 206, 211
 serous, 186
 suppurative (purulent), 187
 swelling, 184, 190, 215
influenza, *169*, 170, 190
 pandemic (1918), 150
inoculation, 24
insulin, 167
Interleukin-5, 61
intermittent fever, 10-11, 15-16, 19-20, 30-2, 39, 129
 and hectic, 32-7
 and Rheumatic fever, 120, 125
lysosomal enzymes, 189-90

James, Samuel, 98-102, 109
jaundice, 115
Jesuit's bark, 125-6
Joachim, Dr. H., 3, 5
Johnson, Thomas, 74

Kalle & Company, 161
Kauppi, M.P.E., 247
keratin, 85
Ketoprofen, *162*
kidney disorders, 115, 166, 186
kinin system, 200
Kolbe, Herman, 134
Kolbe-Schmitt reaction, 134
Kraepelin, E., 257
Kyeldsen, Dr. S.E., 240

Lacey Green, Buckinghamshire, *92*
Lancet, 54, 116, 143, 148, 157, 259
 Lehmann's article (1946), 205
 Reye's paper (1963), *166*
laxative effects of cascara sagrada bark, 89
Laycock, Dr., 54
Leake, Chauncey D., 89-90
Lehmann, Jurgen (1898-1989), 203, 204-5, *205*
Leroux, J., 131, 132

Lester, G, 163
Lettsom, John Coakley (1744-1815), 37-41
leukocytes, 191, *195*
leukocytosis, 185
leukotrienes, 199
Lewis, Thomas, 191
Liber de arte distillandi (Braunschweig), 74
Lintott, G., 157
liver disorders, 166-7, 170
London Pharmacopioiea, 27-37, 126
 Febris Hectica, 32-7
 Febris Intermittens, 30-2
Lowig, K, 132
lymphatics, 189, 193
lymphocytes, 60, 201, 227
lymphocytosis, 185
lymphokines, 199
lymphomas, 61, 64
lysosomes, 198, 199

Macclesfield, Earl of, 92, 97
Maclagan, Douglas, 54
Maclagan, Dr. Thomas (1838-1903), *viii-ix, x*, 50-3, 116-19, 125, 216
 'Rheumatism: its nature, its pathology and its successful treatment', 119-22
macrophages, 185, 189, 190, 196, 201
malaria, 57-8, 99, 122, 126
mandrake plant, 67
Mann, Ralph, 85, 90
mannan binding lectin pathway, 200
margination, 195
marine sponge cells, 222
mast cells, 218
Materia medica (Dioscorides), 67-70, *69*
McConkey, Brian, 211
McGeer, P.L., 259
meadow sweet *(Spiraea ulmaria)*, 89, 131, *132*
meclofenamate, *162*
mediators, 184
 histamine, 193, 194, 199, 219-21
 leukotrienes, 199
 lysosomes, 198, 199
 prostaglandins, 199, 218, 220-1
  coagulation process, 228
  inhibition by aspirin, *223*, 248
  scheme detecting, *220*
 serotonin, 199
Medical Research Council Epidemiology Unit, Cardiff, 235
Medicina Magica (Biedermann), 67
melaena, 159
meloxicam, *224*
membrane attack complex, 189
menadione, 230

Index

meningitis, 57, 190
meningococcal septicaemia, 187
menopausal patients, 34
Merck, 132, 225
mercury, 86, 107, 113
methaemoglobin, 163
methotrexate, 259
methyl salicylate, 131, *133*, 134
micro-organisms
    opsonisation, 197-8
    phagocytosis, 189, 197-8, 198
microbial agents, 198
microbial infections, 183
microcirculation, 191
mitogens, 248
monocytes, 227
monocytosis, 185
mosquitoes, 47-8, 58-9
multi-infarct dementia, 258, 260
'Murder, Magic and Medicine' (Mann), 85
muscle fibres in a normal and inflamed appendix, *182*

N-acetyl p-aminophenol, 163
naproxen, *162*, 164, 224, *224*
narcotics, 74
National Cancer Institute, Maryland, 249, 250
National Health Service, 204-5
National Heart and Lung Institute, Maryland, 243
National Institute of Health and Clinical Excellence (NICE), 224
natural selection, 118
necrosis, 183, 188, *188*, 192, 248
'Neue Kochbuch, fur die Krancken' (Ryff), 79
neuritis, 57
neurofibrillary tangles, 257, *257*
neutrophilia, 185
neutrophils, 189, 222, 227
    cellular exudation and, *194*, 194-6, *195*
    chemotactic factors, 196-7
    polymorphs, role of, 190, *194*, 197-8
Nicholas, George, 149
North General Hospital, Edinburgh, 217-18
NSAIDs *see* anti-inflammatory drugs
Nurse Sykes' powders, *161*

O'Brien, John, 233
oak bark, 101
Observations and Experiments on the Broad-leaved Willow Bark (White), 102-8
Observations on the Bark of a particular species of willow (James), 98-102
oedema, *182*, 184
Office of Epidemiology and Biostatistics, Maryland, 170

oponisation, 189, 197-8
osteoarthritis, 159, 164
osteomyelitis, 115
otitis media, 104
oxicams, 165
oxygen utilisation, 189, 198, 203

Pagenstecher, J, 131, 132
pain, 184, 200, 222, 223
Panadol, 163-4
pancreatic and prostate cancer, 249
pancreatitis, 187
Papyrus Ebers, 2-7
papyrus, medical documentation on, 1-8
Paracelsus (1493-1541), 82, 85-6, 88, 117
paracetamol, *xi,* 161, 163-4, 165, 171-2, 222
    purchases by drugstores, *169, 171*
    rates of mention by age groups by year, *168*
    physicians' mentions, *169*
parasitic infections, 59, 64, 183
pavementing of neutrophils, 195, *196*
penicillin, 62
percardium, inflammation of the, 62
peritoneum, *182*
Peruvian bark, 20
    Heberden on, 29, 31-2, 36-7
    Huxham on, 20, 25
    see also Peruvian Chinchona tree
Peruvian Chinchona tree, *x,* 27, 40, 97
    Cinchona *officinale, 128*
    Cinchona *succiruba,* 128
    James' case notes, 99
    Maclagan, T. J., on, 116, 122, 125-6
    Wellcome on, 127-9
    White on, 108-9
    Wilkinson on, 107-8, 111-12
    see also Peruvian bark; quinine
Peto, R., 237
phagocytosis, 189, 194, 197-8
Pharmacopieia, 82
Phenacetin, 161-2
phenylbutazone, 157-8, 164
Philo of Byzantium, 48
phthisis pulmonalis, 112
physical agents, 183
'Physicall Directory' (Culpeper), 82-3
Physicians' Health Study Research Group (USA), 235-6, 238-9, *241*
'Phytognomonica' (Porta), 86-7
Piper, Priscilla, *xi,* 218-19, *220*
Piria, R., 132
piroxicam, *162*
plants *see* herbs and plants
plasma factors, 199-200
Plasmodium, 58, 122

platelets, 199, 227-9, *228*
    adherence, 233
Platonicus, Apuleius, 70-2
pleural cavitation, 204, *204*
Pliny (23-79 AD), 89
pneumonia (pneumonitis), 181, 193
polymorphs, 185, 190, *195,* 196
    neutrophil polymorphs, 190, *194,* 197-8
polyps (adenomas), 244-5, 250, 252, *252,* 254
    risk reduction looking at aspirin taken, *254,* 254-5
Pott's disease, 115
pregnancy, 34, 64, 101
    fever at delivery, 34, 61
primary prevention project, 241
Proctor, William, 131, 134
propionic acid derivatives, 165
prostaglandins, 199, 218, 220-1
    coagulation process, 228
    inhibition by aspirin, *223,* 248
    scheme detecting, *220*
prostate and pancreatic cancer, 249
proteins, 184-5, 199, 257
    enzymatic, complement activating, 199-200
    fluid exudation and, 192, 193
psoas abscess, 99, 100-1
Puerperal fever, 61
pulmonary embolism, 228-9, 240
pulmonary tuberculosis, 99, 101-2, 106, 113, 115, 185, 200, 202-9
    cavitation, 204, *204*
pulse rate, 14-15, 64
purging, 17, 24, 28
pus, *194,* 204, 248
pyogenic infection, 101, 185
pyrazolones, 165
pyrexia of unknown origin, 55

Q fever, 61-2
quinine, 90, 126
    chemical formula, *125*
    see also Peruvian Chinchona tree

rabbit (aorta) contracting substance (RCS), 220-1
rashes, 202
    erythema marginatum, 62, 215
    in acute inflammation, 183
    in typhoid, 64
    maculopapular, 64
    thurfyl nicotinate induced, 217
    typhus related, 59
    see also skin responses
reactive hyperplasia of the reticulo-endothelial system, 185
Reckitt & Colman, 151, 152-3

recovery by crisis, 10, *11*
rectal cancer, 245-9, 251-6
Rees, W.D.N., 157
Reflections on the General Treatment and Cure of Fevers, (Lettsom), 36, 37-40
resolution by lysis, 10, *11*
respiratory disorders, 114, 166-7, *193, 195*
Reye's syndrome, 62, 166-72
    cases reported (1977-1985), *168*
Reye, Dr R.D.K., *166,* 167, 170
Rheumatic fever, 62-3, 107-8, 116-17, 215-16, 233
    Maclagan on, 119-22, 125
    range of temperature, *124*
    Stricker and Riess's treatment of, 122-3
    see also fevers, types
'Rheumatism: its nature, its pathology and its successful treatment' (Maclagan), *119,* 119-22
rheumatoid arthritis, 157, 201
    Alzheimer's disease trials and, 259
    colorectal cancer trials and, *247,* 247-9
    early and advanced, *216, 217*
    treatment through aspirin, 216-17
    treatment through aspirin derivatives, 202, 209-12
    VIGOR study, 224-5
    see also arthritis
Rickettsia prowazeki organism, 59
rickettsial diseases, 64
    typhus, 28, 51-3, 59, 121
Riddle, Dr. John M, 67
Riess, L., 122-3
rifampicin, 57, 62
rofecoxib (Vioxx), 139-40, 223-5, *224*
Royal Alexandra Hospital, Sydney, 166
Royal College of Physicians, 27, 28, 82
Royal Society, *96-7*
Rufinus, 81-2
Rush, Benjamin (1745-1813), 41-8
Ryff, Walter Hermann (c1500-1548), 78-81

Salasprin, 151
salazopyrin, 210, 211
salicin, 90, 117, 157
    Maclagan on, 123
    graph of results, *118*
    process of first preparation, 131-2, *133,* 135-6
salicylaldehyde, 131, 132, *133*
salicylates, 165-6, 213, 222, 243
    natural occurrences of, 131
    Reye's syndrome and, *167,* 170
    sodium salicylate, 135, 143-4, 157, 203, 222
salicylazosulphapyridine, 210, 211
salicylic acid, 122-3, 147, 157
    action and uses, 213, 217-18
    preparations, 214
    5-aminosalicylic acid, 210-12

Index

4-aminosalicylic acid (PAS), 203-7, *206*
    process of first preparation, 131-2, *133,* 134
    soluble, 213
    sources, natural and artificial, 213
    synthesis, 134, 154-5
        exploitation of, 135
Salix
    S. alba, 110, 130
    S. caprea, 110-12
    S. latifolia, 98, 109-10
Salmonella typhi, 64
Salsalate, *162,* 165
salt, 86
Sanctorius, 48
Sandler, R.S., 251
Scammon, James, 84
scrofula *see* tuberculosis
Secundus, Caius Plinius, 8
Sée, Germain, 108
Semmelweiss, I., (1818-1865), 61
serotonin, 199
sexual characteristics, 206
Shippen, William, 44
side effects
    of aniline by-products, 161-3
    of anti-inflammatory drugs (NSAIDs), 157-8, 162-3, 165
    of aspirin, 229-30
        on gastric mucosa, ix-x, 157, 159, 161, 215, 223
    of cortisone, 202
    Reye's syndrome, 62, 166-72
simples, 70
skin responses
    to salicylic acid, 213
    triple response to injury, 191
    see also rashes
Sloane, Sir Hans, 126
Smith, Professor H.L., 144-5
Smith, Sidney, 202
sodium salicylate, 135, 143-4, 157, 203, 222
Spiraea ulmaria (meadow sweet), 89, 131, *132*
spondylitis, 158
St. John's College, Cambridge, 25-6
St. Mary and St. Nicholas, Church of, Saunderton, *92*
St. Mary, Church of, Charlton-on-Otmoor, *93*
St. Michael, Church of, Horsenden, *92*
St. Nicholas, Church of, Saunderton, *92*
St. Peter, Church of, Drayton, *93, 94, 95*
steriods, 62, 157, 167, 259
Sterling Products, 150, 152
stomach disorders *see* gastro-intestinal disorders
Stone, Edward (1702-1768), *viii, x,* 90-8, 110, 129
    experimentation and letter to the Royal Society, 96-8

streptococcal bacteria, 61, 210
    in Rheumatic fever, 62-3
streptomycin, 57, 203, 204, 207, 208-9
Stricker, S., 122-3, 134
strokes, 235, 236, 237, 238, 239, 240-1
    multi-infarct dementia, 258, 260
subphrenic abcess, 115
sulindac, *162,* 245, 250
sulindac sulphone, 249
sulphasalazine, 211-12
sulphonamides, 203, 210-12
sulphur, 86
suppurative (purulent) inflammation, 187
Sutton, Dr., 122
Svartz, Nanna, 210-11
Swedish drug trials, 207
Sweetnam, P.M., 235
swelling, 184, 190, 215
Sydenham, Dr. Thomas (1634-1689), *14,* 15-17
    Huxham on, 23
Syntex, 164
synthetic production of aspirin, 134
syphilis, 58
systemic effects of inflammation, 185

tannin, 90
temperature *see* body temperature
temporal Arteritis, 22
tenoxicam, *162*
tetracycline, 57, 59
Theophrastus (372-287 BC), 66, 89
thermometers, development of, 48-54
thermoscope, 48
Thom, Robert, 7-8, *67*
Thomas Kerfoot Ltd, 151
thrombin, 227
thromboses, 115, 229, 230-1, 239
Thrombosis Prevention Trial, *241*
thyrotoxicosis, 106
tinnitus, 157, 206
tissue necrosis, 183
Tolmetin, *162*
toxins, 189
Traum, J., 57
'Treatment of acute rheumatism by Salicin, The' (Maclagan), 116
Truelove, L.H., 217
tuberculosis
    clinical drug trials, 203-7
        resistance and combination therapy, 208-9
    intestinal, *207*
    pulmonary, 99, 101-2, 106, 113, 115, 185, 200, 202-9
        cavitation, 204, *204*
tumours *see* cancer

'Twentieth Century Practice. An International Encyclopedia of Modern Medical Science', 123, 125
typhoid, 64-5, 121
typhus, 28, 51-3, 59, 121

ulceration, 201
   gastric and duodenal, 159-60
   in pseudomembranous inflammation, 188
ulcerative colitis, 201, 212
United States of America, 149-50, 163
   Bayer's Rensselaer factory, *143, 150*
   Federal Drugs Administration, 225
   patenting of aspirin, 141-2
   Reye's syndrome cases, *168, 169,* 170-1, *171*
   studies into Alzheimer's disease, 259
   studies into colorectal cancer, 246-7, 249, 250
   and on aspirin use, 254-5
   tests on aspirin usage, 235-6
   tests on haemorrhaging, 229-33, 235
   tuberculosis cases, 203, 208
   Vioxx litigation, 225
urinary disorders, 105
   aetiocholanolone fever, 60
   Blackwater fever, 57
   dropwort and, 84
uterine disorders, 107, 113

vaginal discharge (fluor albus), 107, 113
Vallentine, Dr. Gylfe, 204, 206
Vane, Sir John, *xi,* 218-19, *220, 221*
vascular mortality, 238
vascular system, 189, *195,* 200, 226-7
   cardiovascular mortality, controlled study, 238-9
   changes in vessel calibre, 191
   controlled tests into disease of, 238
   increased permeability, 192-3, 199
   ultrastructural basis of, 193-4
vasodilatation, 191, 199
venules, 195, 226
Vioxx (rofecoxib), 139-40, 223-5, *224*
Virchow, Rudolph, 179, 184
vitamins, 246, *246*
vomiting, 166-7
   of blood, 159, 215

Waddell, W.R., 244-5
Wadham College, Oxford, 91-2, 93-4
Waksman, Selman, 203
Wallenberg, Raoul, 210-11
warfarin, 229, 240-1
   and aspirin reinfarction study (WARIS II), 240
Weiditz, Hans, 76
weight loss, 185
Weiss, Harvey, 233

Weissman, Gerald, 222
Wellcome, Henry, 126-9
Weskcott, Johann Friedrich (1820-1976), 135
White, W., 102-8
Wilkinson, G., 108-12
   case notes, 112-16
willow, 70, 75, 84-5, 88
   astringency of, 89, 98-90
   cited in *The Rufinus herbal,* 81
   common willow, *104*
   Goat broad-leaved willow, *104*
   Salix *alba* (white), 110, 129, 130
   Salix *caprea,* 110-12
   Salix *latifolia,* 98, 109-10
   used by the ancients, 5, 7, 8
   see also willow bark
willow bark, *95*
   harvesting and preparation, 110
   James' case notes, 100-2
   phial of extract, *261*
   Stone's experiment and letter to the Royal Society, 96-8
   'tonic' properties, 108, 111
   used by the ancients for arthritis, 89
   Whites' case notes, 102-8
   Wilkinson's case notes, 112-16
   see also willow
wintergreen, 79-81, 85, 90, 131, *132,* 134, 213
Winthrop, 165
Withering, William (1741-1799), 25, 88, 118, 202
   on the White or Common Willow, 129
Witthauer, Kurt, 140
Wunderlich, Carl, 49

Yale University, 161, 163
yellow fever, 41-7, 65

zoonosis transmissions, 47-8, 61-2, 183
Zyklon B, 152